EARLY MODERN NAVAL HEALTH CARE
IN ENGLAND, 1650–1750

McGILL-QUEEN'S/AMS HEALTHCARE STUDIES IN THE
HISTORY OF MEDICINE, HEALTH, AND SOCIETY

Series editors: J.T.H. Connor and Erika Dyck

This series presents books in the history of medicine, health studies, and social policy, exploring interactions between the institutions, ideas, and practices of medicine and those of society as a whole. To begin to understand these complex relationships and their history is a vital step to ensuring the protection of a fundamental human right: the right to health. Volumes in this series have received financial support to assist publication from Associated Medical Services, Inc. (AMS), a Canadian charitable organization with an impressive history as a catalyst for change in Canadian healthcare. For eighty years, AMS has had a profound impact through its support of the history of medicine and the education of healthcare professionals, and by making strategic investments to address critical issues in our healthcare system. AMS has funded eight chairs in the history of medicine across Canada, is a primary sponsor of many of the country's history of medicine and nursing organizations, and offers fellowships and grants through the AMS History of Medicine and Healthcare Program (www.amshealthcare.ca).

50 *Broken*
Institutions, Families, and the Construction of
Intellectual Disability
Madeline C. Burghardt

51 *Strange Trips*
Science, Culture, and the Regulation of Drugs
Lucas Richert

52 *A New Field in Mind*
A History of Interdisciplinarity in
the Early Brain Sciences
Frank W. Stahnisch

53 *An Ambulance on Safari*
The ANC and the Making of a Health
Department in Exile
Melissa Diane Armstrong

54 *Challenging Choices*
Canada's Population Control in the 1970s
Erika Dyck and Maureen Lux

55 *Foreign Practices*
Immigrant Doctors and the History of
Canadian Medicare
Sasha Mullally and David Wright

56 *Ethnopsychiatry*
Henri F. Ellenberger
Edited by Emmanuel Delille
Translated by Jonathan Kaplansky

57 *In the Public Good*
Eugenics and Law in Ontario
C. Elizabeth Koester

58 *Transforming Medical Education*
Historical Case Studies of Teaching, Learning,
and Belonging in Medicine
Edited by Delia Gavrus and Susan Lamb

59 *Patterns of Plague*
Changing Ideas about Plague in England and
France, 1348–1750
Lori Jones

60 *The Smile Gap*
A History of Oral Health and Social Inequality
Catherine Carstairs

61 *The Boundaries of Medicare*
Public Health Care beyond the Canada Health
Act
Katherine Fierlbeck and
Gregory P. Marchildon

62 *Reimagining Illness*
Women Writers and Medicine in
Eighteenth-Century Britain
Heather Meek

63 *Early Modern Naval Health Care in England,*
1650–1750
Matthew Neufeld

Early Modern Naval Health Care in England, 1650–1750

MATTHEW NEUFELD

McGill-Queen's University Press

Montreal & Kingston · London · Chicago

© McGill-Queen's University Press 2024

ISBN 978-0-2280-2058-5 (cloth)
ISBN 978-0-2280-2059-2 (paper)
ISBN 978-0-2280-2060-8 (ePDF)
ISBN 978-0-2280-2061-5 (ePUB)

Legal deposit second quarter 2024
Bibliothèque nationale du Québec

Printed in Canada on acid-free paper that is 100% ancient forest free (100% post-consumer recycled), processed chlorine free

This book has been published with the help of a grant from the Canadian Federation for the Humanities and Social Sciences, through the Awards to Scholarly Publications Program, using funds provided by the Social Sciences and Humanities Research Council of Canada.

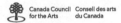

We acknowledge the support of the Canada Council for the Arts.

Nous remercions le Conseil des arts du Canada de son soutien.

McGill-Queen's University Press in Montreal is on land which long served as a site of meeting and exchange amongst Indigenous Peoples, including the Haudenosaunee and Anishinabeg nations. In Kingston it is situated on the territory of the Haudenosaunee and Anishinaabek. We acknowledge and thank the diverse Indigenous Peoples whose footsteps have marked these territories on which peoples of the world now gather.

Library and Archives Canada Cataloguing in Publication

Title: Early modern naval health care in England, 1650-1750 / Matthew Neufeld.
Names: Neufeld, Matthew, author.
Description: Series statement: McGill-Queen's/AMS Healthcare studies in the history of medicine, health, and society ; 63 | Includes bibliographical references and index.
Identifiers: Canadiana (ebook) 20230550568 | Canadiana (print) 20230550509 | ISBN 9780228020615 (EPUB) | ISBN 9780228020608 (ePDF) | ISBN 9780228020585 (cloth) | ISBN 9780228020592 (paper)
Subjects: LCSH: Great Britain. Royal Navy—Medical care—History—17th century. | LCSH: Great Britain. Royal Navy—Medical care—History—18th century. | LCSH: Sailors—Medical care—Great Britain—History—17th century. | LCSH: Sailors—Medical care—Great Britain—History—18th century. | LCSH: Medicine, Naval—Great Britain—History—17th century. | LCSH: Medicine, Naval—Great Britain—History—18th century.
Classification: LCC RC986 .N48 2024 | DDC 616.9/8024094109/032—dc23

Set in 9.5/13 Baskerville 10 Pro
Book design & typesetting by Garet Markvoort, zijn digital

Dedicated to the memory of my grandmothers

Maria Peters Klassen and
Justina [Elizabeth] Hiedebrecht Neufeld

Die Liebe höret nimmer auf

Contents

FIGURES
ix

ACKNOWLEDGMENTS
xi

CHAPTER 1
Introduction: Care Work and Care Workers
in the Early Modern Royal Navy
3

CHAPTER 2
Finding Care for Sick and Injured
Seamen in England, 1650–1688
19

CHAPTER 3
Suffering the System of Care during the
Nine Years' War and After, 1689–1701
45

CHAPTER 4
Securing Care for Seamen during
Queen Anne's War, 1702–1715
69

CHAPTER 5
Naval Health Care during the
Early Georgian Era, 1715–1739
105

CHAPTER 6
Failing and Succeeding to Provide Care
during the War with Spain, 1739–1744
125

CHAPTER 7
Disorders and Due Care for Seamen during
the War against France, 1744–1748
158

CHAPTER 8
Conclusion
187

NOTES
197

BIBLIOGRAPHY
237

INDEX
259

Figures

FIGURE 5.1

Sites of Care, Third Dutch War (1673).
Map by Alan Wobeser and Maria P. Sánchez, HGIS Lab,
University of Saskatchewan. Projection EPSG: 27700.
Source: BL Add. MS 11684.

121

FIGURE 5.2

Sites of Care, King William's War.
Map by Alan Wobeser and Maria P. Sánchez, HGIS Lab,
University of Saskatchewan. Projection EPSG: 27700.
Source: BL Add. MSS 42140 and 28748.

122

FIGURE 5.3

Sites of Care, Queen Anne's War (1712).
Map by Alan Wobeser and Maria P. Sánchez, HGIS Lab,
University of Saskatchewan. Projection EPSG: 27700.
Source: TNA, T1/150/16.

123

FIGURE 5.4

Sites of Care, War with France (1747).
Map by Alan Wobeser and Maria P. Sánchez, HGIS Lab,
University of Saskatchewan. Projection EPSG: 27700.
Sources: NMM, ADM/F/7 and ADM/F/8.

124

Acknowledgments

Financial support for researching and writing this book was provided by the Social Sciences and Humanities Research Council of Canada in the form of a post-doctoral fellowship. The University of Saskatchewan supplied crucial assistance through a President's SSHRC grant in 2012, a New Faculty Recruitment and Retention grant in 2016, and a sabbatical travel grant in 2019. Additional institutional support was offered by the University of Warwick's Centre for the History of Medicine and the University of Manitoba's Institute for the Humanities. I would also like to acknowledge the professional assistance and courtesy I enjoyed while working at the UK National Archives, the National Maritime Museum, the British Library, the London Metropolitan Archives, the Devon Heritage Centre, the Pepys Library of Magdalen College, Cambridge, Carlisle Archive Centre, the Wiltshire and Swindon History Centre, and the Royal Navy Museum. The latter is the only repository I visited that involved walking past a sentry bearing an automatic weapon.

This book's genesis may be traced to the wise advice I received from Professor Mark Knights of Warwick University in late 2008. As the external examiner of my recently defended doctoral thesis, and potential future post-doctoral advisor, Mark suggested that it would be better for me to leave behind the field of social memory and take up a topic related to disabled veterans. I then developed a research program focused on cultural perceptions of wounded soldiers in late-Stuart England. It was while reading petitions from injured seamen at the Devon Heritage Centre in the spring of 2010 that I became interested in how they were cared for, and by whom. The rest became this history.

Since those far-off spring days in Exeter, many people have helped bring this book into being. Nadine Lewycky gave some of the best counsel I ever got on writing for argument as I drafted my first reflections on "casualty care" in the mid-seventeenth-century navy. The late Aaron Graham read through two dense draft chapters and asked excellent questions that helped me improve them. Adrian Wilson of Leeds University likewise read a draft chapter and offered useful criticism. My patient and generous colleagues of the History Department at the University of Saskatchewan at various times read over or heard me present chapters or sections of chapters. I owe special gratitude to Lesley Biggs, Jim Clifford, Geoff Cunfer, Erika Dyck, Chris Kent, and Jim Handy. The maps were produced by the very helpful summer staff at the History Department's HGIS Lab in 2021. During various research and writing phases, I enjoyed the encouragement and assistance of Geoffrey Hudson, Erica Charters, Daniel Baugh, Matthew Dziennik, and James Thomas. The latter pointed me to the Reymes papers at Swindon, which was an enormous help. A number of students, undergraduate and postgraduate, assisted with my research and with organizing the materials that I gathered from the archives. I wish to thank Madeleine Peckham Shakotko, Erin Spinney, Matthew DeClouet, Blaine Wickham, and Daniel Ruten.

Several people graciously offered to read the entire manuscript. Huge thanks in this regard are owed Rilla Friesen, Benjamin Hoy, and Adam Montgomery. I am also very grateful to the two excellent anonymous reviewers secured by McGill-Queen's University Press to adjudicate this book's suitability for publication. Their comments and questions helped to make it so much better. Relatedly, Kyla Madden, my acquisition editor at McGill-Queen's, expertly and with relentless good cheer, guided me through the different stages of submission and revision: thank you so very much.

All these good people did so much to help me research and write this book over the past decade (!), such that I shall be grateful always. Nonetheless, all errors or omissions that may be found in this book are my responsibility alone.

Portions of "The Framework of Casualty Care during the Anglo-Dutch Wars," *War in History* 19, no. 4 (2012): 427–44, appear in chapter two of this book; I am grateful for SAGE Publications's permission to reproduce them. Similarly, I thank Oxford University Press for permission to use material previously published (with Blaine Wickham) in "The State, the People, and the Care of Sick and Injured Sailors in Late Stuart England," *Social History of Medicine* 28, no. 1 (2015): 45–63.

I am deeply thankful for the tireless and generous support of Trudi Neufeld, Christine, Liam, and Brontë Rygiel, and Michael Neufeld over the years it took me to finish this book. As with my previous book,

Acknowledgments xiii

my family formed its spiritual – and so its real – base. Similarly, I am proud to dedicate this book to the memory of two women who had nothing at all to do with maritime matters, save for travelling by ship from Europe to North America a century ago to escape tyranny and persecution. This book is one unlikely offspring of their many labours of love.

In this book, all dates are given, as in the originals, in the Old Style of the Julian calendar, though the new year is taken to have begun on 1 January.

EARLY MODERN NAVAL HEALTH CARE
IN ENGLAND, 1650–1750

CHAPTER 1

Introduction: Care Work and Care Workers in the Early Modern Royal Navy

Wars take lives and destroy the works of human hands. Wars also leave traces on those who survive them. Thus, in January 1674, John Spry, a mariner from Buckland, County Devon, requested relief "as a maimed souldier" at a meeting of magistrates. The previous spring, Spry had been pressed into the Royal Navy of Charles II and served on the *Royal Katherine* in the country's third war against the Dutch Republic. While serving, Spry "was wounded in the shoulder and arme," but having "somewhat recovered" from his wounds, he "was not put off but continued" on board. During a subsequent encounter with Dutch ships, Spry "had his Leggs shattered and much torne with Shott, especially one of them, whereout were taken severall bones and splinters of bones." Although he could now "goe without crutches," Spry often felt "in such great paines and weaknes that hee is hardly able to helpe himself." Fortunately, the Justices of Devon granted him a pension of 50d. per year as a "maymed seaman."[1]

John Spry survived a war at sea, albeit with a much diminished capacity to look after himself, thanks in part to people who attended to his injuries. This book concerns the emergence of a health-care system for Royal Navy seamen, a system built on such "labours of love."[2] It tells a story about the Royal Navy's efforts to find, secure, and order care for its most valuable, if most troublesome, resource: its seamen. Caring for injured seamen invariably involved the navy in ongoing relationships with a crucial contingent of people who provided care work, space for care, or both.

The history of naval health care in early modern England is a story of the changing relationship between people willing to look after men like John Spry (often women in the community, who looked after the seamen in their own homes) and naval officials, especially the commissioners for sick and wounded seamen and their agents. From roughly

1650 to 1700, naval health care on shore was characterized predominantly by the navy's need to *find* sufficient spaces for care, and ordinary people to perform care work. Since the navy did not possess its own places to care for seamen, nor employ its own cohort of care workers, it looked to the people of coastal communities to provide both spaces and people for seamens' treatment and recovery. In attempting to find care on shore, the navy was in an important sense dependent on local communities. Moreover, the navy's relative financial weakness meant that it often struggled mightily to find care workers from coastal communities. Then, from the beginning of the eighteenth century, naval officials sought, at select ports, to *secure* care at spaces operated by hospital contractors, while continuing to find sufficient sites for care and care workers in what were called "town quarters." This shift meant that at certain ports the navy was less dependent on the willingness of local people to provide the space and labour needed to heal seamen. The shift in the navy's emphasis from finding to securing care happened when newly available financial resources coincided with an intention to extend command and control over care work and care spaces. Finally, from 1744, the navy undertook to erect permanent sites for orderly care for sick and injured seamen at Portsmouth and Plymouth naval hospitals. *Ordered care* demanded spaces that fostered healing and recovery while also retaining seamen in naval service. It also meant naval oversight of the conduct of both care workers and seamen in care to expedite their return to active duty.

Histories of medicine concern diseases, the people who suffer them, and those who try to treat and heal them.[3] This book is a history of health care, with a special focus on care work and care workers. Madeleine Bunting was not wrong to characterize care work as "dark matter." It is everywhere and practically invisible.[4] Yet its existence cannot be gainsaid. Care work means attending to a human need in a direct way that usually requires physical contact.[5] A health-care system is one in which people attempt through patterned interactions to match needs for healing and attention with people able to meet them. A health-care system cannot function without care work and care workers.

Today, care work involves direct and intimate labour focused on the body and the body's immediate environment. Care work may or may not be done at home; it may or may not be paid.[6] During the late medieval and early modern periods, caring for someone explicitly involved both corporeal and spiritual labour, both "body work" and attending to the person in need as an embodied soul.[7] For example, caring for sick children at home included feeding, cleaning, watching, visiting, and praying for them.[8] A key continuity in the long history of care work is the reality that, although both men and women historically (and today) have performed it, care work has long been associated with a sexual division of labour and work performed mostly by women.[9] Nonetheless, while care work is often about attending to people's essential needs, and often the most private of body parts, at different times and for various reasons, it becomes an issue of intense public concern.[10] This is especially the case in relation to the history of the Royal Navy, as caring for sick and wounded sailors demanded significant financial resources and many people willing to care.[11]

Care work directed at sick and injured sailors concerned the provision of a bed, clean bedding, regular washing, and food and drink. As early as the sixteenth century, health manuals written for surgeons emphasized the importance of keeping specific body parts clean, including face and hands, eyes, teeth, feet, and head.[12] It would have been care workers who washed the bodies of injured and sick sailors on shore. Similarly, care workers were responsible for washing seamen's clothes (their "slops") and bedding, which was understood to help prevent various fevers and skin ailments. Medical practitioners recommended cleanliness of the body and the clothing covering it as key to restoring people to health.[13] In other words, striving to ensure that naval patients received proper rest and nourishment and maintained a level of personal cleanliness were central to early modern medicine and to naval health care.

Throughout this book I use the term care work because it captures well the continuities between early- and late-modern people who attended to the bodies of the sick and injured (and the disabled and the elderly), whether through washing, feeding, shaving, cutting hair, doing laundry, or changing bedclothes. Much of the literature on care work in modern, developed nations seeks to analyze it in relation to long-standing questions in the history of women's work.[14] These questions include the often-shifting boundaries between domestic duty and paid employment, or else the related dichotomy of private versus public spheres of activity.[15] To what degree was care understood to be one of the obligations that members of a household could expect from each other, therefore rendering care outside the scope of the market?[16] To what extent, why, and at what times did people consider care work to be the sort of labour that requires monetary compensation?[17] Additionally, on which side of the line between profit-driven enterprise and public welfare did communities locate care work?[18]

The English Royal Navy's efforts to find, secure, and order health care for seamen on shore emerged within a broader and longer-term change in the nation's approach to people who were, for a variety of reasons, unable to look after their own needs. During the decades following the dissolution of religious foundations, including many hospitals, under Henry VIII and Edward VI, the question of caring for those unable and/or too poor to look after themselves confronted English communities. The crucial question about care work in England after roughly 1550 was not whether the care provided was formally or informally organized, or paid for by the community or by family and friends, but whether it was voluntary or involuntary.[19] Although parishes and towns were not initially required by law to provide care for the sick poor, in some instances local authorities demanded that the poor look after their own. The reason poor people were made to care for their impecunious neighbours was connected to the changing nature of public relief during the Tudor era.[20] As early as the 1620s, English parishes and towns began to levy rates on households to provide either temporary relief to people out of work or ongoing support for those who were too old, too sick, or else "disenabled" from paid employment.[21]

Poor people who received parochial relief, especially widows, could be expected to look after other poor sick people, either in their homes or in the sick person's own dwelling. In the parish of St Bartholomew's Exchange, London, for example, a woman in receipt of relief who refused to keep a sick person could be denied subsequent benefits.[22] There was clearly a gender component in parish leaders' conception that women on relief needed to be prepared to nurse their sick neighbours. The duties of nurse-keepers were those typically managed by the mistress of a well-functioning household.[23] These duties included making meals, mixing remedies for ailments and salves for sores, and washing clothes and bed linen.[24] Laundry was a particularly important aspect of body care from the sixteenth century, as the focus of cleanliness shifted from bathing the body to changing and washing undergarments.[25]

In some areas of the country, care work directed at the sick poor was a public matter with a gendered dimension: parishes and towns paid for care out of monies raised on the taxpaying public and could occasionally expect women receiving poor relief to tend to the bodily requirements of the sick, infirm, or aged in their midst. Despite the element

Introduction 7

of coercion underlying the expectation to provide care, female care workers – increasingly called nurse keepers, or simply nurses from the early seventeenth century – were almost always paid cash by the parish for their labour. This fact concerning payment for work is important. Compensation meant that care work could also be a by-employment for the poor in receipt of public relief; it was not an unpaid obligation that recipients of relief owed to the community.[26] For example, Andrew Wear's research found that in 1602 a woman in St Bartholomew's, London, Goody Wharton, was paid 2s. 6d. per week to look after one Anne Smith, who was lame.[27] Thus, caring for the sick or disabled poor was, in some places at least, taken as a public responsibility and viewed as a commercial transaction: if you nursed the sick poor, you would get paid to do it. Care for the sick poor at the parochial level was not always so informally organized, however. Other historians of London have argued that, by the middle of the seventeenth century, some districts of the capital had organized a scheme of parochial nursing. Significantly, a few of the parish nurses of St Boltoph Aldgate (c. 1620–1650) and St Martin-in-the-Fields (c. 1650–1725) appear to have created and maintained nursing enterprises; that is, they ran establishments specially designated for the care and cure of homeless people and the sick poor.[28] Looking after poor people's basic needs had become a kind of economic opportunity by the mid-seventeenth century.

What began as an ad-hoc approach by late-Elizabethan parochial officials for dealing with the sick poor – compelling women on relief to care for them, albeit for pay – became systematic at different places during the seventeenth century. Within what became an established practice, certain women operated, sometimes for a number of years, informal enterprises that traded their care labour, or that of their servants, for public funds. What began as an involuntary system of care provision became voluntary as different parishes formalized collection and payment procedures. Additionally, an unintended consequence of England's Poor Laws saw poor-if-enterprising women, particularly widows, looking after their poor sick neighbours as a lucrative, or at least viable, economic endeavour.[29] This development fit within Peter Earle's observation that the period from roughly 1650 to 1750 was the "high point" of women's participation in healing and medical practice, occurring at the same time as domestic healing work – both medical and nursing – was increasingly commercialized. Women were paid to make and administer remedies, to do laundry, and to provide food and lodging for the sick, old and young.[30] Care work, in other words, became imbricated in the expansion of the market.[31] Care work also became a concern for naval officials.

England's early modern naval health-care system arose over the century when the Royal Navy established its global pre-eminence, roughly from 1650 to 1750. Naval health care emerged as an unintended outcome of the country's first maritime war with an economic rival, the Dutch. In September 1653, the Council of State appointed a three-man commission to oversee the onshore provision of care for sick and wounded sailors.[32] They had the responsibility to find suitable physicians, surgeons, and apothecaries on shore. The commissioners also located accommodations at designated ports for sick and injured sailors to receive treatment and recover their health. Disbanded with the coming of peace in 1654, the commission's work set the precedent for the Crown's management of care for seamen. Over the next nine decades, each subsequent maritime conflict saw the creation of a new commission for sick and wounded seamen of the Royal Navy.[33]

Commissioners for hurt and sick seamen were authorized to put them into existing hospitals or elsewhere on the least-expensive terms; to ensure a surgeon or a physician attended the men; and to employ agents at the ports to keep account of the men recovering on shore.[34] Sick and injured sailors were supposed to remain in their sick quarters until they were well enough to rejoin their ships, were discharged as unfit, or were sent to London for treatment at a hospital. Some sailors chose to desert the navy from sick quarters, preferring the higher pay, and lower risk, offered by the merchant marine.[35] The people of coastal towns such as Deal, Plymouth, and Portsmouth provided lodging and basic care for seamen; this practice became known as town quartering. When the care providers, known as quarterers, were not paid regularly or when promised, they protested, and even resisted receiving more sick and hurt men.

Relationships between ordinary people and naval officials structured the system of care for sick and hurt seamen.[36] A key factor driving the structural changes to naval health care was the level of trust between naval officials and the people of coastal communities, especially the women who typically oversaw care spaces and care workers. During the late-seventeenth century, representatives of the navy believed that the care offered in town quarters worked well most of the time.[37] Then, in 1703 and again in 1744, particular officials within the navy lost faith in the people's capacity to provide good care for seamen.

Introduction

In the first instance, the commissioners of sick and wounded seamen distrusted the capacity of care providers – landlandies – to tend adequately to the needs of seamen. As a result, private-contract hospitals at major ports were incorporated into the system. In the second instance, the Admiralty distrusted the willingness of nurses to keep order at Gosport's private-contract hospital. Consequently, permanent naval hospitals were later constructed at Portsmouth and Plymouth.[38] At these two institutions, the navy assumed full authority and control over the space where care work happened, and could monitor the conduct of care workers. Thanks to these structural changes, by the beginning of the Seven Years' War (1754–63), the Royal Navy had a health-care system that was beginning to assume the form that endured well into the twentieth century.

Naval health care had a role in the formation of England's early-modern state, insofar as it was oriented toward warfare.[39] Throughout the period, naval officials found spaces for care and care workers by negotiating various informal and formal partnerships with civilians living in coastal communities. From the beginning of the eighteenth century, officials aspired to, and gradually attained, the goal of ordered care. In other words, naval health care emerged and was transformed through processes of state-directed centralization that were dependent heavily upon informal, local arrangements over care work and sites for care.[40]

For more than a century, historians have argued that war largely explains why, between roughly 1450 and 1750, some European countries effectively "modernized," developing institutions that enabled them to project force across vast distances and to begin to manage the conduct of their subjects.[41] During these centuries, armed forces became more technologically sophisticated, professional, and reliant upon rule-driven bureaucratic institutions.[42] As states employed more officials to oversee more responsibilities, at least two key changes occurred: (1) the distinction between instruments of governance and economic organizations sharpened; and (2) the state overrode its competitors in providing for public order and protecting people from external threats to their security.[43] Thus, warfare spurred social change that laid the foundations for modern political formations.[44]

Before 1640, the Royal Navy was a hybrid of warships owned by the Crown and temporarily mobilized merchant ships owned by individuals or proto-corporations.[45] During the Civil War, the Long Parliament supported a professional army and navy through property and consumption taxes. By 1654, the English navy was able to support two hundred state-owned warships in the final campaign season against the Dutch. The expansion of the number of state-owned ships and the professionalization of the navy's officer corps – reliant on merit rather than birth – both occurring between roughly 1645 and 1665, transformed the relationship between the state and England's maritime communities. As the former assumed responsibility for the security needs of the latter, the social and economic ties between the two became tighter. By the end of the second Dutch war in 1667, England had a professional standing navy.[46]

Warfare concentrated power at the centre of government during the early modern era. However, financially secure and centrally regulated officials and administrators could do only so much on their own.[47] Countries whose public officials and private enterprises co-operated in the procurement of goods and the delivery of services, including England and the Netherlands, generally performed better during interstate conflicts than those where this did not happen. In England, for example, the navy depended on hundreds of contractors to provide goods and services that it simply could not produce from its own resources.[48] Historians have therefore highlighted the salience of personal and contractual relationships for the emergence and effectiveness of the early modern English state and its armed forces.[49] The country's remarkable rise to global naval pre-eminence depended on the formation of productive partnerships between local and private interest groups and the Crown.[50] The second half of the seventeenth century was a crucial period in the construction of a state capable of sustaining expensive and lengthy wars on a global scale.[51] The deployment of both relationally centred and bureaucratically organized modes of operating contributed to England's (later, Great Britain's) martial achievements.[52] Indeed, the importance of co-operative partnerships involving officials and contractors endured well into the eighteenth century.[53] The Royal Navy's reliance on private enterprises to meet many of its demands made the senior armed service financially resilient and fostered its integration into maritime communities and broader society.[54]

Naval health care emerged in a way that afforded officials the opportunity to pursue a braided set of ambitious objectives: saving seamen's lives, saving money, and keeping men in the sea service.[55] Over time, these objectives, which I call the preservative ethos of early modern naval health care, were pursued through ever-more-ordered care: to oversee directly the spaces where men could rest and recover their health, while receiving the attentions of care workers. The aim was to ensure that seamen and care workers comported themselves in ways that aligned with the navy's ongoing need for manpower. Thus, among the possibilities of early modern naval health care lay a crucial ambition to exercise authority and control over an aspect of the social world. In a word, to become modern. Naval health care's emergence did not foreordain its modernization, but without the preservative ethos sitting within its core, the system's eventual modern form is unimaginable.[56]

Modernization theory, for all its faults, remains a useful model for making sense of social change.[57] Of course, no model can ever hope to account for all salient causal mechanisms, especially in what critical realist sociologists rightly call "open systems."[58] A model for explaining change in the world of women and men cannot work like a covering law that algorithmically connects past inputs with present outputs.[59] The unexpected outcomes of actions are not evidence of foresight nor of the typological fulfillment of some earlier phenomenon. Likewise, social change is certainly not always a "good thing," let alone "progress."[60]

Paradox and contradiction crosscut the history of war. Warfare on sea and land demanded the labour power of people willing to kill and other people willing to heal.[61] Although most of the care work demanded by the navy was done by socially and economically disadvantaged people, these workers had a measure of authority while tending sick and injured sailors. The care worker, a nurse, was often in a socially more precarious position than her patient, yet she maintained a degree of control over his health. Temporarily, at least, a woman looking after a man, albeit one in a weakened state, could tell him what to do. A care worker was authorized to refuse sick seamen's requests for spirituous liquors, for example. She could also harm him by failing to provide his prescribed medicine or diet. At the same time, sailors might attempt to undermine a nurse's authority by complaining about her to a hospital official or naval officer. Thus, the relationship between carer and cared for was about much more than an objective (or perceived) socially prescribed power imbalance.

Care work can be demanding. Yet without it there would not have been a naval health care system, with devastating consequences for the navy's capacity to project force at sea. However, it barely features in histories of the Royal Navy during the Age of Sail.[62] When it has, it has too often been judged according to modern standards.[63] In light of periodic calls for permanent hospitals in England for seamen, beginning in the 1650s, the government's decision to build one nearly a century later may appear as the long-overdue fulfillment of an earlier promise.[64] Thankfully, recent scholarship has expanded what we know about naval medicine, both on land and at sea, without judging it according to contemporary practice.[65] Two historians in particular deserve special mention: Patricia Crimmin's essays on the eighteenth-century Sick and Hurt Board deserve a wide readership, as does Kathleen Harland's doctoral thesis on early modern naval hospitals.[66] The latter's research corrected several dubious interpretations put forward in mid-twentieth-century histories about early modern naval medicine, including the fate of the quartering system of onshore care after 1700.[67] Some of what follows departs from their conclusions in significant ways. However, my arguments could not have taken shape but for the opportunity to engage productively with their attempts to build on the first wave of histories concerning naval medicine.

Like other "new" naval histories, this book seeks to put the story of the United Kingdom's senior armed service into dialogue with diverse historical literatures and methodologies.[68] It takes seriously the wide spectrum of medical practitioners at work in early modern England, of whom physicians, surgeons, and apothecaries constituted an important, but by no means monopolistic, fraction. Rather than giving most of its attention to medical professionals, this book strives to recapture the significance of the people who did the majority of caring for injured and sick sailors. The transformation of naval health care between 1650 and 1750 was largely a product of the often fraught and contested relationship between the major purchaser of health care for seamen – the state – and the sellers of care. The majority of the latter were ordinary women and men living in coastal communities.

Sources constrain what historians can construct about past reality. Unquestionably, this book's narrative often represents a view from the centre, a perspective on the past that privileges men with authority and power. While acknowledging that the producers of our sources had self-interested, and at times distorted, points of view, we can affirm that the actions and objects described in these sources correspond to real actions and objects of the past.[69] Thus, while not discounting the limitations of such sources, nor claiming that my reading of them is

Introduction

"unbiased," I hope the story that follows is a valuable and true interpretation of the past. To claim something as true makes it possible for others to point out features of it that are in fact wrong.[70] Indeed, this book will have succeeded if it encourages other historians to prove my story wrong.

Frustratingly, institutional archives do not shed much direct light on the practical realities of care work performed for sick and wounded seamen; that which was most necessary to naval health care is least visible to historians. Much of this book's narrative draws on the sources generated by those who managed care work and care workers, that is, those naval officials, all of them men, who directed and took responsibility for naval health care on shore. More often than not, naval officials recorded where, who, and for how long someone provided care for a sick or wounded sailor. The records shed light on the social breadth of care work, rather than on the actual labour focused on the body (and the person).[71] Sources that do refer to care work directly often derive from third-party observers, such as officers or agents of the sick and wounded commission. In order to attain a modestly objective understanding of early modern care work for seamen, I have sought to triangulate qualitative and quantitative sources. The latter can convey a sense of who cared for whom, where, and for how long. Financial records suggest that naval officials often deemed care to have been secured when seamen were accommodated and provided with food and drink. Care work was concluded when seamen had recovered their health sufficiently to return to duty. In sum, uncovering the history of care work, and naval health care in early modern England, requires reading both what is and what is not represented in numbers, reports, and correspondence. It is helpful, if sobering, to keep in mind that care work and care workers were so important, so vital, to getting sick and wounded seamen back to their ships that naval officials did not think they needed much commentary.

Nonetheless, thanks to the survival of the papers of several commissioners for sick and wounded seamen, we can know a great deal about naval health care in Restoration England.[72] Several tables of quantitative and qualitative data, registers of seamen put ashore, form part of the John Evelyn collection at the British Library and the Bullen Reymes papers held at the Wiltshire and Swindon History Centre. These registers offer truly unparalleled quantitative data about the seamen in care, the people on shore who cared for them, and the cost of care.[73]

Additionally, the correspondence to and from Commissioner Evelyn about the conditions at several coastal communities during the second and third Dutch wars offers vivid descriptions of the conditions of care and the difficulties experienced by care providers. Unfortunately, almost no registers of sick and injured seamen survive from the period after 1688.

The Nine Years' War (1689–1697), initiated by the Glorious Revolution, generated comparatively more sources about naval health care than the wars against the Dutch. These sources include the minutes of the Admiralty lords' meetings, the correspondence of the lords of the Treasury, the papers of the Navy Board collected under its secretary Charles Sergison, and the postwar meeting minutes of the successor to the fourth commission for sick and wounded seamen.[74] By contrast, not a single collection of documents produced or collected by anyone appointed commissioner for sick and wounded seamen during the Nine Years' War survives. My account of naval health care during this conflict and of the experience of finding and giving care for sailors on shore, relies on the qualitative descriptions offered by commissioners for sick and wounded seamen, directed primarily toward the Treasury.

The sources produced by the Admiralty supply most of my evidence for the eighteenth-century half of this book's narrative. Two important collections, non-existent for earlier periods, enrich the source base for understanding naval health care under Queen Anne (1702–14). The meeting minutes of the commissioners for sick and wounded seamen, and the Admiralty's correspondence to the commission, both survive, although with a five-year gap in the former.[75] Nonetheless, as is the case for the fourth commission, there are no extant personal papers from any commissioners serving from 1702 to 1715. This absence might be explained by the fact that the commissioners kept all their papers at their offices, of which most were later transferred to another location. In a letter submitted to the Treasury in the spring of 1714, the commissioners indicated that they possessed forty-two register books of payments at the ports, along with a similar number of books listing payments for prisoners of war.[76] The registers were lost almost certainly because, according to Admiralty Secretary Josiah Burchett, "the Papers belonging to" the sick and wounded commissioners "were accidently burnt" sometime in 1716.[77]

Naval health care between 1715 and 1739 left behind the fewest documentary traces. Correspondence between the Admiralty and the commissioners for sick and hurt sheds some light on care for seamen on shore, with occasional insights afforded by the Admiralty's meeting minutes. My account of care for seamen during the 1740s, and the shifts that accelerated its modernization, during which time Britain made war first on Spain and then on France, relies primarily on the commissioners' meeting minutes and the correspondence between them and the Admiralty.

This book focuses almost exclusively on England, in part because that is where most onshore care occurred, since England was where relations between the people and the navy were most decisive for the system's emergence and transformation.[78] The global or imperial dimensions of naval health care deserve a proper narration, and I look forward to analyses of naval health care *outre-mer* by historians who have greater familiarity with those places. Finally, this book does not concern what in fact most occupied the attention of the commissioners for sick and hurt seamen, namely prisoners of war. The exchange, custody, and care for prisoners take up the bulk of the commissioners' meeting minutes and their correspondence with the Admiralty. The navy's treatment of its prisoners of war is a much understudied aspect of the humanitarian project's history.[79]

This book tells a story of emergence and transformation. It begins in the 1650s and ends roughly a century later. The period covered by this book includes the origin of both the early modern and modern systems of onshore naval health care in England. After 1750, the Royal Navy sought care for sick and wounded seamen in spaces that recalled the circumstances of the Dutch wars, and within institutions that endured well into the twentieth century.[80]

My narration of naval health care's evolution unfolds over six chapters that centre on periods of war or peace. Maritime warfare called forth care on shore such that it had, for the people who organized it, delivered it, and received it, discernable beginnings, middles, and ends.[81]

Chapter two covers the period between 1652 and 1688, the opening of the first Dutch war and the coming of the Glorious Revolution. It traces how the emergent system of naval health care established a successful if also troubled working relationship between the English state and the people of coastal communities. The emergence of naval health care can be connected to the early history of England's fiscal-naval state. Emergent naval health care also belongs to the history of public relief and of care as a kind of paid labour.

Chapter three provides an overview of the system during the Nine Years' War and its immediate aftermath. It emphasizes continuity in the midst of significant political and fiscal change during the 1690s, and the tremendous financial challenges that confronted the system's managers and the people at the ports. Given the strains placed on the English state during that war, the fact that naval health care did not collapse represented a kind of success. The system managed to meet the challenge of nearly a decade of war, thanks to the country's fiscal revolution.

The Nine Years' War also witnessed a number of proposals to improve naval health care composed by people adjacent to the naval administration. During Queen Anne's War, the subject of chapter four, administrators themselves took up the task of reform. The fifth commission for sick and wounded seamen, preferring to work with a handful of hospital contractors rather than a multitude of mostly female care providers, introduced hospitals for sick and injured seamen at several ports. There was better care for seamen during this war, at least until 1709–10, because there was money to pay for it. The relatively consistent availability of money for care of seamen was itself the result of greater trust between the political nation and the Crown, forged during the 1690s. Thus, public credit instruments sustained naval health care at the same time as its administrators restricted the number of trusted care providers. Queen Anne's War also saw for the first time the formation of a sustained objective within the sick and wounded service. As mentioned earlier, I have called the articulated ambition to save seamen's lives, to save the Crown money, and to keep seamen from fleeing the service, the preservative ethic.[82]

The Treaty of Utrecht (1713) that ended Great Britain's war with France produced roughly a quarter-century of general peace in Europe. Chapter five, which is concerned with the years 1715 to 1739, shows the persistence of the system of care, and of care for seamen ashore, even in the absence of warfare. Certain aspects of naval health care during this period stayed the same, and others changed, both to the good. The state saw fit to continue investing in care for seamen, including officers and infrastructure, despite the absence of war. Officers and administrators addressed the problem of returning sick or injured men into active service. Moreover, naval officials bestowed greater levels of trust on ordinary people who provided care on shore. This renewal of trust would provide crucial for the biggest challenge to confront the system: war with Spain and the typhus epidemic, the Great Sickness, of 1739 to 1742.

Histories of naval health care in England generally portray onshore care during the war against Spain, which began in 1739, as exceedingly poor. While acknowledging that the conditions in which seamen were supposed to heal at Gosport and Plymouth provoked serious complaints about overcrowding and filth, chapter six, which focuses on Britain's war with Spain, shows that care on shore did improve from 1742 to 1744. The chapter also revisits the significance of the Admiralty's 1741 request for three permanent royal naval hospitals, which did not succeed. I argue that, while the Admiralty presented a portrait of domestic onshore care that delinquent local providers seriously endangered, the commissioners for the sick and wounded continued to believe in the value of the status quo. The commissioners' positive assessment of the quality of care provision on shore, and of the ability of local people to provide good care when asked, casts doubt on the inevitability of the navy's shift to permanent, navy-run hospitals.

The book's final substantive chapter (chapter seven) attends to naval health care ashore during Georgian Britain's first war with France, from 1744 to 1748. Two seemingly contrasting themes tie the final part of the story together. First, the circumstances surrounding the 1744 Admiralty-led proposal to construct permanent Royal Navy hospitals. This chapter will show that the decision to erect Haslar hospital resulted not from historical or medical necessity but rather from the rhetorical mobilization of an acute breakdown of orderly care at Gosport's contract hospital for seamen, also known as Forton Hospital. Blame for the breakdown of order at Forton fell unfairly on its largely female workforce. Thus, as had been the case four decades earlier, a breakdown in trust between the officials seeking care and the people providing it propelled structural change to the system of naval health care. Part of the explanation for that breakdown lies in the fact that most of the care workers were female, and were regarded as – by nature – more prone to disorder than men. Thus, greater naval oversight of care work would reduce the chances of disorderly conduct at naval hospitals by both patients and nurses. Second, although the Admiralty's proposal succeeded, leading to a massive public investment in health-care infrastructure in the form of Haslar naval hospital, onshore care for seamen after 1745 reached peak performance. This accomplishment emerged from the potent combination of financial stability and due care from the people at the ports, especially the women working as care providers and care workers. Thus, female labour both underpinned early modern naval health care and played a significant role in fostering its transformation.

Women were responsible for much of what naval health care did right during the later half of the 1740s, and in previous conflicts. At the time, this truth was not acknowledged widely. This book aims in part to right that wrong.

CHAPTER 2

Finding Care for Sick and Injured Seamen in England, 1650–1688

By the outbreak of the first Dutch war in 1652, the English state possessed a standing navy.[1] At the war's end, it had produced the first draft of a permanent system for the onshore care of sick and wounded navy sailors.[2] In part, the origin of this system for care stemmed from contingent factors. The war witnessed an unprecedented demand for care on shore, because it was fought in home waters, and over several seasons.[3] Naval health care in England also emerged as a product of several existing schemes for relieving people in need: the parochially based system for providing care for the sick poor through rates on local households; the navy's provision of surgeons on ships during wartime; the county pension scheme for the support of disabled former sailors.

The navy of the 1650s recognized its responsibility to provide medical assistance to wounded and sick seamen. The scope of this task during the first Dutch war, however, required the navy to turn to the people for help. Naval health care initially was focused on finding space in which seamen could rest and be treated, and finding people who could attend to their needs while they recovered. In other words, during the war the navy presented to coastal communities a huge demand for accommodation, or care space, and for care work. For the most part, the people, many of whom were women, responded to the demand for care willingly, and as an economic opportunity for their households or enterprises. However, there were times during the Dutch wars when the navy applied direct pressure on local governors and ordinary people to find space and care workers for sailors. Such episodes revealed the navy's desperation, which was born of the immediacy and unpredictability of naval operations, and the Restoration regime's financial problems. The difficulties the navy had in finding care during the second and third Dutch wars also reflected the fact that paying the charge for seamen's accommodation and care could be a low priority for government ministers. Despite having the fiscal capacity to float sizable navies

20 Early Modern Naval Health Care in England

after 1650, late-seventeenth-century English governments, whether republican or monarchical, tended to take their time attending to the real cost of caring for seamen.[4]

This chapter will argue that the system fostered a periodically troubled but mostly successful relationship between the English state and the people of coastal communities. Emergent naval health care in Restoration England was grounded on interactions between a few naval officials trying to find care spaces and care workers for seamen, and many ordinary people, mostly women, who answered the demand for space and labour. Because the navy choose not to prioritize paying for care during wartime, a kind of moral economy between naval officials and ordinary people developed.[5] People received sick and hurt seamen and cared for them on credit, in the belief that the navy would honour its debts in a reasonably short period of time. When local people perceived that the navy was too slow in honouring its obligation to settle its accounts with people of coastal communities, they could assert a moral right to protest. In other words, what they owed to each other by virtue of their relationship framed their interactions more than determining an appropriate price for care work. Naval officials knew that the system of care would collapse if people refused to work with them, and a sure-fire reason not to provide care for seamen was outstanding debts of payment (arrears). Thus, most of the difficulties between the people and the navy over the burden of care centred on when compensation happened, not its cost nor how the navy managed the system.

During the Dutch wars, when most action occurred in the North Sea and the Channel, many sick and wounded received care along the southeast coast, especially in Essex and Kent. Portsmouth and Gosport became centres for care by the second Dutch war, while Plymouth assumed importance once the French navy became the chief adversary from 1689. Generally, the chief centres for care were found near the mouth of the Medway, the town of Deal (the meeting point of the North Sea and the English Channel), Portsmouth and Gosport, and Plymouth.[6]

Naval health care in coastal communities occurred almost entirely in the homes or outbuildings belonging to ordinary people, or in the public houses. Women performed most of the basic care work and often made up the majority of people who provided accommodation or "town quarters" to seamen.[7] Admittedly, men also performed care work at this time, pre-eminently on board ship, but also ashore. For example, a 1674 petition to the navy for payment from fifteen self-declared nurses of Deal (Kent) included two men.[8] More strikingly, at least to post-Nightingale sensibilities, a 1676 petition from seventy-one self-declared nurses from Dover lists only twenty-six women.[9] Nonetheless, naval officials usually described care providers or care givers as women, widows or landladies. And usually, the officials were not wrong to do so. An undated petition in the Evelyn papers from sometime during the third Dutch war, submitted by the people of Sandwich and Deal who had "cherished and maintained" a great number of sick and injured seamen, listed forty-six signatories, all but one of which was a typical female name.[10]

The emergence of a system for naval health care in England occurred as part of a multi-generational process by which the state's capacity to extract resources in order to wage war expanded and intensified.[11] The process of state formation operated at multiple levels, both top-down and bottom-up. It succeeded when officials developed workable and effective relationships with local officials and local people that satisfied the expectations of all concerned. In other words, state formation depended on the nature, frequency, and the quality of the interactions between officials representing the state and elements of the people.[12]

Naval health care worked as a consequence of co-operative monetary and moral relationships. Over the course of the Restoration era, naval officials came to trust care providers – those who provided accommodation – and care workers to look after sick and injured men so that they would heal and, if not severely disabled, then return to active duty.[13] Care providers and care workers trusted the navy to seek first their co-operation and, if necessary, to demand their assistance with proper authorization. The care providers also, naturally, trusted that the navy would pay them for their accommodation, and would compensate care workers for their labour. When the care workers of Deal and other coastal communities protested to commissioners, it was in part to invoke the moral economy underpinning the system of naval health care. The system could only function when both the navy's care managers and the care workers met their obligations to each other. Thus, maintaining right relations with care workers enabled the navy to fulfill the sailors' expectation that they would be cared for.

Dealings between the people and the state in the formative years of naval health care could be fraught with tension and frustration, particularly when care providers became convinced that the government had betrayed their trust. However, the responses of overworked and harried naval officials to the complaints from people should not lead us to conclude that the earliest system of naval health care in England did not work. Naval officials were hopeful that, with adequate funding and honest interactions, the system would serve the state well for the future.

Early-modern naval health care was a relatively successful new service that built on established practices of naval medicine and relief for disabled ex-servicemen. It is therefore useful to sketch out briefly the shape of these schemes as they existed around 1650.

WAR, MEDICINE, AND RELIEF IN EARLY MODERN ENGLAND

It was long believed that war provided excellent training for surgeons. The increased use of gunpowder weapons after 1500 presented battlefield surgeons with many more cases of compound fractures, burns, and gunshot wounds.[14] Before firearms, compound fractures were unusual, because hand-held weapons could not generate sufficient kinetic force to break bones in several places. When a bone was broken, it normally broke in one place, making it relatively easy to set. Classical physicians considered compound fractures generally fatal and recommended amputation as the only treatment. Ambroise Paré, who served in French armies during the sixteenth century, wrote several popular medical treatises based on his experience that advocated for new approaches for treating wounds and performing battlefield amputations. Paré advised the use of vascular ligature instead of cauterization to stop bleeding, which was especially helpful.[15] He also discussed injuries from mines and burning or exploding missiles, which blew up or burnt up many soldiers.[16] Richard Wiseman, an English surgeon who served during the Civil War, developed a method for finding and removing bullets that mitigated the risk of the wound becoming infected.[17] Clearly, early modern surgeons developed empirically grounded approaches to war-related injuries that saved lives.

Surgeons were trained as apprentices of Master surgeons for seven years. They needed to practise their craft a further seven years before they qualified as a Master themselves. Surgical knowledge was empirical. Apprentices learned how to prepare bandages, clean and dress wounds, let blood, lance boils, and employ methods for incision, extirpation, and stitching.[18]

However, most soldiers and sailors who died in war fell from disease, not combat-induced wounds or injuries. This was the case even after the advent of gunships transformed maritime warfare.[19] Shipboard conditions played a role in seamen's morbidity, but a ship's destination and the duration of the voyage were more significant factors for rates of sickness. The shorter the distance sailed, the lower the chances of seamen catching a disease and dying. Early voyages to the Indian Ocean and Caribbean had terribly high mortality rates. Scurvy was the biggest killer on long-distance voyages – unsurprising given the lack of fruits and vegetables. The sickness usually started to appear after a month or two at sea.[20] A lack of vitamin B also affected seamen's health, causing fatigue, depression, and memory loss. Dysentery, known to contemporaries as the "bloody flux," was another unpleasant product of consuming tainted water. Sailors were also susceptible to typhus, sometimes called "ship fever." Carried by lice embedded in unwashed clothes, the disease was particularly terrible during the early phases of naval wars, when thousands of pressed (conscripted) seamen crowded onto ships. Sailors on ships that plied tropical waters, whether in America or Africa, succumbed often to malaria and yellow fever.

On board ship, employers, including the Royal Navy, had a customary obligation to care for ill, injured, or wounded sailors (the Laws of Oléron).[21] When it was possible, ship owners and the navy preferred to remove sick or wounded from the ship. But during the late-Elizabethan and early-Stuart periods, naval seamen could expect a surgeon on board to provide first assistance. Surgeons were paid according to the number of men they treated. This put them in the awkward position of having to maintain their professional reputations as healers, while profiting the most from voyages with high mortality. Shipboard surgeons were not able to do much to treat the diseases that killed most sailors, such as scurvy or fever. They did help the injured or wounded, although at times the treatments did more harm than good.

There were a few attempts to improve what we might call hygiene on ships. Most of the changes happened on merchant ships, many of which carried cannons and served in the navy in wartime. Soap accompanied sailors to West Africa. The navy provided clothes, "slops," to some men, and encouraged them to keep them clean. However, the fact that the state could conscript or press men into naval service meant that it had less incentive to implement and bear the cost of improved sanitary conditions. Nonetheless, from the middle of seventeenth century, the Crown began to take better care of sick and injured seamen.[22] Seriously injured men had been able to count on the Crown from the 1590s.

The two main sources of relief for disabled navy seamen were Chatham's Chest and the county pension scheme.[23] Both originated in the late-Elizabethan period, and both aimed to provide financial support to former sailors who had been disabled because of their service. Originally, Chatham's Chest was funded from voluntary deductions of 6d. per month from Royal Navy seamen's pay; from 1619, the deductions became compulsory. Over time, the administrators invested surplus funds in land as a way to increase its value. To qualify for a pension, ex-sailors had to have paid into the Chest and been wounded or hurt abroad in naval service. The level of the pension benefit was supposed to reflect the nature of the injury. A lost limb meant a man got over £6 a year for life. Loss of an eye was worth £5 per year.[24] By contrast, the county pension scheme was supported from rates assessed on parishes by local magistrates. Initially, former seamen who petitioned for a pension needed to demonstrate that their inability to look after themselves stemmed from a war-related injury. However, by the outbreak of the Civil War, ex-sailors in need because of old age also were granted pensions. This suggests that, in the context of the county pension scheme, the meaning of disability had expanded during the first half of the seventeenth century to include the inability to look after oneself or one's family because of age. In other words, elderly veterans were deemed worthy of relief by virtue of having served the Crown in war.

Paternalism and reciprocity underpinned Chatham's Chest and the county pension scheme. The Crown and the gentry recognized that former seamen belonged to a distinct community of service, and that the honour of the Crown required that they be shown a fit measure of material compensation as a sign of gratitude. Rewarding disabled seamen was an opportunity for the men who ran England's counties and parishes to show charity to a deserving sort of poor person, while holding up before the public the cause of his disability – loyal service to the Crown.[25] Additionally, the "better sort" understood that disabled former seamen needed to be seen to be well treated in order that others would be more willing to join the navy in the future. Not for the last time, war-related disability was both defined and deemed meritorious insofar as it conformed to the state's manpower requirements.[26]

Thus, by the beginning of the first Dutch war in 1652, the English state had long acknowledged its duty to care for demobilized seamen disabled in the course of naval service. During the war, it recognized that it had a similar duty to ensure that those still in its service received adequate care for injuries and sicknesses.

CONSTRUCTING A SYSTEM FOR CARE

When the first Anglo-Dutch War broke out in 1652, the politicians and officials responsible for the Commonwealth's navy did not immediately think about what to do for sick and injured sailors. During the initial season of combat, the Republic's Council of State instructed the leaders of port towns that received sick and hurt men, primarily in Hampshire and East Anglia, to make their own arrangements for accommodating sailors. In this war, and subsequent maritime conflicts, the communities most burdened with care depended on the primary theatre of operations. The expenses that local authorities incurred caring for sick and injured sailors were to be submitted to the navy and subsequently reimbursed.[27] As the war entered its second year, however, it was clear to some naval commanders that relying entirely on local authorities to manage the care of sick and injured was neither medically effective nor politically wise. Officials from Ipswich, for example, sent a letter to the Commonwealth's committee for affairs of the navy about the sick and wounded set down in Suffolk. The town's bailiffs complained that the surgeons sent to them from London wanted the seamen moved into the town's hospital, even though to do so would, the bailiffs argued, endanger the health of the surrounding households, and especially the children who attended the hospital's free school.[28] A regime barely three years old, and unpopular with most people, could ill afford to have its method for treating sick and injured sailors perceived as a kind of public-health risk. Additionally, the navy's manpower requirements would be much harder to meet if it could not provide seamen with basic medical care.

Responding to concerns from the navy and local officials, the Council of State ordered members of the navy commission, the panel of officials responsible for administering dockyards, to correspond better with authorities along the coast over the needs of accommodating the sick and injured. The commissioners were also told to inquire about the possibility of using space in any of London's hospitals for naval casualties.[29] However, these matters only added to the workload of the commissioners without improving conditions for wounded or sick seamen, or for the townspeople accommodating them. In February 1653, Francis Willoughby, a commissioner based at Portsmouth, reported that there were many sick and injured sailors there who were in need of relief. Without some form of assistance, it would difficult, Willoughby argued, to encourage others to "hazard lives and limbs" for the regime.

The following month, a group of officers petitioned the Admirals concerning the relief of sailors' widows and disabled mariners "as a service to the public good and incitation" to others to serve the Commonwealth.[30] The notion that providing care to casualties of war was a way for the people to encourage servicemen in their duty was not limited to naval officials. For example, the bailiffs of Ipswich instructed the constables of Ingatestone to accommodate sick and wounded men up to one night "for the better Incouragem[en]t of them and others Employed in the service."[31]

At some point between the spring and late summer of 1653, the navy commission sent the Admiralty a proposal for organizing the treatment of sick and injured seamen on shore. The commissioners suggested creating another commission whose sole duty would be to oversee the care of sailors. The three-member board would work to locate space for naval casualties in England's hospitals. If the country's hospitals could not accommodate the seamen, the officials would look for places for them "at the most reasonable costs attainable, due respect being had to the condition and state of the diseased parties." The commissioners would be empowered to direct local authorities at the ports to find accommodation, called "quarters," for sick and hurt men, and to hire surgeons, physicians, and apothecaries to give treatment.[32] Thus envisioned, the navy would have an agency responsible for finding sites of care, and care workers. The navy would not, however, get into the business of overseeing care directly.

The proposal for a new commission evidently was sent up from the Admiralty to the Council of State, but nothing happened. Then in the autumn the navy commission complained directly to the Council of State. They claimed that it was impossible for them to manage the sick and wounded, widows of dead servicemen and disabled seamen, while also running the dockyards and maintaining the fleet. Nor did it help matters that their office was engulfed with the "lamentable cries" of widows and disabled seamen.[33] Evidently, this time the regime's chief executives decided to act. Within ten days the Council of State had appointed the first commission for supervising the relief of sick and wounded sailors, along with widows and orphans. The tasks assigned to the four-man commission, including Samuel Ward, Joseph Larke, Samuel Cooper, and Methuselah Turner, were essentially identical to those proposed by the navy commissioners.[34]

One striking feature of the proposal underlying the first English governmental agency responsible for naval health care was where it envisioned care would occur. The proposal's framers wanted the sick and injured to be accommodated and treated in the first instance at hospitals. The prioritization of care for sailors at hospitals, in 1654 and afterwards, probably partly reflected the sense among leading government figures that hospitals as institutions would offer the injured or sick "real relief and cure."[35] The "hospitals-first" plan likewise implies that officials were confident that the country's residential long-term-care infrastructure could suffice for treating the casualties of naval warfare.[36] Indeed, during the first Dutch war, many naval and military casualties were cared for at London's hospitals, St Bartholomew's and St Thomas's, as well as at Ely House and the Savoy Hospital.[37] However, it became evident very soon that the government could not rely on existing hospitals, most of which were tiny and located inland, to lodge the sick and injured.[38] Later in the century, the Royal Navy's practice of directing London's hospitals to receive sick and injured sailors created tension between the Crown and City.[39] The governors of the great hospitals did not think they needed to help the navy when its demand for care prevented the hospitals from caring for the sick poor of London.

Additionally, at least one person was bold enough to suggest during the first Dutch war that what the navy needed for its casualties was a building dedicated to treating them. Dr Daniel Whistler, an energetic "roving medical agent," suggested in March 1653 that a hospital at Portsmouth would offer better care and save more money than treating men at scattered dwellings throughout coastal communities. He posited that a well-situated building would save the seamen having to wait a long time outdoors before finding accommodation. Better provisions of medicine, food, and nursing would be at hand, and "the thronging of weak men into poor, stifling houses" with their attendant "temptations to drink" better avoided. Whistler also suggested that "the expense of one man" lodged in a private house "would pay for two in a hospital."[40] At the emergence of naval health care, both existing and imagined hospitals were part of official discussions about the proper methods of managing care work and the resources – human and material – necessary to undertake it.

The first commission for sick and wounded sailors continued working after the war with the Dutch ended. From the surviving records, it is evident that the commissioners were for the most part busy adjudicating the claims for compensation from sailors' widows and paying communities or individuals for providing quarters and care to sick and injured sailors.[41] During the seventeenth century, disabled mariners could apply for public relief, in the form of pensions, either from county quarter sessions courts or else from Chatham's Chest.[42]

The chief significance of the English Republic's commission for sick and wounded sailors is the fact that it became the pattern for similar bodies that were instituted in all subsequent naval wars until the Napoleonic era.[43] The commission for sick and wounded was an office for healing and care in a service dedicated to fighting. All commissioners for sick and wounded seamen were primarily administrators who sought to manage care work that took place in coastal communities. They received their authority from the state, and then the Crown, as falling under a public, then royal, duty of care for seamen. After the restoration of the monarchy, royal authorization meant that the commission for sick and wounded operated as part of the navy, yet not entirely under the Admiralty's jurisdiction.

Restoration-era commissioners' duties were set out in Instructions that were enrolled into the register of the privy council and publicized for the information of captains and naval officers.[44] These instructions set out where the commissioners were to find care providers, what sort of care providers were to be sought, who was to find care providers, and the sort of care that was to be offered. Additionally, each commissioner was ordered to ensure the provision of quarters (the lodgings) and care for sick and wounded men set ashore within a specific region.[45] For example, during the second Dutch war, John Evelyn had oversight for Kent and Sussex, Sir Thomas Clifford was responsible for Devon and Cornwall, Bullen Reymes had authority in Dorset and Hampshire, and William Doyley looked after Norfolk and Suffolk.[46] In 1664, the privy council designated five coastal communities as reception points for casualties; in 1672 the number rose to fifteen.[47] While the commission was responsible for finding and appointing the physicians, surgeons, and nurses who would perform the necessary care and cure tasks, local officials, including mayors, bailiffs, and corporation officers were ordered to "take care and provide for good quarters and billeting of all Sick and Wounded" men.[48] It was also the commissioners' responsibility, through their agents in the ports, to ensure that, once cured, sailors were put back on naval vessels. For their work, commissioners received £300 per year. By comparison, the navy's able seamen received 24s. per month, about 95 per cent less.[49]

The privy council's 1672 Instructions were essentially the same as those issued eight years previously, but with a few significant additions.

The number of ports designated to receive sick and injured men tripled, a change probably intended to spread out the burden of care more fairly along the coast and to make it easier for the commission to work with local authorities in finding care providers. The second addition was an order to the commissioners to submit quarterly reports to the privy council about all the sick and wounded ashore. This order placed a much heavier burden of responsibility on the commissioners' agents at the ports, since they were the ones charged with keeping account of the care business. It is probably also the case that this order motivated Commissioner Reymes's detailed instructions to his agent-deputy at Portsmouth, Samuel Williams.[50] Williams was expected to watch over and keep records about sick and injured sailors. This meant monitoring their progress, so that recovered men did not stay in quarters longer than was necessary. Malingering meant lost money and labour that was desperately needed on ships. Williams was instructed to get intelligence occasionally from the local Clerk of Cheque, an agent of the Navy Board, about the allocation of men on ships. He was also responsible for reporting to Reymes about the state of affairs of the sick and wounded at Portsmouth and environs.

Commissioner Reymes's instructions likewise shed a bit of light on what constituted, in the eyes of naval officials, proper care spaces and care work. Reymes ordered Williams find sailors "good quarters" and to ensure that they received so-called "necessaries for cure," including diet, lodging, fire, candles, and nurses. Seamen were to be properly sheltered from the elements, fed, rested, warm, with access to sufficient illumination and someone to attend to their needs.

Williams's responsibilities put him in contact with, and necessitated him to form relationships with, many different sorts of people: with the mayor or other local officials to find quarters and with surgeons and surgeon's mates, directing them to injured men and paying them an allowance. Williams also had to relate to many – potentially hundreds – of quarterers who lodged sailors during their recovery. And if a sailor had died in care, Williams had to find a gravedigger and a clergyman to give the man a Christian burial.

The instructions for managing care from the privy council of Charles II, and from Reymes to his deputies or agents, envisioned a regular system of accounting for money and men. For example, sick or hurt sailors who were set ashore were supposed to provide Williams with a certificate signed by two superior officers and the ship's purser or deputy, and/or the ship's surgeon. The certificate authenticated that the man was either sick or injured in the king's service. Although the Instructions do not say, we can infer that the deputy was supposed to keep these documents until the man was healed and back on a ship, or else discharged. Williams was required to write once per week to Commissioner Reymes at his office in Westminster, "or oftener if there be occasion," giving Reymes information about local situations and the cost of quartering sailors, their cure, deaths and burials, discharges and desertions, officials who were not co-operating, surgeons' negligence, or anyone concealing a cured sailor. Reymes also wanted Williams to "take note of seamen whose wounds are slight or sickness inconsiderable and record their names and place set down." Not only was Williams supposed to find help for men in desperate need, he had to watch out for potential frauds.

Thus, the agent for sick and wounded seamen at Portsmouth was supposed to provide once-weekly reports, both qualitative and quantitative, about the local operation of the naval health service. We know from the correspondence preserved in the Evelyn papers that deputies did write in to report on the local situation, very often to complain about either lack of quarters or, more worrying for them, a lack of money to pay quarterers. The commissioners or their agents were to discharge – that is, to pay off – the cost of quartering sick and wounded men directly to quarterers or local officials. The rate for quartering sick and hurt men was set at 7s. per man per week.[51] This amount is comparable roughly to 4 per cent of the annual spending on food for a pauper family of five (£9 14s.).[52]

Although the Instructions do not call for it, deputies such as Williams entered information about sick seamen into an account book.[53] How exactly deputies acquired the data is not clear. Presumably, deputies such as Williams depended on quarterers for information about the sailors they housed. The survival of the Westminster account books suggests that agents drew up rough record sheets, and then sent copies to the commissioners at Westminster. Other clerks transferred the information from these record sheets into account books. Additionally, since an agent was supposed to pay surgeons and their mates for cure (6s. 8d. per man), Williams received some kind of paper invoice for services rendered, which might or might not in turn have generated a paper receipt for payment from surgeons.

All the paper technologies and forms of data management that deputies were required to employ – certificates from the sick and injured, regular letters and reports to the commissioners, account books – concerned the whereabouts of the navy's most crucial human resource: sailors. Because the navy so often lacked manpower, the fear of malingering remained high throughout a conflict. This fear produced ongoing questions, including those about whether the men set ashore were really sick or injured? Where were sailors once they were landed? Were there problems finding a place to lodge them in the community, and had they returned to their ship once discharged? These were important questions from the navy's perspective, and they mean that the medical or care-work relationships between surgeons and sailors, between nurses and sailors, between quarterers and sailors, between nurses and surgeons, were off the books of the sick and wounded's "man in Portsmouth." There is very little information about these relationships in the surviving sources. What the extant accounting records do show, along with significant financial data, is the fact that, from the earliest period of naval health care, the management of care was about healing and attending to human resources. In other words, managing naval health care was about knowing as best as possible where sailors were, as well as how healthy they were, or were not.

The Instructions and other orders from the highest officials suggest that the king's council and the Admiralty wanted to develop co-operative relationships with the people who would quarter and care for the sick and wounded along the coast. Thus, in January 1665, before hostilities with the Dutch again commenced in earnest, commissioner Reymes wrote to the constables of Fareham requesting a list of houses, rooms, and beds "fit to receive and lodge sick and wounded men."[54] Seven years later, the governors of the Isle of Wight and all other civil and military officials of Hampshire received a general order from the king to "assist commissioner Reymes," who had been appointed "out of care for the seamen and encouragement of all seamen" to provide the sick and injured with quarters and accommodation.[55]

Obviously, if the local authorities chose not to co-operate with the commissioners, the system would collapse. Unfortunately, at times the leading figures and officials of coastal communities were indeed not willing to help the commissioners or their agents to locate fit quarters for sick sailors. For example, in the terrible autumn of 1665, as London and much of the southeast endured a deadly outbreak of the plague, John Evelyn complained to the privy council that he was not getting the help he required at the ports to accommodate diseased seamen. The council responded by reminding justices of the peace, mayors, bailiffs, and constables that they were required to assist sick and injured seamen by "providing [them] with such convenient Quarters, Lodging and attendance as their necessity shall require." The order encouraged local authorities to "give particular Demonstration in this sad time of sickness of your care and Zeal for His Majesty's service by helping these persons."[56] This appeal to the authorities' enthusiasm for naval casualties during a time of great national suffering suggests that the government recognized that it could not simply compel them to care, particularly in difficult times. This was the case not just for the authorities: local people needed to be convinced that they too had a stake in the health of the navy's sailors.

Once they disembarked, most sick and injured sailors were accommodated and cared for in an inn or someone's home. When many men were set ashore at once, almost any shelter sufficed as a space for care. On 26 September 1665, for example, 350 men were brought up to Gravesend, forcing the commission's agent to put three hundred of them in one building, probably a barn.[57] In practice, fit quarters meant alehouses, inns, and the homes of such people as were willing and able to provide shelter and food for hurt and sick men. Naval health care under the restored monarchy would rise or fall based on the readiness of many ordinary people to form working relationships with the navy – and many were indeed willing. At the beginning of the third Dutch war, an agent at Deal reported that, not only were "our cleanly nurses houses ... redy now to receive" the sick and hurt men, the nurses "here flock about me to receive them."[58] Nonetheless, during the second and third Dutch wars, commissioners for sick and wounded sailors sometimes had to rely on a combination of coercion and willingness from the people of England's coastal communities.

THE DEBT FOR CARE

During the second and third Dutch wars, the emerging system of naval health care encountered difficulties, because it was chronically short of money.[59] This is in contrast to the prevailing situation during the first Dutch war, when the Commonwealth's chief problem was coordinating care rather than paying for it. Arrears of pay for the quarters of sick and wounded seamen was a recurring issue for the regime of Charles II, especially during and after the second Dutch war.[60] The ordinary people on whom the Royal Navy relied to provide care for sick and injured seamen during the king's wars with the Dutch often had to wait a long time for compensation. Some communities refused to take in more sick

Finding Care for Sick and Injured Seamen in England 33

and injured sailors until the old debt for care was settled. However, an unwillingness on the part of ordinary people to extend care on credit to the navy's sailors does not mean that the earliest system of naval health care was fatally flawed. Both parties had reason to be impatient with the other: the state over the reluctance of some communities to provide care; the people over the time it took for the state to pay them.

Arrears of pay for quarters was a recurring and chronic issue during the Dutch wars, and the size of the arrears was often large. The commission for the sick and hurt was reportedly £9,000 in debt in February 1666.[61] At the conclusion of the first season of the third Dutch war (autumn of 1672), the quarterers at Dover had not been paid £700 for the care and cure of 546 seamen over the previous spring.[62] Care providers and workers, local officials and the agents of the commission all agreed that the navy was woefully slow in settling accounts for quartering and looking after seamen. Official tardiness was a common complaint across the period. In 1653, the bailiffs of Ipswich, Aldborough, Southwold, and Dunwich complained to the navy about not yet being paid. Over twenty years later, the town of Southwold petitioned the privy council concerning the £1,700 still owed them "for the entertainment of sick and wounded seamen and soldiers" during the third Dutch war.[63] In mid-August 1665, Commissioner Bullen Reymes declared that his debt for quarters and care for both sick and hurt servicemen and prisoners of war was over £1,000, yet since June he had not got "a farding of the King's money."[64] Similar frustrations were expressed during the third Dutch war. Samuel Pepys's brother-in-law Balthasar St Michael, was very disturbed by his owing the "poor nurses" of Deal £100 by May 1673. That same month, the complaints of the quarterers in Dover, evidently bursting with sick and maimed men, were "soe extreame" that the agent feared he could no longer pacify the people without a speedy supply of money.[65] At the end of 1674, Evelyn calculated his arrears for quarterers in Kent together totalled £15,377. Indeed, nearly half (48 per cent) of the total care cost during the third Dutch war was owed to the communities of the southeast.[66] No doubt Evelyn and his agents would have been aghast to learn that, at the beginning of summer 1673, the amount the government owed to those who quartered sick and wounded sailors represented over one-quarter (27 per cent) of the regime's annual debt.[67]

The relationship between the navy and the care providers of coastal communities broke down when the people felt sufficiently aggrieved by the state's delay in paying for accommodation and care work. In response, the people would either make extra demands on the commissioners for sick and hurt or simply refuse to look after the sick and hurt. The commission's agent at Gravesend during the third Dutch war, Robert Birstall, claimed that his superiors "well know that most of the people who bee willing to take in any men, are soe miserably poore, that they cannot provide for them, without money aforehand, and from time to time, soe long as they keep them."[68] Such concerns went back to the beginning of the navy's reliance on the local people to provide care. During the first Dutch war, Generals George Monck and William Penn were afraid that unpaid arrears could lead Suffolk towns to take a pay-first, quarter-later approach, with obviously unpleasant consequences for the regime and its sick and wounded seamen.[69] In January 1665, the people of Deal were reluctant to take in sick mariners without assurances that they would be paid for quarters quickly. The parishes next to Erith refused to receive any hurt and sick men, despite that town being full, because they were not included in the privy council's warrant for quartering. This refusal can probably be explained partly by a fear that payment could be delayed a long while.[70] By the autumn of 1665, Evelyn reported that the mayor of Rochester had confirmed that local publicans had sworn to evict the sick and hurt sailors staying at their establishments unless they saw money very soon. Some of them, the mayor also indicated, were making unfavourable comparisons between the monarchical regime's management of care provision and the Republic's.[71]

Resistance to quartering was more marked in Kent during the third Dutch war. The agent at Margate claimed that he had to break open the door of one alehouse keeper who refused to admit another sick man unless the agent "would pay the ould quarter furst." The landlords of Gravesend on three occasions threatened to turn sick sailors out onto the streets unless they were paid for quartering in seven days.[72] From Gravesend, the commission's agent reported that an alehouse keeper named Ralph Bailey, "married to a pore widow that kept the ale house before and did willingly quarter several men," had recently "shut his door against [a sailor] and would not let him in unless I would pay the ould quarter of[f] first." Agent Glover reportedly broke down Bailey's door to let the sailor in. He defended his action against "proud saucey" Bailey because Glover was worried that Bailey's reluctance would "like one infected sheep spoile the whole stock" of potential quarterers.[73] A similar refusal to quarter men reported by the commission's agent at Faversham prompted fears that a "universall defection and absolute

Finding Care for Sick and Injured Seamen in England   35

refusal" to quarter casualties "would blossom" across the county unless money was made available to settle the "vast arrears for sick and wounded."[74] At the same time, the agent at Deal reported that nurses and sailors were both suffering from arrears of pay. "They and their sick seamen lie in the streets," he told Commissioner Evelyn, "an epitome of the town's general lamentation."[75] Consequently, Evelyn was prepared to force the reluctant residents of Deal to quarter more men until Pepys dissuaded him for the sake of his personal safety and the honour of the king's service.[76]

The reluctance and outright resistance to receiving large numbers of sick and hurt men that naval officials experienced during the third Dutch war makes sense, not only for the burden that caring for seamen placed on local resources, and the delays of payment, but also for the threat quartering diseased naval servicemen posed to the health of their hosts. Surgeon Hannan at Deal told Evelyn that the "nurses have also got their share of sickness, for there are few houses where they quartered that have escaped and still our town remains very sickly."[77] It is therefore not surprising that one sailor was reported to have died in the streets of Chatham after being turned out by a landlord who believed the man had contracted the plague. The people of Gravesend, confronted with one hundred seamen dropped into their midst in "unspeakable misery for want of clothes," refused to accommodate them "if they be not allowed fresh clothes and sweet shift" without which they would "not annoy themselves nor infect their houses to the indangering of their lives."[78]

However, resistance to care provision, such as that demonstrated in Kent in the 1670s, was an exceptional response to the strain that sick and hurt men put on to local communities.[79] For the most part, the surviving sources of the commissioners for sick and hurt suggest that, during the Dutch wars, naval officials could count on individuals within coastal communities to take up the work of providing care for sick and hurt seamen. The high degree of compliance and even willingness to care for servicemen, which is evident in the records from Portsmouth during the second Dutch war, indicates that enough people saw care work as more of an opportunity than a burden. The case of the parishes adjacent to Erith – who would not quarter men without a warrant – points to a long-standing concern over the legality of an official obligation, not necessarily to a refusal to receive large numbers of sick men. The perception of legitimacy was always a crucial variable in civilian-military relations, of which the navy and senior government officials were aware.[80] On at least two occasions during the third Dutch war, the privy council addressed this concern by issuing additional warrants of assistance to communities in Kent: Margate in May and Greenwich/Deptford in September 1673.[81] It was not the fact of being told they must co-operate with the navy that sometimes angered the people in coastal communities, but the manner in which they were told. The people were mostly willing to work to care, and naturally wanted to get paid, the sooner the better. The longer they had to wait, the greater the chances that impatience would turn to protest.

DEALING WITH CLAMOUR

In the spring of 1665, Bullen Reymes, commissioner for sick and wounded seamen for Hampshire and Dorset, sent a letter to his fellow commissioner John Evelyn, in which Reymes tried to convey the intense pressure he felt from impatient local care providers. "It seems the other day," he wrote,

> some women had gott a whisper amongst them as if the Commissioner (meaning me) [was] going to London the next day; this did so alarum them, as betime the next morning my dore was so beset, as when I came down the stairs to goe abroad, my entry was barricaded with 20 or thirty of the sharpest tonged women, charging me with an outcry, or rather a iangling (for an outcry, there may be harmony) of their several wants and necessities, and all at once, and that they must have their mony and would have their mony before I went.

Reymes went on to claim that another "Squadron" of women confronted him as he went out into the street, while he was "all this while in the midest of them crying and Praying them to have patience a little longer." Only the promise not to leave the town until the women were paid for caring for sick and injured sailors calmed down the demonstrators.[82]

Protest from dissatisfied care providers was an unpleasant means, for naval officials, by which people who had or were looking after sick and injured seamen demanded their just compensation. In the autumn of 1672 Evelyn was very concerned that a lack of steady money to discharge the "great Arrears owing" (about £3,000) to communities in Kent with "neere 3000 sick creatures dispers'd amongst them" would

Finding Care for Sick and Injured Seamen in England

produce troublesome clamours.[83] By March 1673, the arrears for quartering in Kent and Sussex were so high (about £9,000), that Evelyn's agents were "no longer able to support the clamour and threats."[84] Care providers also protested when the commission for sick and hurt's local agents failed to uphold the moral authority of their offices.[85] For example, the two agents in Kent who reported the greatest incidences of clamour during the third war, Robert Birstall at Gravesend and Balthasar St Michael at Deal, were also accused of cheating care workers.[86] The nurses of Deal petitioned Evelyn twice (September 1673 and 1674) to investigate their allegations that St Michael was withholding the funds owed to them. They accused St Michael of paying them 5s. 4d. per man per week, instead of the 7s. per week allowed by the king. The "smallness of the pay," was ruining financially the nurses who were required to extend their credit to take care of sick and hurt men. More importantly, the nurses pointed out that St Michael's alleged embezzlement was fatally undermining the system for finding and managing care work. St Michael's malfeasance would, the petitioners claimed, "deterre others that would willingly provide for such persons did they not think themselves abused by him." The second petition accused St Michael of keeping back even more money from Deal's nurses (1s. per man per day), and of threatening to withhold greater sums should they complain to Commissioner Evelyn. This petition was signed by fifteen people, twelve of whom were women.[87]

Unsurprisingly, the commissioners did not relish dealing with "clamorous" care providers. It is significant that the second notable plan for a naval hospital (infirmary), drawn up by Evelyn in 1666, included among its benefits the total cure of what the commissioner called "the altogether intollerable clamor and difficulties of rude and ungratefull people; their Landlords and Nurses, raysed by their poverty upon the least obstruction of constant and weekly payes."[88] By contrast, Dr Daniel Whistler's case for a permanent naval hospital, put to Henry Vane in March 1653, did not include stopping the clamour of local people as one of its advantages.[89] Read against the grain, Evelyn's plan implies that constant and regular payments would have stopped all complaints, and made his job that much easier to do. Especially during during the fallout from the Plague, Evelyn would have preferred to avoid dealing with ordinary people providing care. Indeed, one of Evelyn's agents in Kent, Robert Birstall, claimed that his regular weekly payments to carers to buy food for their lodgers stopped their otherwise "very clamorous and impatient demands for due payment."[90] Yet his small disbursements evidently did not go far enough for some of Gravesend's care providers. Their credit, he reported, had been so extended in caring for sick and hurt men that they lost their goods and even their homes.[91] For such people, the navy's inability and unwillingness to honour the debt for care was catastrophic. The navy had broken trust with them in delaying payment for care, with potentially harmful consequences for seamen's health and naval strategy, for how could a great navy succeed if it lacked a functioning system of care?

The navy's inability to compensate care workers in a timely fashion sometimes compelled coastal communities to prioritize the health of one group or one person against another's. The high cost of caring for sick and hurt sailors during the wars made the burden of postwar relief more onerous. In some cases, the county pension scheme's requirement to support ex-servicemen, whether Civil War veterans or disabled Dutch-war seamen, caused county communities to reduce the number of "king's pensioners" on the county roll. For example, Gravesend, which we have seen bore a heavy burden of casualty care in both the second and third Dutch wars, sought and was granted an exemption from the county pension scheme by the East Kent Bench.[92] Clearly, the magistrates of east Kent believed it was unjust for the Crown to expect places along the coast both to shelter sick seamen during wartime and provide ongoing relief to disabled Civil War veterans. At least some disabled Dutch-war veterans were encouraged to re-enlist as cooks or to seek accommodation at cathedrals with royal foundations because they had a more difficult time securing county pensions than wounded Civil War veterans.[93] Discouraging seamen from applying for relief under the county pension scheme was an unhappy, if unintended, legacy of the state not allocating enough funds to naval casualties during its naval wars.

While local authorities were not always generous or sympathetic to wounded and sick seamen, and commissioners such as Reymes and Evelyn had to withstand demonstrations from "clamouring" women, the naval officials were generally sensitive to care providers' justified demands and worked to satisfy them whenever possible. The Restoration monarchy seems to have understood that without the space and work such people provided, the Royal Navy's sick and hurt would receive no care, at tremendous cost to the service's ability to function and to the state's strategic ambitions.

During the third Dutch war, senior government officials were reminded in clear terms of the importance of maintaining and, if neces-

Finding Care for Sick and Injured Seamen in England   39

sary, restoring the trust of care providers. In August 1673, the Admiralty recommended to the Treasury that money for sick and hurt arrears be paid promptly, both to bolster the morale of servicemen who might soon find themselves needing care, and for the encouragement "of those housekeepers and others upon whose credit His Majesty's Service must in a great measure inevitably depend for the entertainment of them." Unless concrete steps were taken swiftly, the people could not acquire the credit they required to carry on providing care for sick and wounded men.[94] Early the following year, in a joint letter submitted to the Treasury, the commissioners for sick and hurt expressed their dismay that only £1,000 had been set aside to pay for the seamen's sick and hurt quarters, when the total amount owing was closer to £20,000. Such a miniscule sum would, they argued, simply enrage the people of the ports, with an "evil consequence whereof cannot be sufficiently forseen."[95] In the war's immediate aftermath, evidence mounted of the damage caused by not directing payment to care providers. A representative of the nurses at Deal, Charity Pinder, reminded commissioner Evelyn in a petition presented to him in February 1675 that he had suggested to her that "wee might have our money about midsummer last." Half a year on, and no money received, Pinder claimed that she and other nurses "are run so farr in debt upon the account of the said sick men that if some very speedy course be not taken we are all undone and ruined."[96]

Within months of Pinder's petition, a period when financial retrenchment was the government's top priority, Lord Treasurer Danby took significant steps to meet the arrears of the "sick and wounded service." In July of 1675, Danby ordered a full account of all the monies still owing for quarters in Kent, probably to prepare for paying off the care providers.[97] In 1676, Danby sent Richard Gibson, one of Pepys's clerks, to visit the ports where men had been quartered during the last war to determine exactly how much remained unpaid for the accommodation and cure of sick and hurt seamen.[98] Danby subsequently put Gibson in charge of paying off the remaining debt for care, and over the next two years he issued several orders to eliminate it.[99] Indeed, toward the very end of his tenure as Lord Treasurer, Danby ordered £600 directed toward arrears for sick and wounded quarters, adding, "not to make any failure or delay, it being of greatest consequence to His Majesty's Service."[100] Unfortunately, the state's debt for care remained after Danby was forced out of office in 1679. Faversham's inhabitants claimed they were still owed £900 in May 1679. Two months later, their request was seconded by the Navy Commission, which argued again that settling the debt speedily would "be of advantage to the King's service."[101]

That autumn the towns of Rochester, Chatham, Milton, and Strood stated they were still short over £5,200.[102] The towns of Gosport and Portsmouth petitioned King James II for the cost of sick and hurt quarters in May 1685, "the only debt remaining unpaid for service of like nature." The order to pay the town its arrears, £718, was sent over to the Treasury in December 1686.[103] But it was not until the spring of 1689, as England was on the verge of beginning its longest foreign war in a century, that officials from fourteen coastal communities certified that Richard Gibson had "Publickly, Fairly and Faithfully, discharged all *Arrears* of Quarters" due for caring for the navy's sick and wounded seamen "in the last *Dutch War*."[104] From the time of Charity Pinder's petition in 1675, fifteen years had passed for the Royal Navy to make good the trust of the many local care providers who had attended to the needs of sick and wounded seamen.

During the three Dutch wars, the navy needed coastal communities to provide accommodation and care workers, often in great numbers and with very short notice. In general, the people responded to the sick and injured with compassion. Their first priority was to provide shelter, food, and people to attend to men's basic needs. However, the costs incurred looking after seamen, which they paid out of pocket, became heavier the longer people had to wait for compensation. For example, in the summer of 1653, one Ipswich official addressed General Monck after the town had received "A Thousand poore sick and wounded Souldiers and Seamen" whose "Loud cries cannot but move all Christian harts." Unfortunately, the townspeople were subsequently compelled to "expresse [their] inability of Relivinge them, wee have expended all the moneyes wee could com[m]and or entreat for."[105] The later and similarly heart-wrenching pleas of commissioners such as Reymes and Evelyn to their superiors in the navy and to the Treasury, and the attention of a Lord Treasurer such as Danby, show that senior officials recognized that they could not take care providers and care workers for granted. The emerging fiscal-naval state did eventually honour its moral and monetary obligation to care providers, but in its own time and at great cost to many ordinary people. Almost everyone involved recognized that the problem of arrears was the system's biggest challenge.[106] Reporting to Treasurer Danby about "the sick and wounded seamen in the several ports of England," Richard

Gibson noted that "the payments which have been made to any of [the] Ports, have been generally late, arbitrary, uncertaine and private." This reality caused "the ruin of many poor families," which in turn generated a "prejudice to His Majesty's Service, which ... maybe found attends with very ill effects to his service upon any future occasion."[107] In Gibson's judgment, which was not unique, the government needed to apply itself more to the needs of the people who cared for seamen if it hoped to have a navy that was strategically effective. Experience had also shown that, when the state was too slow in honouring its debts, or allowed its officials to cheat the care providers, the people could and would demonstrate vehemently and noisily, and even leave the sick and hurt to suffer in the street.

Naval health care during the Dutch wars placed a heavy burden on the people of coastal communities. The navy's reliance on people's willingness to provide care on credit led to the ruin of some poor families and enterprises. However, the fact that resistance and refusal to care were rare suggests that the commissioners, their agents, and ultimately the government succeeded in establishing productive relationships with enough people, such that the system of care never collapsed. Almost always, the navy was able to find care for seamen, often under extremely difficult circumstances.

AN EARLY MODERN SYSTEM FOR HEALTH CARE

The emergent system of naval health care had serious flaws. A framework that was supposed to heal and cure was the source of trouble and tribulation for many ordinary people, including seamen. Nonetheless, the fact that the system was invented and then reconstituted twice in 1664 and 1672 was a significant achievement for the Commonwealth and then the Restoration monarchy. Modern people, who are accustomed to living in societies in which new institutions and public agencies emerge (and sometime collapse) on an almost daily basis, should credit their predecessor's ability to erect similar, if simpler, organizations in very different governmental, social, and economic circumstances.[108] In a largely agrarian and subsistence economy such as mid-seventeenth-century England's, it was always going to be difficult to organize the provision of accommodation, and to locate willing care workers, for thousands of sick and injured men. Care work is by its very nature difficult to scale up- and outward, since one person can provide a reasonable level of attention at one time to one other person only.

This fact meant that the navy's demand for care work would necessarily involve many hundreds of care providers and care workers needing compensation. Considering the extant modes of communication and transportation, for an agency of three to four men, supported by at most forty-two surgeons and clerks in fifteen communities spread along hundreds of miles of coastline, and working together with dozens of county magistrates and other local officials, it was a minor administrative wonder that care providers were found and subsequently paid.[109] From an early modern perspective, the Royal Navy's first system of health care worked, if not always well and certainly never without painful breakdowns.

This first system of naval health care worked because it established patterns of interpersonal interaction between the state and ordinary people, in which both parties accrued benefits and had an interest in the relationship's survival into the future. Indeed, Royal Navy officials could be, or at least could claim to be, very concerned with maintaining good relations with care providers along the coast of England, particularly through prompt (or prompt as possible) payment of debts. For example, in 1688 the navy's surgeon-general, James Pearse, reported to the Admiralty that it was his practice to visit the quarterers annually. During his visits, Pearse would "pay the landladys myself to see that they have right done them by my deputies, and by this punctual payment and kind words to the people I perceive such an Interest in them, that upon any greater occasion there will be no want of Quarters."[110] A lack of quarterers was certainly not in the Royal Navy's interest, so Pearse's expression should not be read as wholly self-serving. Furthermore, naval officials did not seem to think that the demands of care providers were unjust or unreasonable, despite often being voiced by women. Female and male care providers were sometimes impatient with public officials, but they were willing to work with them to provide and give care to sick and injured seamen. Indeed, doing care work for the navy created mutually beneficial relationships between the fiscal-naval state and many English subjects living in coastal communities.

Providing care to sick and injured seamen gave significant numbers of people along the country's coasts a reason to want the state – and by extension the Royal Navy – to succeed in managing its resources and paying its bills.[111] Unfortunately for many providers of care, the late-Stuart Royal Navy, although expanding and modernizing, was constantly broke, sometimes desperately. This was particularly the case toward the end of the third Dutch war.[112] However, the fact that the

Royal Navy periodically delayed or deferred payment to civilian carers of sick or wounded men was a step better than persuading or coercing local populations to assume the whole cost of looking after incapacitated servicemen, as, for example, had happened in parts of France during the Thirty Years War.[113] If judged by contemporary standards, early English naval health care was not an inherently oppressive imposition of the strong upon the weak.

It is significant that the emergent system of naval health care in England was grounded not on new institutions, but rather on patterned interactions between officials and people. Other major powers, including Spain and France, had constructed at least one permanent naval hospital by 1670.[114] This was not the case in England, where the majority of onshore care continued to be performed by local people throughout the seventeenth century.[115] Considering that it was a system in its infancy, the fact that it did not collapse should be taken as a mark of success.

Naval health care in England was more organized and better managed under the commissions for sick and hurt in large part because naval officials and care providers learned what the other party needed and expected. The system worked to the extent that it did because it echoed earlier and effective approaches taken by the state to extend its capacity to govern. Along with the creation of a few crucial institutions to execute policy and preserve law and order, the regimes of Henry VIII and Elizabeth increased the number of offices through which their power and policies were upheld and even extended. The active participation of increasing numbers of upstanding propertied men in governance enabled the Tudors and early Stuarts to govern successfully, at least until 1640.[116] The key to active local participation in royal governance was the mutual benefit that office-holding offered: office holders' honour, credit, and status within their locality were enhanced in exchange for upholding the Crown's authority. Similarly, the navy chose to organize a framework for health care that relied upon large numbers of local people to do the hands-on work of looking after the welfare of sick and hurt servicemen, rather than establishing one or more institutions that would have been managed by a few professionals, as in the hospitals proposed by Whistler and Evelyn. And the commission for sick and wounded found enough people in coastal communities who were willing to care on credit for the navy's hurt and sick, particularly those most prone to make money from nursing the sick – widows. Care providers were not state servants in the same way as were a constable or county magistrate. However, providing caring for sick and hurt seamen put care providers in a relationship with state officials that relied on assumptions of mutual (if unequal) benefit and effective performance. In that sense, there was structural analogy between the role of a care provider and a justice of the peace.[117] Thus, care in the community at the command of the commissions for sick and hurt is an apt descriptor of naval health care as it emerged during the Republic and Restoration eras.

Thus far, the story of naval health care suggests that the benefits and detriments of taking up care work were differentially distributed. Naval officials, and many care providers, were men, while women made up most of the care workers. This reality fostered a particular dynamic: public officials were reliant upon many women to look after seamen so that the monarch could pursue his foreign policy. The sexual division of this dynamic would be a source of concern for the administrators of naval health care, a concern that propelled at different times the system's most significant transformations.

CHAPTER 3

Suffering the System of Care during the Nine Years' War and After, 1689–1701

The Glorious Revolution of 1688–1689 resulted in a long and very expensive war.[1] On average, over forty thousand men served in the Royal Navy annually between 1689 and 1697. By 1695, the largest portion of government spending went to the navy.[2] Care for sick and injured seamen happened in contexts that were qualitatively and quantitatively different to those of the Restoration era.[3] Numbers never speak for themselves, but representations of the magnitude of the debts naval health care incurred, conveyed in letters to the Treasury and statements to Parliament, generate a stark, if not sharp, image of the cost of preserving seamen's lives during the 1690s.[4] At the end of 1690, the navy had spent £28,950 on service to the sick and wounded, and was indebted to the people of coastal communities in the amount of £3,479.[5] By comparison, the total cost of the sick and hurt service during the second Dutch war was reportedly £18,000.[6] Less than three years into the war, the debt of the sick and hurt service was reportedly approaching £37,000, nearly double its total charge during the 1664 to 1667 conflict.[7] A year after the end of the Nine Years' War, the outstanding debt for the sick and hurt service, £61,102, was more than three times the total cost of care during the second Dutch war.[8]

The English state faced incredible financial pressures during the 1690s.[9] The Treasury could not afford to provide funds to all governmental departments on the same basis or at the same time.[10] Bills from suppliers of goods to the navy bore interest, so they tended to be paid off first.[11] This reality helps explain why the navy often chose to pay for care last. Care costs were also relatively tiny when compared to other naval expenses. Between 1689 and 1693, the money the navy's treasurer allocated to pay for health care never represented more than 3 per cent of total disbursements.[12] In 1690, £25,000 was allocated to the sick and wounded office from £904,000 in total. The same amount was allocated in 1693, plus an additional £19,000 for Chatham's Chest. Yet the total amount of naval expenditure that year was over £1.9 million. Thus, the combined amount of money directed to the care, cure, and welfare of seamen that year equalled 2.3 per cent of the navy's annual spending.

Unfortunately, as we have seen, many of the people who provided space for care and who attended to the needs of sailors on shore experienced tremendous hardship as they waited for the navy to compensate them.[13] Naval officials aware of the circumstances facing many care providers along the coast sent heart-wrenching pleas for money to the Treasury. Sometimes, care providers expressed their frustration at not getting paid by refusing to offer accommodation for seamen. Nonetheless, the system of care did not break down or stop working, despite the financial struggles King William's regime confronted. The patience of care providers and care workers prevented naval health care from total collapse during the Nine Years' War.

The war placed unprecedented demands on the nation's human and material resources. Annual English public spending before 1688 was on average about £2 million, whereas from 1689 to 1702 it was around £72 million.[14] The documentary sources that remain from the navy's health care system shed important light on the heavy burden borne by ordinary people who offered space and attention to sick and injured seamen during the 1690s. The care providers' plight prompted the commissioners for sick and wounded to become their advocates to the Treasury. In a sense, naval officials negotiated with the regime on behalf of the people who cared for seamen. During the Nine Years' War, the commissioners represented carers to the state as much as they represented the state to the people.

The difficult circumstances of the 1690s also prompted officials to envision a more organized system for care on shore. The demand for care placed on the people of Plymouth occasioned the first hospital dedicated to seamen in England. Plans were issued to improve naval health care by making it better able to save money and preserve manpower. The high monetary cost of care also spurred new efforts to extend the navy's credit. These developments reflected a broader culture of governmental improvement and heightened accountability to the people that eventually helped to stabilize the political nation, and set up naval health care to do better by the care providers in the next long and expensive war.

The System of Care during the Nine Years' War

A NEW ARRANGEMENT AT PLYMOUTH

The fourth commission for sick and wounded seamen was appointed in July 1689.[15] Its members – Thomas Addison, Edward Leigh, John Starkey, and Anthony Shepherd – were appointed because of their political connections and administrative capabilities. Addison, for example, was a business partner of Sir John Lowther of Whitehaven, one of the commissioners of the Admiralty.[16] Commissioners were supposed to seek room for sick and injured sailors at hospitals, or if these did not have room, at places deemed appropriate by the Admiralty. As will be evident below, most sick and injured seamen were accommodated and cared for in town quarters, almost always in inns or people's homes. For example, a surgeon engaged by the commissioners for sick and wounded at Deal, Josias Nicholes, evidently ran a hospital for seamen in "the house called The Black Dog," with space for at least a dozen men.[17] At one coastal community, local initiative led to the creation of new hospital dedicated to the needs of navy seamen. The hospital represented an innovation in the provision of care space, while continuing to rely mostly on care work performed by women.

Plymouth got a naval hospital because George Dickinson, the town's agent for sick and wounded seamen, determined that concentrating men in one place would save money and result in better care.[18] Dickinson accepted the post of agent shortly after the November 1688 revolution.[19] He claimed that had consulted his predecessor, a man named Mr Vallack, for advice on whom to employ as a surgeon for the seamen set ashore at the town. One of names Vallack forwarded was Mr Berry, whose brother was a local attorney. The agent subsequently appointed Berry as one of the two surgeons engaged in treating seamen set ashore. By Christmas 1688, many injured and sick men had been disembarked, and Berry had become ill while treating them. He left town to recover. During Berry's absence, Dickinson undertook an assessment of the cost for care in the town. He concluded that the amount paid to surgeons, "6:8 a head," and the "12 pence a day for each mans dyet," was an "extravagant charge to the King." Moreover, the current arrangements meant that seamen were "butt indifferentlie accommodated, more specially when any quantity was sent ashore." After consulting again with Vallack and another surgeon, Dickinson proposed to the commissioners that a hospital for seamen "would be very commodious," to which they consented.[20]

Agent Dickinson was not the first naval official to propose a hospital for seamen. He was, however, the first to convince his superiors that such a structure was worthwhile. It is possible that Dickinson's idea won approval because he emphasized its potential to save money, upward of "two hundred and eighty pounds one Q[uarte]r for two surgeons." Probably his proposal also stood a stronger chance of success because he forwarded it at the beginning of the war. Whether it was his timing or his concern for thrift that got Plymouth a hospital for seamen, the fact that a hospital would reduce the uncertainty of finding accommodations for men when many were needed on short notice was important to the navy. A hospital at Plymouth reduced the navy's need to negotiate with people willing to provide accommodation to seamen. Thus, the hospital was a step in the direction of the rationalization of care space that everyone welcomed.

At least some people of Plymouth thought Dickinson's naval hospital was an attempt to enrich himself and rob ordinary people of the opportunity to profit from providing accommodation and care work for seamen. Dickinson eventually faced "obstructions and difficulties" from his colleagues, not the least of them from Mr Berry. The surgeon's "carridge" at the hospital eventually became so intolerable that Dickinson reported Berry as a "turbulent person and an Obstructor of the King's business." Berry was dismissed, but not before declaring publicly to one of the commissioners visiting Plymouth that Dickinson "had cheated the people that Quartered the Seamen." In his response to Berry's charge of defrauding local care providers, Dickinson claimed that he had used a town crier to summon all people who had cared for seamen to visit him at the hospital, with a commissioner for sick and wounded in attendance, to claim reimbursement for any outstanding debts. "Several people did appear to Commissioner Elder," Dickinson later wrote, "and owned the sums paid them and it appeared there was noe more charged to the king's books then they owed to have rec[eive]d."[21] Another former surgeon, John Leakie, asserted that Dickinson paid the people who had quartered seamen less than was due to them in order for the agent to reduce the supply of carers and boost the number of men staying at the hospital. Rather than paying the people 7s. per week per man, he paid 5s. 6d., keeping back 2s. 6d. "This so discouraged the people who quarter the men," Leakie declared in a subsequent statement to the commissioners for sick and wounded, "that they did not care to entertain them any more." For his part, Leakie claimed that a public promise made by him to the people

The System of Care during the Nine Years' War   49

to pay quarterers the established 7s. per week for each seaman they lodged had raised the number of available care spaces from 126 to 1,700. The "grand effect" of Leakie's undertaking to pay the people of Plymouth and environs "nothing but their just due" was the reason, he claimed, "that when the grand fleet was off Torbay he was able to quarter 2100 sick men ashore."[22]

The correspondence of the commissioners for the sick and wounded make it clear that the hospital at Plymouth did not assume a monopoly over care for sick and wounded seamen during the Nine Years' War.[23] Sailors were lodged and treated either at the hospital or at other available accommodations in the town. It would have made sense for Dickinson, the initial sponsor of the hospital, to make it the care space of first resort at Plymouth. It also makes sense that some quarterers who had counted on the additional income from accommodating sick and wounded seamen might have resented the hospital. Additionally, as the agent responsible for managing the hospital, Dickinson would have had opportunities to overcharge the navy for the cost of care and supplies. An Admiralty-led investigation of affairs at Plymouth did find that the commissioners for sick and wounded had shown "partiality" to Dickinson, despite some irregularities in how he accounted for the cost of the hospital.[24] In other words, the hospital, while seeming to address one set of problems – seamen accommodated randomly throughout the town, at a greater cost to the navy – complicated the relationship between the navy and care providers and raised the potential for the misuse of naval resources by agents. Nonetheless, the hospital continued to operate throughout and even after the Nine Years' War.[25]

Plymouth naval hospital represented an innovation in the provision of care space during the Nine Years' War. However, the institution relied on the same pool of people to attend to the needs of the sick and wounded sailors as provided care in town quarters. Agent Dickinson's and surgeon Berry's dispute reached a high point in the spring of 1692 over the latter's reaction to the presence of two male nurses employed at the hospital. Dickinson claimed that at one point in the hospital's early operation, there had been such a shortage of nurses to attend the men in care that he had approached two recovered sailors, Francis Champainge and Edward Gillett to "act in that capacity ... by reason they had seen the manner of attendance" that nurses normally performed. The two men had been "very serviceable in that place" and according to the agent "did more than four women, and gave greater satisfaction to the sick." Upon seeing the men nursing the sailors at the hospital, surgeon Berry at first had said nothing, but when he finally asked Dickinson what these men were doing, "it was answered that they were such as were appointed and acted as Nurses because there was a great want of good women."[26] This exchange suggests that care work on shore was viewed as a mostly female activity by naval officials, albeit one that some men evidently could do better than women.[27] Female labour would remain an essential aspect of naval health care during the late-seventeenth century.

Plymouth's naval hospital was the first but not the most famous new space for care founded during the 1690s. Greenwich naval hospital, founded in 1694, offered a place for the relief of elderly and disabled seamen.[28] The promise of Greenwich for seamen, of a place at a long-term-care institution as a reward for service, was meant to induce otherwise reluctant men to enlist.[29] Greenwich hospital did not become a place to preserve the lives of seamen to get them back on ships.[30]

The geographic scope of the naval health care system expanded considerably during the Nine Years' War. Care provision for sick and injured seamen was also organized for the first time in the waters of the West Indies and western Mediterranean.[31] In the summer of 1695, the privy council received a request from the Admiralty to direct the commissioners for sick and wounded to care for seamen "put on shore in the straights and other places abroad." One commissioner travelled with the Mediterranean fleet "for taking care of the sick and wounded seamen in those parts."[32] Nonetheless, the burden of care in the West Indies and Mediterranean relative to onshore care in England does not seem to have been substantial.[33] A postwar financial statements suggests that the charge for care provision in the whole of the West Indies, £878, was comparable to that owed at Deptford (£626) and Dartmouth (£751). By comparison, the outstanding debts at major ports such as Rochester (£3,509) and Portsmouth (£3,428) were much higher.[34]

THE HEAVY BURDEN OF CARE

Summary financial statements offer a tiny window into the tremendous exertion of ordinary people along England's southeast and south coasts to care for the navy's sick and injured sailors. The Treasury papers show with greater clarity the burden of care borne by coastal communities during the 1690s. These sources also convey how close the system for care came to collapse. As was the case during the Dutch wars, extending care on credit sometimes annihilated the resources of households, with similar destructive consequences extending out to the victual traders and onward to the producers who supplied them. Considering the financial crises of 1693–94, with the loss of the Smyrna fleet (one of whose consequences was the creation of the Bank of England), and the profound economic contraction caused by the recoinage of 1696, it is a secular wonder that the system of naval health care survived to 1697. The relatively frequent reports of resistance during the summer of 1697 suggests that the system might not have survived a major fleet engagement along the lines of Beachy Head that year, let alone another year or two of combat.[35]

The Treasury received just over 130 requests for money from the commissioners or the Admiralty during and after the Nine Years' War.[36] Many of these pleas for payment contain descriptions of suffering seamen and care providers, and not a few reports of impending and outright resistance to quartering – and, by extension, refusals to care for the sick and wounded. Unquestionably, the burden of providing care space and care work for seamen on credit was heavier for many people in some years than in others. Partly, this was the result of factors external to the system of naval health care, such as the incidence of a major sea battle. Partly the uneven nature of the burden was a function of financial realities that were inherent in the navy's approach to paying its bills at a time of national economic distress.[37] What follows is an attempt to portray how the navy's demand for care space and care work made the lives of many hundreds of ordinary people close to unbearable.

The experience of the people who cared, compared over the years, varied from not bad to very bad. Four years, 1692, 1695, 1696, and 1698, seem to have been moderately successful: there are reports of suffering, but not of resistance. The years 1694 and 1701 witnessed reports of both great suffering and resistance to quartering. The years with the highest total reports of resistance to quartering and carers in distress – the very worst of the bad years – were 1690, 1693, 1697, and 1699. The year 1691 is the dark one within the sources. The Treasury papers have no reports from the commissioners. The Admiralty's meeting minutes note that £1,000 per week of £3,000 weekly spending was allocated to the sick and wounded service. The only other mention of naval health care in the Admiralty minutes from 1691 was an order for the commissioners for sick and wounded to examine the cost of compensating seamen who transported themselves from Weymouth to Plymouth for treatment.[38]

The year in which the care system provoked the fewest complaints witnessed a decisive set of major sea battles between the English and French navies. These occurred in late May and early June 1692 off

Barfleur and La Hougue. The commissioners and the Admiralty had anticipated an engagement and took steps to ensure the service for sick and hurt men was ready. In early May, the commissioners wrote to the Treasury that money was needed soon, because they did not know when the surgeons would be required at ports and especially in order "to encourage the people to entertain the seamen on shore."[39] A week later, the commissioners asked again for money to answer the cries of the "necessitous clamourous people." Without funds available to pay off at least some of the existing arrears, the commissioners claimed that they would not be able to discharge their credit, "and the seamen would not be quartered nor could they be carried on the hospital at Plymouth."[40] Around the same time, the Admiralty promised Admiral Russell that they would write to the council about the arrears due for quartering men at Portsmouth and Gosport.[41] Evidently, the situation at Portsmouth concerning the outstanding debt for care was so bad that the commissioners had to tell the locals, then "vehemently pressing for arrears," that the Treasury had "already ordered money for that end," which was a patently untrue statement.[42] The pleas of the commissioners, and perhaps news of the battles off the coast of Normandy, appear to have had some consequence with the Treasury. On 3 June 1692, they ordered £2,000 per month for ten months for the sick and wounded service. This was certainly nowhere near the amount the commissioners had requested, but it might have kept just enough money flowing down to the people caring at the ports that the Treasury papers do not contain reports of outright resistance to quartering sick and hurt seamen over the rest of the year.[43]

After the summer of 1692, the navy of Louis XIV was not again assembled as a prelude to an invasion attempt. Instead, for the remainder of the conflict, the French regime encouraged privateers to prosecute *guerre de course*, systematic attacks on English and Dutch mercantile shipping.[44] This policy produced deadly and nearly catastrophically expensive consequences for the English economy and the war effort. Close to four thousand English mercantile ships were lost to the French.[45] Letters from the commissioners for sick and wounded within the Treasury papers suggest that thousands of English sailors were lost to the Royal Navy as prisoners, or killed, sick, or wounded. For example, in June 1695 the commissioners claimed that the arrears for care costs from the start of the war to 31 December 1693 were close to £30,000, with the amount outstanding from 1694 at just over £13,000. The fact that the Treasury had paid £29,000 over the previous

The System of Care during the Nine Years' War 53

year might explain why there are no reports of suffering or resistance to quartering at the ports in 1695, although the commissioners did warn in January that, unless the arrears at the ports were paid "forthwith," no quarters for seamen would be found. The largest issue of money from the Treasury to the sick and wounded service in 1695 was only £6,000.[46]

Similarly, the commissioners brought the suffering of seamen to the Treasury's attention months after the war's end. In January 1698, many "poor creatures" with "lingering distempers" were reliant for care upon people of coastal communities who themselves were "utterly disabled for want of money."[47] By year's end, the debt of care was so large and overdue in parts of the country that, without immediate redress, "the cries of the people would," the commissioners for sick and wounded claimed, "grow intolerable."[48]

There are reports in 1694 and 1701 of both great suffering and resistance to quartering men. For example, early in 1694 the commissioners for the sick and wounded reported on the "miserable conditions of the poor people" at several key reception centres, including Rochester, Plymouth, Portsmouth, and Deal. The response of the Treasury was to issue £1,200 to the commissioners.[49] The commissioners subsequently pleaded for £2,000 per month, without which they "should not be able to quarter a man at any of the ports." The request was not answered.[50] Two weeks later, the commissioners claimed that quarterers had pre-emptively refused to take in sick and wounded sailors.[51] By the mid-point of the year, the commissioners, having been ordered by the king to travel to the ports to make sure provisions for seamen were in place, requested £10,000 to "pay part of the Portsmouth" quarterers cost, since that was a place "where seamen must be entertained." The Treasury responded by issuing £2,000.[52] Days later, the commissioners again sent a warning about the "cold reception" that sick and wounded could expect unless the people at the ports received at least £8,000 to pay off the outstanding (to June 1693) debt for care at ports. This time the Treasury issued half of what the commissioners requested.[53] By the end of August, the commissioners claimed that they had "in some small measure" managed to "assuage the cries of the poor people at Portsmouth, Gosport, and Dartmouth," but at communities in Kent, including Rochester, Deal, Dover, and Chatham, the people "were constantly crying to them."[54]

Evidently, the commissioners had to practise a sort of financial triage in disbursing monies to care providers at the ports. Their correspondence does not offer clues about the extent to which local factors, including pressure from care providers, influenced the choice of whom to pay first. Given the increasing importance of southern and western ports in the war against France, probably care providers at ports such as Plymouth and Portsmouth received greater priority when they complained than the communities in Kent.[55]

The relative neglect experienced by care providers in Kent is evident from postwar requests for payment. By 1701, the sick and wounded service was under the oversight of two members of the Navy Board. An agent, Edward St Leger, reported to the board in March that it was very difficult for him to find quarters for seamen at Deal, and that he expected the situation to get worse. "The tradesmen that formerly credited the nurses," he wrote, "are now unable not having received but one third of their old arrears."[56] Another agent based at Rochester reported on the serious difficulties facing the nurses of that town, as represented to him by several determined women. In early June "several of our chief Nurses came in earnest" and told agent Dr Robert Cony that "I must provide other quarters for the sick and wounded seamen for they could entertain them no longer." Their sudden resolution stemmed from the fact that "they had great sums due to them and of a long standing." Additionally, "several of the Nurses and their families had already been ruined by it. That they found that they must inevitably follow, since they understand the Parliament took no care of them." These care providers claimed that they expected the "Brewers, Butchers, Bakers" to whom they were indebted to demand payment at any time, with catastrophic consequences for the care providers' households.[57] As during the Dutch wars, the Crown's tardiness in settling its debt for care, and taking advantage of ordinary people's credit, threatened the economic stability of care providers, care workers, and their suppliers.

The navy's demands for care space and care work sometimes threatened to undermine the social, economic, and moral fabric of coastal communities. The first year of the war was evidently horrific for seamen and carers alike. For example, the commissioners complained to the Admiralty that the commander of HMS *Monmouth* had put eighty seamen on shore at Gosport without "the least notice to their agents or Chyrgeons there" and thus exposed the lives of his men by leaving them on the beach.[58] By the end of January 1690, the residents of neighbouring Portsmouth had refused to receive any more sick and injured without some payment toward the £20,000 owed them for

The System of Care during the Nine Years' War   55

care.[59] The Admiralty was evidently so concerned by this development that the lords twice wrote to the Treasury requesting money to cover the already massive arrears of care costs.[60] The "great want of money" for the sick and wounded service,[61] and the desire of the commissioners to reduce the burden of care at the ports might explain why, toward the end of 1690, seamen were sent to London for treatment at the city's two great treatment hospitals, St Bartholomew's and St Thomas's. As reported by Dr Lower to the Admiralty, one result of this decision was that "some of the wounded men were suffered to lye two days on Tower Hills till there were maggots in their wounds."[62]

Treasury papers suggest that in 1693 the navy's practice of demanding care and delaying payment as long as possible caused immense hardship. Seamen put ashore at Portsmouth and the West that spring were lodged in miserable conditions, while, during the autumn, some sick and injured seamen set down in Kent were simply ignored. Resistance to the accommodation of sick and wounded seamen reached a level not reported since the end of the third Dutch war. In March 1693, the commissioners wrote the Treasury office that Portsmouth's residents were owed £12,000 and had already sworn not to receive any more men until their arrears were paid. "That which is most lamentable," the commissioners wrote, "and so ill resented by the members of parliament for the several ports is the dayly Complaints and most miserable out-Cryes of the poor needy people, who with the Provisions made for themselves and Children, so readily Entertained and took care of all the Sick as well as the Wounded Seamen." The commissioners noted with deep feeling the disappointment of many people "for whose good service to the publick, instead of being satisfied, members of the best Nurses and honest house keepers have had their Goods distrained" and lost to their creditors. Consequently, nurses' and landladies' "houses [are] broke up, Their ffamilies dispersed and Ruined, and many of them sent to Gaol."[63] These reports of people losing their liberty for unpaid debts incurred in assisting the navy are singularly remarkable. They reveal the extent to which the regime's financial difficulties were borne unfairly by ordinary people. It is doubtful that naval health care could have survived very long had such conditions become widespread.

In April 1693, the commissioners ventilated their concerns about the situation at Gosport. They reported that their agent could not find space to accommodate the many sick and injured sailors already on shore and those waiting to disembark. Local tradesmen had informed

56   Early Modern Naval Health Care in England

Gosport's care-space providers (landladies) that "they should take no more men, for that they can let them have no more goods, they themselves have neither money nor credit in the country to buy more ... so that people that would take men into their houses, have not wherewith to subsist them."[64] In May 1693, the commissioners for the sick and wounded pleaded for money to supply the quarterers of the western ports. The threat of suffering and death was again linked to a lack of money. If the people were not supplied, the "sick and wounded now and soon to be set onshore must unavoidably perish," while the local care providers and suppliers "groan under intollerable Pressures."[65] A week later, both the commission for sick and wounded and the Admiralty wrote to the Treasury that agents of the service could no longer procure quarters for sailors set ashore, especially at the western ports. The towns of Portsmouth, Gosport, and Dartmouth had about six hundred men, but "the people who used to receive them [were] totally disabled by want of arrears."[66] The Admiralty related that news from Portsmouth was that "nurses doe absolutely refuse to receive any more sick and wounded men until their arrears are paid, as being no longer able to keep them."[67] Subsequent to these alarming reports, the commissioners explained to the Treasury that the "poor people" at the ports refused to care for seamen, because those who had cared for men the previous spring after the battle of Barfleur were still not in course to be paid.[68]

The devastating social and economic consequences of the navy's seeking care for seamen on credit were unmissable in 1693.[69] The Treasury had only so much money it could distribute for the care providers at any one time. These punctual disbursements did not match the cost of those demands on local supplies of labour, goods, and services, especially since they too were acquired on credit. It did not take long for local fiduciary and provisioning resources to become overwhelmed. As the quarterers of Rochester and Chatham who refused to supply care reckoned, "they and their families are like to starve, and they had better let the sick men die without, than hunger them within."[70]

The last year of the Nine Years' War was also one of the worst for the people upon whom the system of naval health care depended. In January 1697, Plymouth and Harwich made known their refusal to care on account of the outstanding arrears for quarters.[71] "The unthinking people will," the commissioners reported, "neither have further patience nor pitty, But have driven away our Officers from Plymouth for fear of being imprisoned where things are very unsettled." At Harwich, the

The System of Care during the Nine Years' War 57

people told local magistrates that "they neither can nor will entertain any more [seamen] till the Arrears due for Quarters there be paid in full."[72] That spring, the inhabitants of Dartmouth evidently also had had enough of asking the commissioners for sick and wounded seamen for money; they went directly to the Treasury lords with a petition for payment.[73] Fifty widows and other residents of Dartmouth reminded the Treasury that they had cared in their houses for fifteen hundred men, and had taken good care of them, at the cost of much credit "which hath reduced [them] to great penury and [they] must inevitably perish with their children unless His Majesty pay for the sick and wounded men."[74] In June 1697, Admiral Sir George Rooke, commander of the fleet, wrote to the Admiralty about the "want of Quarters for sick and wounded seamen."[75] The commissioners subsequently reported that there was no hope of finding places onshore for seamen "without a supply of money."[76] On 22 June, the Treasury received three separate statements about the need for money to encourage people to care for seamen: one from the Duke of Shrewsbury, who was one of the secretaries of state, another one from the Admiralty, and a third from the commissioners for sick and wounded. According to the latter, the situation was bad at Portsmouth and Gosport, while, in Dover, their agent had not managed to "get one poor sick man lodged, till the people were moved with his begging to be carried aboard to die."[77] In response to the triple request, the Treasury issued £5,000 for the sick and wounded service from £25,000 in Exchequer bills.[78] This amount might have "stopt the cryes at Portsmouth, Deal and most other ports," but not the complaints from Rochester.[79]

The frustrations of many ordinary people of coastal communities continued well into the postwar period. In May 1699, one Ann Payment and other food suppliers from Weymouth, Melcombe Regis, and Dorset petitioned the Treasury for a total of £151 owed to them for entertaining sick and wounded seamen.[80] The same month, the privy council received a petition from the "Innholders, victuallers, and other poor inhabitants" of Dartmouth, most of whom were "aged and infirm" and who were due, they claimed, £1,500 for accommodating sailors during the war.[81] These petitioners also declared that waiting for reimbursement had impoverished many of them, they "not being able to work by reason of their great Ages and Infirmities." A few months later, the former commissioners for sick and wounded sailors told the Treasury that they could "not find words" to express the poor people's resentment at being "kept out of their money." The commissioners were referring to the overall outstanding debt for care, which in autumn 1699 was just over £61,000.[82]

Considering the financial constraints under which the English state operated during the Nine Years' War, and the difficult choices that the Treasury confronted concerning the allocation of scarce resources, it is no surprise that care providers often waited a very long time for payment. Resistance to quartering also makes sense considering the heavy burden of care placed on people by the government of King William. Yet, the system of naval health care did not collapse. A larger state, with more ways to raise revenue and more options for securing credit, helped the navy's system of onshore health care avoid total breakdown.[83]

ESTABLISHING A NEW FISCAL BASE FOR NAVAL HEALTH CARE

England's naval health care system came close to failure during the Nine Years' War in the face of periodic labour shortages ("a dearth of good women," in agent Dickinson's words) and insufficient financial liquidity. The former problem was directly related to the latter. People at a given port could be willing in mind but unable in body to offer space and care for seamen because their household's credit had been shredded to bits by outstanding navy debts. The governments of King William did take important steps toward addressing the sources of the endemic bottlenecks between demand for care and the supply of care workers. Fiscal innovations and new monetary instruments, enabled by the Parliament, helped the navy's health care system stagger toward the Peace of Ryswick in September 1697 without collapsing. The additional revenue streams also proved that the king's government was keen to pay the cost for onshore care for seamen more quickly than had been possible before.

One fiscal expedient involved an ancient form of accounting for payment. In June 1696, hundreds of sick and wounded seamen and prisoners of war languished in and around Plymouth, which threatened to overwhelm the people.[84] In response, the Treasury authorized the commissioners for sick and wounded to raise money to pay for care space by discounting the cost of an established credit mechanism, known as a tally.[85] Notched pieces of wood that were split in half, tallies were a way to account for and transfer credit obligations. Most often issued by the Exchequer, a tally was comparable to a modern investment certificate with a guaranteed rate of interest.[86] The Treasury had been able to issue £15,000 for the sick and wounded service earlier in the spring of 1696, and then another £4,000 later that summer.[87] However, selling tallies at a discount did not achieve what the Treasury hoped. By late October 1696, the commissioners reported that, without money to defray their daily charges from the people, "they were threatened at the ports that the prisoners of war must be set at liberty and the seamen starved."[88]

Other financial innovations proved more lasting and more decisive for the short- and medium-term survival of onshore naval health care: the Bank of England and its bills, revenue from lottery tickets, and revenue from a duty on silk.[89] The Bank for the first time united debt and cash creation, with awesome consequences for the government's capacity to borrow and for the liquidity of the economy.[90] Within two years, the Bank of England's bills were used to transfer money from the commission for prize ships to the sick and wounded service, and later directly from the Treasury to the commission for sick and wounded seamen's receiver.[91] During the final summer of the war, the Treasury appropriated proportions of the sale of malt lottery tickets toward the debt for sick and wounded care: roughly £6,700 in July 1697 and another £5,000 in early September.[92] And with the debt remaining for the care of seamen reaching over £60,000 two years after the end of the war,[93] in 1700 Parliament directed that £20,000 from a new duty on wrought silk be paid to the sick and wounded service.[94] Parliament subsequently earmarked £20,000 toward the sick and wounded debt from duties levied on French goods and shipping, as well as India silk.[95] Remarkably, considering the burden that the financial constraints put on the care providers only five years earlier, the Treasury was, in essence, able to pay off all remaining debts for the sick and wounded charge in the summer of 1702, a few months after the outbreak of Queen Anne's war with France.[96]

The new fiscal instruments that the Treasury could employ toward settling the Crown's debt for care were products of England's post-Revolution fiscal and constitutional settlement, and the continued growth of its foreign trade.[97] The system of naval health care operated in much the same way during and immediately after the Nine Years' War as it had from 1650 to 1688, but the mode of supplying its material base was significantly altered. So too were the fiduciary contexts in which it had to be organized and effectuated.

In marked contrast to Charles II's governments, naval health care during and after the Nine Year's War was subject to close inspection. The fact that the war was the longest and most expensive naval war to date meant officials were under tremendous pressure to keep naval

60   Early Modern Naval Health Care in England

health care working. The commissioners, like most other spending departments, came under greater scrutiny to account for their money rightly.[98] The war's duration also gave the commissioners and other officials of the navy time to experiment, to try new methods to prevent catastrophe, or to slow down the effects of entropy. Some reforms were implemented in reaction to mistakes of organization or planning. Others were simply a response to changed realities.

ACCOUNTING FOR MEN AND COSTS

Greater public expenditure and new fiscal instruments spurred a drive to greater public accountability during the 1690s.[99] For the first time in the domain of naval health care, regular attempts at accurate reporting of both the number of men in care and the cost of their cure were merged with an ambitious attempt to know where a healthy stock of seamen could be found.[100] The Admiralty consistently demanded accounts from the commissioners for the sick and wounded concerning the disposition of the seamen,[101] the charge of their care,[102] and the number of prisoners of war.[103] The Treasury likewise regularly asked for statements of account from the commissioners.[104] The Admiralty's repository of accountings from the commissioners has not survived to the present, but there are several extant financial statements that were deposited with the Treasury,[105] as well as ad-hoc reports to the secretary of state.[106] The managers of the naval health care evidently kept up their accounts and submitted them to oversight, if not always as quickly as was desired.[107] At the end of the war, the commissioners were ordered to "make up" all their accounts and transfer their records to their successors.[108]

Tracking the cost of care became a significant concern of the commissioners' administrative superiors during the Nine Years' War. In the summer of 1693, the Navy Board wrote to the commissioners, because it appeared that the account books sent up from sick and hurt agents at the ports, in which the length of seamen's time in care was recorded, did not match the data in the reports of the ships' surgeons. Normally, a cured seaman's name was to be removed from the agent's account book on the day of the sailor's discharge from his accommodation. "It is absolutely necessary," the board declared, for the agents' books to be "so correctly prepared as to the time of the [seamen's] being received into and Discharged from Sick Quarters ... for their doing Right to their Majesties."[109] The period of time a seamen spent in care had implications for how much the navy owed care providers. This concern for correct reporting was reiterated six months later, after the board claimed that "there are many errors discovered of several men being born longer in sick quarters than they ought to be." However, the board found that it "seems almost to be a practice in the ports for the surgeons or those Intrusted to take care of sick men to bear them in Quarters after they are returned to their ships, thereby increasing their Majesties charge on the account of the sick and wounded."[110] This statement implied the board's belief that at least some of the agents for sick and wounded seamen in coastal communities were deliberately falsifying their accounts to defraud the navy. Eventually, a former clerk of the commissioners, Samuel Baston, went public with an allegation of corruption in the sick and wounded service.[111] Yet, the privy council did not find the commission's accounting methods secretive or misleading, as had been claimed. The privy council simply ordered the commissioners to use more care in monitoring the accuracy of the agents' books and records.[112]

Financial accountability depended on accurate financial records. However, accountability encompassed more than the trustworthiness of the account books. Naval health care relied on the fostering of trust between naval officials and the people who provided care spaces and care work for sick and injured seamen. This fact is clear from a remarkable postwar financial statement of the outstanding debt for care. In the statement's preamble, the former commissioners, Thomas Addison, Anthony Shepherd, and David Elder, explained why they went to the ports in person to pay the town quarters.[113] At the beginning of the war, the Admiralty had related that "those who were in our situation in the Dutch Wars had been so unkind to the subject and chargable to the Kingdom that we were not to follow any method or precedent of theirs." The commissioners had gone "into the ports to pay the town quarters," a method commanded by the "necessity of the service" and to "enable the Poor Quarterers to take in Sick Men." Paying people in person for caring for seamen would, they hoped, encourage the people to undertake similar work in the future.

Despite the tremendous burdens placed on care providers and care workers during the 1690s, despite the numerous instances in which ordinary people refused to take on additional seamen, the system for care did not crumble. Financial expedients in part help to explain the resilience of naval health care during a very difficult decade. At least as important, however, was the people's willingness to trust that the navy would fulfill its obligation. Without that trust the system would not have survived. It was at times strained to the limit, but it did not break.

THE EMERGENCE OF THE PRESERVATIVE ETHIC
IN NAVAL HEALTH CARE

Officials within and without the navy's health care administration responded to the challenges of the Nine Years' War with plans to improve it. An improved system for care would embody a braided ethic of preservation: the saving of seamen's lives, their labour, and the Crown's money.

The challenges facing naval health care at the end of 1690 prompted a re-assessment. Shortly after the battle of Beachy Head (June 1690), the Admiralty had ordered the commissioners to "give account of what methods they have taken about the care of sick and wounded men."[114] Whatever account the commissioners had been able to convey, a few months later the Admiralty decided that matters had not improved, and ordered a discussion of alterations in the work of the commission for sick and wounded.[115] This judgment evidently meshed with the king's. In early December, William III ordered an "examination and enquiry how the commission for sick and wounded seamen have executed their office," the exercise of which had provoked "many complaints of the commissioners ill management and neglect."[116] Richard Lower, a physician, was very soon thereafter requested to "propose in writing in what manner he thinks it will be best to have [the service] managed."[117] Lower probably already had some ideas about what was needed to better the navy's sick and hurt service when he met the Admiralty. Five days after he was asked to submit a review, Lower presented a proposal for "more effectual care of the sick and wounded seamen."[118] Effectively, the physician suggested that the path to better care for sailors was greater expenditure on buildings and a larger number of care managers. His plan was to preserve the honour of the Crown by saving lives, saving public money, and making it difficult for men to refuse to fight.

The key problems that Dr Lower identified in his report were too many men lost to death and too much debt owed to care providers along the coast. Lower estimated that the total debt for care was close to £50,000. He proposed as his cost-saving solution the conversion of five existing structures into hospitals for receiving up to five hundred men each. These places, along with Plymouth's recently established hospital,

The System of Care during the Nine Years' War 63

would provide care for twenty-thousand seamen "using utmost industry and skill to receive and speedily send abord all such seamen as shall be putt ashore." Lower's plan would cost £29,900 per year, the largest portion of which (£20,000) was provisioning the men with food.[119] Each hospital would have a permanent staff of eleven medical and support personnel, and a flexible staff of nurses: one nurse to every twenty sick men and ten wounded men.[120] On average, this ratio of nurses to patients implied roughly twenty-three nurses working at each hospital treating two hundred and fifty men. Each nurse would be paid 6d. per day.[121] By way of comparison, quarterers could expect 12d. per man per day, of which 4d. was for care costs. "The whole work" of the hospitals, Lower declared, "could be performed by 3/5th part of the charge (commuting the value of so many able seamen's lives) as by the present commission of sick and wounded seamen have done." Probably Lower envisioned a good deal of the cost saving would come from the reduced cost of care work. A landlady responsible for ten seamen could charge the navy six times more for care costs than one nurse looking after ten to twenty men per day at one of the proposed hospitals.[122]

Dr Lower's proposal did not entirely persuade the king or the Admiralty, but the privy council did reconstitute the commission for sick and wounded in February 1691.[123] The commission grew from four to five members, and one newly appointed commissioner was Dr James Welwood, one of Queen Mary's physicians. This was the first time a medical practitioner had served on the commission.

A subsequent review of the sick and wounded service generated an additional set of directions meant to help the commissioners address the changed geopolitical context of the navy's operations during the Nine Years' War. In September 1695, the privy council ordered the Admiralty to consider the commissioners' salaries and the service more broadly. The report submitted to the council in December reflected the thinking of the Navy Board, since the latter had presented its own assessment of the service in October.[124] The seventeen recommendations centred on ways to better preserve seamen through greater accountability and improved manpower management.

The 1695 proposal emphasized the potential of paper-based technologies to help the navy manage its human resources more effectively. For example, the commissioners for sick and wounded would be required to correspond regularly with ships' captains with information about the men in care ashore. The commissioners would have this information from the registers that the clerks and agents at the ports would maintain on "the circumstances of each man." Additional data about the seamen in care, including a sailor's ship number, would be recorded on the ticket issued by the ship's surgeon or purser and presented to the sick and wounded agent on shore. No man would be received into sick quarters without such a ticket signed by someone from the ship, nor could he be discharged from quarters without another certificate from an agent indicating the dates of release and the ship's name to which the man was to return. Clearly, some naval officials believed that paper-based numerical data concerning the sailors was a useful tool for managing a growing health care service for seamen.[125]

In the world envisioned by the proposals, gathering more quantitative and qualitative data about sick and wounded men punctually collected and shared between officials of the sick and wounded service and officers of ships would keep more men in the navy. A better-managed system for care, so argued the proposals, would lose fewer men to death and desertion. A better service would also cost more money in the form of higher salaries for the commissioners and more agents at coastal communities employed or engaged by contract. Although, the proposals of December 1695 did not win the privy council's approval,[126] the idea of using record-keeping in the form of a registry for seamen to ease the navy's manning problem did win Admiralty approval by the end of the decade.[127]

The next significant evaluation of naval health care occurred under very different circumstances and without a commission for sick and wounded. Nine months after the Peace of Ryswick, the privy council, acting on the Admiralty's advice, dissolved the fourth commission for sick and wounded seamen. At the same time, the council requested recommendations for "a method for the care of sick and wounded seamen now in time of Peace."[128] The Admiralty did not propose putting naval health care under the direction of a surgeon-general, as happened after the third Dutch war. Instead, the management of care for sailors was transferred over to the recently selected Registry of Seamen.[129] Soon after this decision, the Admiralty directed the Navy Board to draw up another set of "proper Instructions" concerning the sick and wounded service.[130] There are good grounds to believe that these instructions were drafted and submitted to the commissioners of the registry by mid-July 1698.[131]

The Instructions of July 1698 were the first to offer a peacetime plan for naval health care.[132] They differ in significant ways from the instructions generated by privy councils for the Nine Years' War and the wars

The System of Care during the Nine Years' War 65

against the Dutch. The 1698 Instructions reviewed what had worked in the past, while suggesting changes to provide more effectual service. The focus of the 1698 Instructions was on procedures, ways to make the service better without necessarily relying on a continuity of personnel. There was also a recognition in them that, even in a time of fiscal and operational retrenchment, the procedures for managing care and the means of keeping officials accountable could be – and so should be – improved. In short, the 1698 draught suggested that the key to a more effectual system of naval health care was to enhance its procedures of measurement and strengthen its oversight of seamen.

An administratively thickened sick and wounded service would have more information, show more care in tangible ways, employ more elaborate methods, and work more systematically. The system would retain more qualitative data. Agents at the ports would have to maintain multiple registers of information, including a Book of Quarterers with men's names, their ships' numbers, numbers of days in quarters, and the amount of money owed to care providers. From these registers, every three months agents would prepare Quarter Books, in which they would record payments to care providers. Copies of these records of payment and the books of quarterers' names were to be sent to both the registry commissioners and the treasurer of the navy.[133] The clerks' records were to be cross-referenced with warrants issued to sailors to seek care – smart tickets – from ships' officers. The practice of corresponding with ships' captains as to which of their men were "Dead, Run [deserted], or still in Quarters or Discharged" was to continue, in order to "do right to both His Majesty and the [seamen]."[134] The registry commissioners themselves were to cross-reference the monthly accounts of men in care sent by agents at the ports and submit a general account of the sick and wounded ashore to the Admiralty. A third strand of paper-bound data transmission between ship and port and London would, per the Instructions, best serve the honour of the Crown and the health of seamen.[135] Other instructions elaborated more complex procedures, such as the directions on the method for returning recovered men to ships. Agents were also directed for the first time to watch out for "any men set ashore who are not sick or could have been treated on their ship."[136]

Additional directions show a desire to systematize relations between the health care system and local people – both governing authorities and care providers – while also allowing for greater operational flexibility. For example, the manner of making payments to care providers was explicitly to follow the Navy Board's method of paying bills in course, made from the quarterly account books in the presence of the commissioners.[137] Care sites were to be procured with the assistance of local magistrates in such a way as to reduce the commissioners' reliance on orders-in-council. Indeed, the registry commissioners were directed to inquire into the method of care at the port and then to impress upon the Admiralty the necessity of implementing the local regulations.[138]

The 1698 Draught Instructions showed more concern than previous directives for seamen's corporal condition. Care on shore was explicitly about more than finding accommodation and people to attend to men in need. Agents of the sick and wounded service were ordered to ensure that seamen set ashore without clothes were "provided shirts, drawers, stockings and shoes as shall be absolutely necessary," if also "as cheaply as possible." The agents would also be expected to find out why ships' captains had set their sick and wounded on shore without bedding or clothes.[139]

The Draught Instructions represented a significant conceptual reconfiguration of the sick and wounded service during the post–Nine Years' War era. The system as envisioned by the postwar Navy Board would have done more than its precursors, and more effectually, in an era of restraint. It remained a system of the mind, however, because the commission itself was massively retrenched, for financial and probably also political reasons, in mid-1699.[140] The probability that the Draught Instruction's vision of robustly accountable service could be implemented diminished to next to nil with two part-time officials from the Navy Board and two clerks responsible for its implementation. Such a tiny body could not hope to implement the vision outlined in the Instructions.[141] Nonetheless, the 1698 Draught Instruction's innovative approach to naval health care is evident when it is compared to a rival contemporary proposal.

In June 1698, three former commissioners, David Elder, Christopher Kirkby, and Thomas Addison submitted a "state of their office" to the Treasury.[142] The statement was both an account of the outstanding debts for care and a proposal that the commissioners take up their former role in the future. They recalled that when they were first appointed (July 1689), they had encountered resistance to quartering the sick and wounded. They had addressed this problem by travelling to the ports to pay off the old debts for care, especially to "the most necessitious," in part by "borrowing and laying down what (they) could obtain to Encourage the quarterers to receave the seamen, whose service then was, and still is, of such use to these Kingdoms." The commissioners now stood £60,000 in debt, "gained upon the poor willing people to serve the King and preserve his Subjects." It was obviously in the interest of the Crown, they said, to see that right was done to the carers, to see them "justly paid, and their [the commissioners'] own obligations discharged." The request for money was followed by five recommendations for frugal, effective continuance of the health care system in peacetime. The key to good service to seamen and care providers, according to the former commissioners, was to ensure a continuity of senior personnel. Under the first proposal, two ex-commissioners would continue to serve as correspondents with surgeons at the ports, while a third would travel to the ports. Visiting the ports and "seeing the quarterers justly paid [would] readily recover seamens health and strength, content the persons that quarter them, prevent all just complaints, preserve the reputation of the service, and save the publique" much more money than the commissioners' salaries. The fourth proposal would have the commissioners also acting as inspectors of naval hospitals built at major reception centres, should the king decide to construct them. Implementing these proposals would "ensure better readiness for war" and save the state £3,000 per year. According to the former commissioners, the role of the service to the sick and wounded was to uphold the prince's honour by restoring the seamen's health, paying the care providers, and preventing undue losses to the Treasury, the very themes that had animated Dr Lower's review of the service nearly a decade earlier.[143] Unlike the Navy Board's contemporaneous improvement scheme, however, neither the methods of data collection nor transmission would be altered.

This post-hoc review of the commissioners' performance managing naval health care during the 1690s is important, not only for articulating the need for the service for the sick and wounded to maintain good relationships with care providers. Right relations between the naval officials, the sailors in need of care, and the people underpinned the system during King William's War as it had under Cromwell and King Charles II. After the most expensive war in over a hundred years, and at a time of profound monetary and fiscal innovation, naval health care was still understood by senior officials to run primarily on fostering and maintaining trust between the people and the state.

Naval health care in England was undoubtedly affected by the consequences of the Glorious Revolution, including the enormous expansion of the navy. But there was more continuity than change in the system during the post-Revolutionary conflict, particularly and most importantly in the modes of managing care provision and delivery of care work. The Nine Years' War severely tested the people's capacity to provide care on credit. Nonetheless, the system of naval health care survived to the end of the conflict. There was, however, much more discussion of ways to improve the system of care. Plans and proposals for a better sick and wounded service reflected the broader political and cultural impetus to innovate and find ways to be more effective with limited resources during unprecedented martial, financial, and economic challenges. The more officials began to think about how best to preserve seamen for the navy, the more attention they gave to the state of the care spaces and the condition of the care workers.

CHAPTER 4

Securing Care for Seamen during
Queen Anne's War, 1702–1715

The system of health care for sick and injured seamen was reformed and improved during Queen Anne's War. At select ports, naval health care officials endeavoured to secure care space by instituting contracts for hospitals, while continuing to find sufficient sites for care and care workers at town quarters.[1] The shift of emphasis from simply finding care to finding and securing it stemmed from the congruence of newly available financial resources with an ambition to extend command and control over care work and care spaces. On the whole, naval health care performed better between the beginning and end of Queen Anne's War than it had during the 1690s because there was more money to fund it.[2] The navy's service for sick and wounded sailors, the contemporary name for naval health care administration, surmounted a serious financial challenge thanks to a fiscal innovation that encouraged a wide public of investors to trust in the future earnings of the South Seas trade.[3] The relatively consistent availability of money for the care of seamen was the result of greater trust between the political nation and the Crown, forged during the 1690s.[4]

By contrast, the fifth commission for sick and hurt seamen worked to centralize care at several ports, because its members lost confidence in the dispersed and lightly supervised system that it had inherited. In their view, naval health care in 1702 relied too much on inadequately managed care providers, many of whom were women. The commissioners preferred to work together with a handful of hospital contractors, known as undertakers. The deficiencies of the inherited system of health care, so the commissioners intimated, were largely the failures of unsupervised care providers to deliver the kind of care that would preserve men and money for the Royal Navy.[5] Thus, to better secure proper care for seamen, certain ports witnessed a centralization of care space at privately contracted hospitals. Paradoxically, broadly based public credit technologies sustained naval health care at the same time as naval officials deliberately reduced the number of trusted care providers and sites for care at select ports.

This chapter begins with a brief overview of the naval health care establishment: that is, the commissioners, the instructions under which they operated, and the places along the coast where care for seamen was provided. In order to gauge how much naval health care improved, the chapter also examines the overall and regional burdens of care. The following section shows that, despite the heavy demand for care spaces and care work, naval health care on shore was more ordered at the start of the eighteenth century than previously. Ordered care on shore is evident in steps taken to secure its financial support, increase its financial accountability, manage more effectively its manpower, and maintain productive relationships with care providers. The most significant step toward more ordered care occurred with the drive at four ports to centralize care work at private-contract hospitals. According to the commissioners, the quality of care for seamen would improve. In other words, fewer care spaces would translate into better care work. Thus, the establishment of contract naval hospitals at the so-called great ports signalled quantitative and qualitative shifts of emphasis within the administration of naval health care. In order to save men and money, the sick and wounded service moved from finding as much care space and as many care workers as possible to finding and securing care work via the centralization of care space at select ports.

THE ESTABLISHMENT FOR CARE

The fifth commission for sick and wounded stands apart from its seventeenth-century predecessors in several important ways, not the least of which were its successful centralization of care space at key ports and its relations with care providers. In June 1702, the privy council appointed Colonel Henry Lee, Philip Herbert, Dr Richard Adams, Dr William Sherrard, and Dr Charles Morley to the commission.[6] For the first time, the Admiralty sent the commissioners their guiding Instructions. In what was probably also an unprecedented move, the commissioners were sent a copy of the Instructions within a week of taking office "to consider thereof and represent what additions and alterations they judge convenient."[7] From the beginning, the commissioners were encouraged to think of ways to change the system for care to make it better.

The commission for the first time had five instead of four members; it continued managing the sick and wounded, and prisoner of war, services with that complement until February 1713. Its period in office was longer than any previous board.[8] Two additional points are worth noting. First, unlike previous commissions for sick and hurt seamen, physicians composed the majority of its membership over most of its existence (1702 to 1706; 1707 to 1713). There were never fewer than two physicians on the commission. From 1707 to 1713, four of the five members were physicians.[9] Second, two men, Philip Herbert and Dr Richard Adams, served continually as commissioners from the spring of 1702 until April 1715. The combination of men with similar professional backgrounds, serving together for over a decade, made the fifth commission easily the most formidable overseer of naval health care during the late-Stuart era.

Nonetheless, the establishment for naval health care from 1702 to 1713, consisting of agents at coastal communities and the central office (for the commissioners and their clerks) at Westminster, largely replicated the one in place during the Nine Years' War. For example, in July 1698, the month King William ordered the sick and wounded service retrenched, there were twenty-three coastal communities in England at which sailors received care and twenty-two surgeons appointed to act as agents for the sick and wounded at these communities. At five places, Rochester, Deal, Portsmouth, Gosport, and Plymouth, the navy paid a surgeon a salary to oversee the provision of care for sailors; each of these five communities, save Gosport, also had a salaried physician to assist with the treatment of the sick and wounded.[10] Four years later, roughly the same number of places, twenty-four, were designated to receive seamen.[11] Non-salaried surgeons at nineteen ports were to receive, as during the previous war, 6s. 8d. per head for cure. Similarly, surgeons often served as local agents for procuring care space and paying for it, except where the commissioners appointed an agent. The four ports assigned agents were Rochester, Gosport, Deal, and Plymouth.[12] The last of these four great ports already possessed a hospital for seamen; the other three would soon have their own.

The Instructions issued to the commissioners on 20 June 1702 show elements of change and continuity with earlier ones.[13] The content suggests that they were indebted almost entirely to the draft prepared by the Navy Board in the summer of 1698.[14] The 1702 Instructions have twenty-four articles, twenty of which are identical to the earlier document. Likewise significant is the contrast between the 1702 Instructions and the set issued twelve years earlier.[15] Eight of the 1702 articles find echoes in the 1689 document, ranging from keeping an office, putting men in hospitals, preparing accommodations on shore, keeping accounts of men at the ports, and managing prisoners.[16] However, the 1702 Instructions envisioned no role for the commissioners in postwar relief: there is no discussion of helping seamen's widows or orphans,[17] nor any connection to Chatham's Chest.[18] Almost certainly, the impending completion of Greenwich naval hospital for aged and disabled seamen explains the shift to naval health care as concerned with treatment and recovery for service.[19]

The 1702 Instructions proposed a much more paper-driven process of quantitative and qualitative data collection than previously was in place. The naval health care establishment consisted of twenty-four towns that were designated to provide care space for seamen, plus an office with a staff of eight at Westminster.[20] The eighth article, which directed the commissioners' local agents to keep a book of names of seamen at the ports, and an example of what its register should look like also included a blank form of the "Quartersbook" in which data from the former (the Book of Names) was to be entered. Article twelve of the Instructions required local agents to record alleged sick frauds; the method for reporting such cases was laid out in article fifteen. The nineteenth article provided a method for receiving money and making payments; the twenty-first outlined a way to get legal authority from the Admiralty to quarter men where no previous warrant was in force. Article thirteen described the method for agents to keep monthly accounts of men under care in town quarters; these monthly accounts were to be cross-referenced with separately prepared quarterly accounts "as a further caution against any mistakes or abuses therein."[21]

Additionally, for the first time several articles of the Instructions related to the conditions of care, presumably as a way to check on the quality of care work. An agent, officer, or surgeon was to visit men staying in town quarters daily. Officials were ordered to ensure that the seamen "be supplyed while they continue there, with Medicines, Dyett and other Accommodations of all sorts, necessary and proper for men in their condition." Agents were ordered to inspect the clothes and bedding with which sailors arrived on shore. In cases where it was necessary, agents were to supply seamen in sick quarters with clothes "for their Preservation," including "Shirts, Drawers, Shooes, Stockings and the like," while also "takeing care to doe it as cheap as possible."[22] Herewith, the Admiralty outlines both the importance of proper bedding, clothes, food, and medicines for the recovery of seamen's health. Cleanliness, diet, and warmth were foundational to good care, provided they were acquired at as little cost to the navy as possible.

The preservation of men and money underpinned the 1702 Instructions and the work of the commissioners for sick and wounded. Toward the end of Queen Anne's War, commissioners Herbert and Adams recalled that they "proposed such alterations, in the manner of providing for all the sick and wounded seamen, as have been a saving of many thousands of pounds per annum, as well as the loss of multitudes of Her Majesties subjects."[23] The commissioners' reforms were, in this view, a fulfillment of their Instructions' preservative ethos – work undertaken to save men while also saving money during another extremely expensive war.

THE FINANCIAL BURDEN OF CARE

Correspondence between the commissioners for sick and wounded and the Treasury provides a broad overview of where and when the burden of care fell heaviest, and how the navy managed it. The cost of onshore care for seamen in England during Queen Anne's War was unprecedented. The period between 1702 and 1710 saw a significant rise in the cost of care compared to the Nine Years' War, despite the lack of any sea battles approaching the scale of Beachy Head or La Hougue.[24] Part of the increase in the charge seems to be explained largely by two factors: the increased cost of keeping prisoners in custody and the added cost, in comparison to the 1690s, of care at foreign ports. Remarkably, toward the end of Queen Anne's War, for the first time ever more money was owed for care performed outside Britain than along its coast. In a 1708 statement, the total debt amounted to £49,224, of which £12,188 was incurred overseas. In comparison, in June 1711 foreign care costs represented 19.5 per cent of the total charge (£8,900 of £45,600). The bulk of the foreign cost derived from the hospitals at Lisbon, Port Mahon, Jamaica, and from prisoner custody charges at places such as Malaga, Bilbao, Boston, New York, and the Channel Islands.[25]

The commissioners' correspondence with the Treasury, consisting primarily of financial statements and pleas for money, do not always provide a breakdown of the particular charges for care at different places. For example, a meeting minute of 30 April 1709 noted that one years' cost for care at the great ports and two years at the lesser ports was £13,000.[26] However, there are a few statements that offer snapshots of the regional burden of care cost at various places around the country. For example, a statement of the money owed for care at home (English) ports at Michaelmas 1708 listed twenty-three places: seventeen were owed £1,000 or less. Of the remaining six, less than £2,000 was due at Deal, Woolwich, and Harwich (respectively £1,266, £1,296, and £1,555), while the sums needed to settle the debts at Rochester, Plymouth, and Gosport (respectively £4,606, £5,199, £7,714), all three with a hospital, were substantially higher.[27] Most parts of the English coastline, south, southwest, east, and northeast, probably entertained sick and wounded seamen at least once. Although most of the work to restore seamen to health happened at places with private-contract hospitals, sailors were looked after at communities not envisioned in 1702. Communities in Cornwall,[28] Scotland,[29] East Anglia,[30] and Somerset also provided care for navy sailors.[31]

Before surveying the costs incurred by sick and wounded seamen, it is worth pointing out two significant contextual factors. First, the interlude of peace prior to the conflict was the shortest – four years – of any naval war since 1650. Second, the war preceding the outbreak in 1702 already had been the most costly for the navy's sick and wounded service. A general account submitted to Parliament by two commissioners from the fourth commission (active during the Nine Years' War) showed that the total charge of naval health care and custodial oversight for the years 1689 to 1699 was £317,914. Of this amount, care for the sick and injured stood at £185,334 (58.3 per cent), and £61,834 for prisoners (19.5 per cent).[32] By comparison, the cost for sick and wounded care between 1702 and 1707 was reported to be £257,337, which, even if including custody charges for prisoners, was £10,000 higher than the charge of the previous decade.[33]

The unparalleled size of the debt owed by the navy for care is evident from an accounting of navy treasurer Sir Thomas Littleton's imprest charge on the commission's account between July 1702 and September 1709, £409,091, which represented an increase of 28.7 per cent over the cost of care during the whole of the Nine Years' War.[34] The costs of care grew even as the Earl of Oxford, Robert Harley, worked for peace and a way to solve the kingdom's fiscal challenges. Between the spring and autumn of 1711, the commission for sick and wounded incurred £19,250 worth of charges at domestic ports.[35] The following summer, the domestic charges amounted to £39,137.[36] Two statements from 1713 show a reduction in the commission's debt and a sharp decline in the debt of care overseas.[37] Never before had people cared for seamen at so many different places.

The charges for sick and wounded care were, as had been the case during the 1690s, punctually uneven. Numbers gathered from the commissioners' correspondence with the Treasury suggest two peaks of very high costs, 1702 to 1703 and 1711 to 1712, and several troughs. The case for a twin-peaks view of the punctual burden of care is correlated by the spending burden per annual quarter, provided by a number of financial statements. For example, the amount of the charge on the service between 30 September and 31 December 1702 was £21,077, a sum that the commissioners noted was high because of the cost of caring for soldiers from the Vigo campaign, and nearly four thousand prisoners.[38] The spring and autumn (or Ladyday and Michaelmas) quarters of 1711 saw a debt of roughly £16,000.[39] By the following summer, the cost of care per yearly quarter had dropped to just over £10,000.[40] There is also a correlation between the number of pleas sent from the commissioners to the Treasury, and the stated debt levels. The greater the need for money, the more requests were sent, as generally had also been the case during the Nine Years' War. By my reckoning, twelve requests (memorials) were sent from the commissioners in 1703, nine in 1704, and no more than five per year thereafter until 1710.[41] Then in 1711 the commission issued twelve pleas for payments, and another eight the following year.

However, the fiscal abyss did not swallow up the service for sick and wounded.[42] Between February and May 1713, the commission's debt dropped from £35,569 to £24,770.[43] At the end of 1714, months prior to the peace-time retrenchment, the debt for the period from September 1713 to October 1714 stood at £5,945, the lowest in over a decade.[44]

The rhetoric employed by the commissioners for sick and wounded in their requests to the Treasury overall was less urgent and pitiful than that used by their predecessors during the 1690s. There is a sense of persistent, sometimes profound, concern underlying the statements and memorials, but before 1711 there are very few pleas evincing panic or impending collapse. The difference in tone between the two sets of documents could be explained partly by the different personalities populating the commissions of the 1690s and 1700s. But more than temperamental contrasts may account for the mood of calm that prevails over the commissioners' requests for money, even in the worst of circumstances. Prior to 1711, the commission for sick and wounded could expect on average between three and four payments per calendar year.[45] At other times, the amounts issued from the Treasury came very close to meeting the board's demands. In 1707 the sick and wounded service received just over £35,000;[46] within eight months it got another £23,000.[47] Then, from the summer of 1710 until the autumn of 1711, the sick and wounded service received no money.[48] This lack of funds was comparatively unprecedented and caused the hospital contractors then operating to threaten the shuttering of their operations.

The commission's papers suggest that 1711 was the hospital contractors' *annus horribilis*. The same was true for many town quarterers. The hospital contractors carried their concerns about not getting paid to the Admiralty, claiming that the great arrears of pay threatened not only their credit, but the system of naval health care, with "disappointment."[49] By May of that year, the lack of compensation for care meant that the contractors could not "proceed to carry on the service."[50] The following month, the commissioners issued a statement outlining the seriousness of the situation at the great ports. Over £71,000 in debt, the commissioners claimed to have received one payment of £20,000 over the previous twelve months. Their hospital contractors faced "insuperable difficulties," because their contracts with the commission afforded them no interest, which was not the case for contractors engaged to the Navy or Victualling Boards. Consequently, to "service the Publick," the contractors themselves were compelled to borrow money at interest, since "the nature of the service demands ready money." Unless their plight was "immediately relieved," claimed the board, the contractors would not only lose money on their contracts for hospital care, but "must be inevitably ruined." Indeed, the commissioners reported that the hospital at Deal was already shuttered, and "the rest have stated they must do the same, so the seamen will be expected to perish in the streets." Adding another grim reality to this terrible prospect, the commissioners explained that, at the lesser ports, its officials "are arrested by the Quarterers for what is due them from the Government."[51] This was precisely the reverse of the situation at some ports during the previous war, when indebted quarterers lost their liberty. Unsurprisingly, Deal and Gosport's hospital contractors took it upon themselves to petition the Lord Treasurer several weeks later.[52] In late September 1711, the four hospital contractors met the commissioners to declare that, if they were not relieved within thirty days, they would "shutt up the Doors" of their establishments.[53]

The recently appointed Tory Treasurer relieved the debts for sailors' care dating from Michaelmas 1711 by virtue of his fiscal-commercial innovation, the South Sea Company. This measure alone did not, however, end the hospital contractors' financial difficulties. In February 1713, the commissioners again related to the Treasurer the "Extream Hardships" under which the hospital contractors had suffered since the autumn of 1711. "Most of them," the commissioners claimed, "having then desired to quit their Employment to prevent their utter ruin, but were prevailed upon to proceed," with the expectation that they would be paid regularly. Moreover, the commissioners' request reflected the geographical stratification of naval health care during the war. The commissioners pleaded for money to support the sick and wounded service "where it is ongoing, vizt the four great ports in England and Port Mahon."[54]

Naval health care at the turn of the eighteenth century was not free of the financial strains that had nearly undermined it during the 1690s. But the financial records suggest that a system collapse threatened only once, when the Tory ministry strove for peace between 1711 and 1713. The otherwise relatively steady performance of the sick and injured service, from a financial perspective, owed much to fiscal expedients manufactured during the 1690s, including the civil list,[55] the land tax,[56] the malt tax,[57] and later the great Tory public-private partnership, the South Sea Company.[58] The Treasury's ability for most of the war, and after, to fund care for seamen was evident indirectly in Robert Harley's willingness, from the spring of 1714, to pay the commission's agent at Port Mahon in money, not South Sea stock.[59] By acknowledging that care overseas could not operate on credit instruments or promises of corporate wealth, the Lord Treasurer also admitted to having the cash to pay for it.

By the conclusion of Queen Anne's War, the Crown possessed the financial instruments it needed to fund, through taxation and borrowing, a massively expensive military and naval war. In the 1620s, the navy of the queen's grandfather had not been able to feed its sailors or supply them with enough ladders to take one small island. By 1715, the Royal Navy possessed the organizational capacity and money to feed, supply, and care for tens of thousands of seamen.[60] This capacity emerged from the financial revolution of the preceding two decades. The landlords and merchants represented in England's parliament came to trust their government to spend vast sums of money that they had agreed to pay. Without this high level of trust between the governed and the government, the navy and its health care could not have performed to the extent that they did during Queen Anne's War.[61]

The consistency with which the state was able to discharge the financial burden of care correlates with a comparative absence of reports of resistance to quartering men. There were times during the conflict when care providers and their suppliers had enough of waiting for payment. But there are fewer such incidents appearing in the records of Queen Anne's War than in previous conflicts. It might be the case that the fifth commission chose not to record reports of reluctance or resistance to care, although its reaction to Portsmouth's landladies in August 1704, as we shall see, suggests a board not shy of naming and shaming those whom it deemed a danger to the provision of good care.

Between 1703 and 1713, payments to town quarterers occurred at the ports.[62] Following the postwar retrenchment, payments were issued at the commissioners' office in Westminster "to ease the charge of travelling."[63] During the war, the commissioners worked together with local authorities to publicize impending payments. For example, in spring 1706, the commissioners wrote to Plymouth's mayor to inform him that one of them would come down "to pay the Debt contracted upon the account of the office." The mayor was to "give publick notice thereof that all there who have given credit to the service may receive their just demands."[64] The commissioners also attempted to inform the people of their method for payment. Midway through the war, the commissioners ordered their agent at Deptford to post up a letter, which stated "whatever men are quartered without having a ticket from the agent, will not be allowed by the Board."[65]

The commissioners evidently followed the navy practice of paying care providers "in course" – but often in spirit, not always in fact. Beginning in the Restoration period, the Navy Board had issued to contractors numbered series of bills, payments for which were announced punctually in the London *Gazette*.[66] In the case of the commission for sick and wounded, local agents issued tickets to seamen bound for quarters on shore (quarters tickets). These tickets were "vouchers by which money expended on the provisions for the sick and wounded is demanded." To be honoured, the tickets had to be endorsed by the recipient, either a hospital contractor or quarterer who provided space in town.[67] At least twice the commissioners indicated that their creditors would be paid in an order or "course" as enabled by the receipt of funds from the Treasury. Thus, three men of Great Yarmouth were, for example, to be "paid in course,"[68] as were the "Inhabitants of Weymouth praying for payment of Quarters to enable them to settle with their Creditors."[69] Yet, in a 1711 reply to a request from the Lord Treasurer for an "Exact

Account" of money "due in the Sick and Wounded office upon Bills in Course," the commissioners' answer was "We never made out any bills in course, or bearing Interest." Rather, per their Instructions, they "pay by our books" and settle, adjust, and clear them "as money [came] in from the Treasury."[70] It might be the case that paying "in course" in the minds of the commissioners meant something like "in good time" and "when we get round to it," depending on the circumstances.

It appears that the commissioners sometimes prioritized the debts incurred at the great ports ahead of the lesser ports. For instance, the minutes of a meeting of May 1706 directed the commissioners' treasurer to pay the amounts owed on the accounts of the hospital contractors at Gosport, Rochester, Deal, and the town quarters at Hull.[71] At that time, the commission was twelve months in arrears of paying its bills, twice as long as the Navy Board thought was appropriate for the service.[72] In the spring of 1712, three ports in Kent that did not have a hospital – Dover, Margate, and Sheerness – had been waiting three years for monies owed for care performed between January and September 1709.[73] There is additional evidence that suggests the commissioners at times chose to clear debts at certain places ahead of others. Minutes of a meeting of June 1708 show the commissioners resolving that, "as soon as money upon the last memorial is rec[eive]d, we pay in the first place the foreign bills of exchange, then the Quarters."[74] Nonetheless, the commissioners did not always favour their relations with hospital contractors over town quarterers at the lesser ports. There were periods, it seems, when care providers at small ports got payments before hospital contractors did. For example, in summer 1709, the commissioners told the Treasury that payment of £10,000 would be helpful for the hospital contractors, since it would bring their compensation in line with payments made already at small ports. This would be, they suggested, "of great service and encouragement to the undertakers for the hospitals."[75] The agent at Plymouth once complained to the Admiralty about "the Delay of payment" there.[76] At ports both great and small, working for and crediting the sick and wounded service required large reserves of patience and trust from care providers.

MANAGING MONEY AND MANPOWER

Distributing money in a more or less timely fashion was crucial for an effective system of naval health care. As naval health care's chief administrators, the commissioners trusted their local agents and medical officials to account for their use of resources, even as the commissioners themselves were required to produce financial reports for their superiors. The commissioners' financial statements of account to the Admiralty, to Parliament, and to the Treasury suggest that naval health care during Queen's Anne's War was more ordered. Paper technologies helped to foster stronger relationships between the commissioners and their agents at coastal communities.

Throughout the war, the Admiralty Board, whether appointed by Whig or Tory ministries, seems to have trusted the commission for sick and wounded's dealings with care providers. Rarely did the Admiralty demand that the commissioners account for their expenses.[77] In one case, the demand to account was probably the result of a staff turnover. In 1714, in the aftermath of George I's accession, the newly appointed Admiralty demanded that the retrenched commission "give an account of the debt due at each port," and what the commissioners had done "toward making up their accounts."[78] The sick and wounded commissioners had to account to parliament's commission for public accounts. Relations between the two commissions, the latter under the direction of the future Lord Treasurer, Robert Harley, were good, at least during the war's early years, 1702 to 1704. Harley had served on the public accounts commission when it conducted an investigation of the accounts of Plymouth naval hospital and its agent, George Dickinson, back in 1695.[79] Therefore, Harley might have thought that he had good reason to request to see duplicate copies of the commissioners' quarterly account books,[80] and certificates on accounts of payments.[81] Harley's requests appear at times to have exasperated the commissioners, as when, for example, they explained to him that their accounts were not ready for Harley's inspection because of "a considerable payment lately made in Kent."[82] But the commissioners did not refuse to take advice on how their might improve their accounting practices. For example, at the suggestion of parliament's public-accounts commission, the sick and wounded commissioners resolved to require quarterers at the ports to sign the seamen's tickets "by way of receipt," and then to hand in the signed tickets as vouchers, along with the quarterers' pay books for quarters.[83] This practice promised to lessen the opportunities for fraud by, for example, paying out money to non-existent quarterers, or for a period of time longer than seamen were actually in care. Following the lapse of the public-accounts commission in the spring of 1704, the sick and wounded commissioners made several presentations to a committee of the House of Commons about the state of their service and its debt.[84]

Most often, the commissioners had to account to the Treasury for how they managed the cost of onshore care. The Treasury's main interest was to ensure that the money it issued to government branches such as the navy did not exceed the sums voted by parliament or were used for other, non-authorized, purposes.[85] The Lords of the Treasury did not always trust that the commissioners' requests for money were legitimate, particularly during the first peak period of high charges. Secretary Lowdnes reported to Lord Treasurer Godolphin in the late summer of 1703 that the £6,599 due on the service for 1702 was "Extravagant," since the "annual expence of the sick and wounded and prisoners in the last Warr is completly doubled in this."[86] Godolphin had evidently earlier expressed some concern about this development. He had written to the Navy Board in July 1703 about the commissioners' management of their business. The Navy Board's subsequent audit of financial statements implied that the commissioners' approach to ordinary care providers – the town quarterers – was costing the service more money than was necessary.

According to the Navy Board's calculations, it had issued about £35,000 per year to the sick and wounded commission during the Nine Years' War. Since the outbreak of war in the spring of 1702 and the middle of 1703, the sick and wounded service had received £31,016, and generated debts amounting to £41,034, for a composite charge on the navy of £72,050. Some of the difference in cost might have been explained, the Navy Board surmised, by the "Number of men put on shore" and the number of prisoners.[87] Significantly, the Navy Board could not believe the commissioners' claim that their credit with care providers was already in danger due to delays in paying them. "That the People who entertain the sick and wounded will not stay Three Months for their payments seems," the Navy Board confessed, "to be very extraordinary." Up to six months' arrears had been the norm during the peace of 1697 to 1702, when two members of the Navy Board had run the sick and wounded service. Arrears in pay had run even longer during the previous war. Nonetheless, the Navy Board acknowledged that "it is absolutely necessary that the Debt of the Sick and Wounded should not exceed 6 mo[nth]s, so that the poor Men may be better take care of."[88]

The Navy Board's report to the Treasury in the summer of 1703 implied that the commissioners had problems controlling their spending and difficulties relating to the people of the ports. Yet, despite his awareness of the sick and wounded service's "present expences being extravagant," Godolphin did not advise the commissioners to change their way of managing money nor their way of relating to the people. He recommended rather the practice of "good husbandry ... and putt them in mind of the Account."[89]

Thus, early in the war, the Lord Treasurer trusted the commissioners of sick and wounded seamen to become better managers of money. The commissioners, for their part, took the recommendation to heart. Two months later, in the autumn of 1703, they proposed a centralization of care space at three ports. Private-contract hospitals, they claimed, would both lower the cost of care at the great ports and reduce the service's dependence on ordinary people, who, they would allege, did not have the seamen's best interests at heart. Having escaped sanction from their superiors, the commissioners for sick and wounded were unable to extend a similar measure of good faith to the people of coastal communities.

The fifth commission was different from its predecessors in seeking systematically to discover problems with agents' financial accounting before they provoked complaints or public scandals. The commissioners wrote to an agent, Mr Bredall, "to advise him of some few errors and mistakes" in his July 1703 accounts.[90] At times, the commissioners were unwilling to pass an agent's accounts until "one of the Board [came] down to clear off" the quarterers books in person.[91] Newly appointed agents received instructions "to send up accounts of all prisoners and sick and wounded in the post according to a Prescribed form," as "oft as any alterations are made in their numbers."[92] Likewise, in the autumn of 1711, the commissioners issued a circular directive to agents "to be very exact and constant in returning their monthly abstracts, in order to enable the Board to make their demand upon the Treasury."[93] Reminders about expected procedures occasionally were issued down to the ports, such as the missive sent to all agents in the spring of 1705 "that all Invoices sent to the Board be signed by both the Physician and a surgeon."[94] "Her Majesties service under their care," the commissioners declared, should not be "subject to abuses either with the number of seamen or the time of their subsistence."[95] The commissioners examined their agents' account books for any suspicious irregularities. For example, agent Langley at Harwich was reprimanded in spring 1706 for leaving two discharged seamen on his quarterers' books "for a considerable time after they were discharged."[96] Had the discrepancy not been noticed, the navy would have been charged extra for the cost of their care. Similarly, officials who made up their own rules faced sanctions. A year following his first reprimand, agent Langley was sent a letter stating the commissioners' displeasure "that he concerns himself in the payment of any Quarterers contrary to his Instructions." Additional complaints "of that nature" would lead to Langley's dismissal.[97] A general letter of warning from the autumn of 1710 suggests that some agents developed accounting habits the commissioners were keen to eliminate. For example, if the agents did not "constantly take care to send up with their monthly accounts what are their contingencies or whether they have any (as has been formerly ordered) the Board will appoint others in their stead."[98] The commissioners at times also cross-checked the number of men recorded in quarterers' books with related records. For example, the commissioners ordered one of their clerks to copy "names of the men sett ashore in the hospital at Jamaica given Mr Churchill that he may compare it with the Victualling account sent over" by the agent, one Mr Gyde.[99]

The fifth commission's most notable innovation in managing the conduct of agents at the ports, highlighted by Admiralty secretary Thomas Corbett decades later, began in the summer of 1705.[100] Commissioner William Churchill was appointed "to Cheque and make up the Accounts of [the sick and wounded] Office, and Muster the Sick & Wounded Seamen and Prisoners at the severall Out Ports" at least four times per year.[101] Additionally, Churchill was required by the Admiralty to "enquire diligently how the Undertakers and officers of the hospitals do perform their contracts and duties," in order to alert the commissioners and the Admiralty "to abuses or corruption."[102] Churchill's appointment ended in 1707 with his departure from the commission for a seat in parliament,[103] but the method of sending a commissioner to the ports "to inspect the service and pay the Quarters" continued.[104] As we will see below, the practice of sending a commissioner to inspect agents' financial records, the conditions of the care spaces, and the quality of care work within them, helped to raise standards of care for seamen over the course of the eighteenth century.

Managing the financial resources underpinning naval health care was never simply about keeping track of money; it also involved monitoring manpower. After a year of war, the Admiralty obligated the commissioners for sick and wounded to account monthly for the disposition of seamen, "what such men are on shore in England, or how many dye or are Discharged or Run from their Quarters."[105] The commissioners' response to the Admiralty's directive included devising a new form of paper discharge certificate that surgeons were to give to seamen, who in turn were to hand in the certificate to the agent, and then the agent was to "keep and produce" as a voucher.[106] Subsequently, hospital contractors, or undertakers, were sent blank forms "to keep Account of the Entry and discharge etc of the Sick and Wounded."[107]

The commissioners' instructions to agents at coastal communities emphasized the collection and transmission of information to save money and preserve men for the navy. Without consistent interactions between agents, medical officers, and seamen, it was impossible to gather accurate data.[108] This is evident in the November 1703 instructions to Dr Haveland of Plymouth, the one site that had a hospital at the start of Queen Anne's War. The commissioners wanted the agent to gather data about seamen and to confirm it via regular inspections in order to stop men from deserting and "to prevent complaints of their [the commissioners'] neglect in that part of their duty." For example, since the navy bore the charge of replacing seamen's garments, the commissioners directed Haveland to inform them about captains who sent sick men ashore without clothes. The agent was to ensure that the sick and wounded were distributed in a coastal community in an orderly and convenient manner, preferably near to his house and not at public houses. Placing the seamen thus would make the twice-weekly mustering in the presence of physicians or surgeons easier to do. Additionally, every Monday morning, the agent was expected to submit a form, either to the physician or the surgeon, on which data concerning the ships, men's names, length of time in care, nature of the disease, and status, were recorded. Medical officers would give the agent orders on when the seamen were to be removed from quarters.[109]

Paper technologies such as discharge forms and tickets for provisioning not only enabled the men who administered naval health care to monitor where its human resources were and in what condition, but also to nudge them toward the path of obedience. Later in the war, the commissioners reminded one of their agents, Mr Aldrich, that "in case the sick men who are set a shore don't quarter where he shall order them, they are to have no Quartering tickets at all made out."[110] Forms such as quartering tickets were like doors that opened up and closed down access to resources, and both freed and constrained men's movements.[111] Which of these effects the form had depended on the information it conveyed, true or false.

Both the Admiralty and the commissioners were concerned to stop men staying in care longer than necessary. The Admiralty directed the commissioners to tell their agents "that care be taken they bee not kept in Quarters longer than is necessary, that we the Public may not only be saved as to the Expence, but have the benefit of their Service."[112] The commissioners responded to this directive with the introduction of the aforementioned discharge certificates, which surgeons and physicians were to pass over to agents. Additionally, quartering tickets were to be examined with the quarter books to "prevent any connivances between the Agents and Quarterers as to the time of their Discharge." Sometimes agents such as Langley of Harwich had to be reminded to record properly what happened to men in care, and when they abandoned it without permission. Thus, the commissioners insisted that Langley note that "if the men will not return to their own ships they must be made Run."[113] A sailor "made Run" had the letter R placed next to his name in the ship's paybook, which stopped him from collecting his wages. The commissioners at times directed ships' captains to find out from agents about seamen's whereabouts.[114] The commissioners, in turn, sent up information that shaped Admiralty policy, as when the Admiralty ordered Vice-Admiral Graydon to "send orders to ships commanders [that] they cause their men to be sent directly to their quarters" in order to avoid the "irregularity of putting such sick and wounded ashore at Chatham."[115] Good communication between the commissioners and the fighting arm of the navy supported their mutual aim of manpower management. Thus, in early 1706, the Admiralty took account of a report from the commission's agents at Gosport concerning seamen who had recovered their health. Thereafter, the agents along the coast were "not to discharge any of the sick and wounded under their care, from time to time, till they have first acquainted the Commander in Chief at Spithead, who will send Boats from there."[116]

Managing sailors who were receiving care on shore also meant mustering them. Mustering was an important preservative tool, intended to prevent the loss of men and money. Men who were lodged at town quarters or at hospitals, or even waiting for admission to a London hospital, were to be mustered regularly. The inspection could be performed by medical officers, such as the surgeon at Rochester, or men hired specifically to count the number of men in care.[117] The commissioners for sick and wounded got permission to employ a man to muster the sick at Harwich in the autumn of 1706.[118] Another way to keep agents honest was through medical officials informing on their colleagues at the ports. Surgeons and physicians were to "have liberty to make Enquiries to prevent any undue Practice," and "report frauds" to the commissioners.[119]

The actions of informants and the practice of cross-checking agents' account books helped the commissioners, in theory, to reduce the incidence of seamen colluding with dishonest officials to deprive the navy of money and manpower. Sometimes the commissioners knew enough about what was going on at the ports to order particular agents to get seamen off their books when they were cured or deemed incurable.[120] For example, the Gosport agent, Mr Levermore, was directed to attend to the case of one Jonathan Arrowsmyth from "Gosport Hospital, where he has been a long time sick."[121] Checking agents' accounts prompted general directions to agents about being more careful not to overburden the care providers. A review of the accounts of quarterers for the great ports at the end of 1705 suggested that "the seamen have continued very long in Quarters, though the nature of their Distempers do generally terminate in a few days." A circular order was sent out, reminding agents "to expedite the care of those that are or shall be under their care, that the Queen may sooner have the benefit of the seamen's service, and not put to extravagant expence." Seamen suffering from chronic diseases were to be sent to one of London's great hospitals. But this practice did not mean, so the commissioners pointed out, sending "them that they may probably dye upon the road."[122] The fact that extraordinarily long stays in care were a problem at places with hospitals was not, perhaps for obvious reasons, noted in the minutes. Consciously or not, the commissioners probably did not wish to concede that its centralization of care the previous year had not diminished the moral hazards intrinsic to taking care of seamen. Whatever the nature of the disease or injury, the longer seamen were kept on a care provider's books, the greater his or her financial payoff – at a higher cost to the navy.

The commissioners' determination to preserve human and material resources for the navy did not inure its members from acts of mercy, nor were the commissioners focused on sailors only as means to an end. For example, the officials at Rochester were informed that the commissioners expected "their utmost care of the men and the expence of medicines" and that the truly unwell seamen should be sent up to London "when fit to travel" only.[123] Saving money did not in this instance justify condemning men to death by an arduous journey by road. Moreover, the commissioners sought to protect from impressment those sailors who fetched and carried the "sick and wounded to and from the Ships."[124] An incident in early 1711 involving a press master "impressing men from the Hospitals before they are cured" prompted a complaint from the commission to the Admiralty.[125]

In practice, the sick and wounded service lost both money and men, sometimes in spectacular fashion. For example, the captain of the *Tilbury* reported that "the men he put ashore" at Sheerness in the spring of 1706 "were all gone from their quarters and noe care was taken of them."[126] Over an eighteen-month period midway through the conflict, the great port of Plymouth was the site of a struggle over moving men from the hospital back onto naval vessels. An official at Plymouth dockyard, H. Walker, reported to the Admiralty that the sick men sent to the hospital were, upon their recovery, "not only not discharged into the Ships from whence they are set ashore," which was against the general orders, "but into none else, and soe never return into the Service ... which proves the loss of many men." The Admiralty ordered the commissioners to direct their officials at Plymouth to give Walker "an account from time to time, what men are fitt to be discharged from the Hospital, that they may be sent aboard such Ships, as may want them." Several days later, the Admiralty told the commissioners to give Walker "an account of the Sick men ... that he may send them aboard Ship as proposed."[127] The commissioners then directed their medical officials and agents at Plymouth to "comply with the Admiralty's directive."[128] A subsequent complaint from a Captain Hanway at Plymouth, that "several of his men sett sick ashore there are discharged and lost to him, not knowing where they are," prompted the commissioners to order their agents not to "discharge [seamen] till the Captains have notice to whom they belong or the superintendent" of the dockyard.[129]

Whatever the effectiveness of the orders aimed at better accounting of and communicating about men discharged from Plymouth hospital, however, desertions were a problem there again at the end of 1709. The commissioners for sick and wounded were ordered to report to the Admiralty about "how the seamens desertion from Plymouth Hospitall which Lord Dursley complains of may be prevented for the future."[130] The answer would involve coordinated action and communication. "For the time being," ordered the Admiralty, ships' officers would go ashore "when the sick and wounded are mustered," to receive the discharged men. The superintendent of the dockyard (Walker) was directed "to take care for the Dispersal of the seamen through Quarters." The commissioners would "give an Account of the Muster Days" to the port's Flag Officer or superintendent, "and take care to prevent the

88   Early Modern Naval Health Care in England

men from Deserting their Quarters."[131] Evidently, ships' officers were disinclined to go ashore to collect their men, prompting the commissioners to complain.[132] Obviously, methods of accounting for men and measures for communicating their whereabouts were effective only so long as officials were willing to carry them out.

Overall, it appears that when officials were accused of derelictions of duty, the board took the charges seriously. For example, surgeon Greenwood of Sandwich was examined by the commissioners twice, once at Westminster and again on site, for "claims of neglecting his duty," frequent absences, and refusing to give seamen their medicines.[133] When a surgeon had been deemed incompetent or negligent, he could be discharged, as happened at Fareham in 1704.[134] Similarly, failure to follow even "one part of [his] Instructions," in connection with paying quarterers, could be grounds for dismissing an agent.[135]

Agents who worked well made the commissioner's interactions with the people of the ports that much easier. Generally, it appears that the commissioners strove to do right by care providers, or at least to play by its own rules in its interactions with them. For example, in early 1704, an agent was instructed not to quarter any more sailors "in those Houses where they are suffered to run in debt beyond the Queen's allowance of 12d per day," since that money was to be paid to "those who produce the quartering tickets."[136] Before the establishment of private-contract hospitals, the commissioners received a letter from Deptford's long-term quarterers asking for preferential treatment in the assignment of space in which to care for sick and wounded seamen. The commissioners concurred, resolving "that the surgeon at Deptford be directed as far as it is within the service to have particular regard to those who have been longest Employed and been at most Charge in maintaining provision for the service."[137] An agent working around Newcastle was reprimanded because he "had refused to satisfy some Quarterers, who had received sick and wounded seamen by direction of the Mayor" but baulked at the agent's offer to pay them 5s. per week instead of the regulated amount of 7s. The commissioners promised the mayor that they would "see to the Quarterers full satisfaction as soon as they have money."[138] The commissioners evidently believed that the "People will be glad to Quarter" seamen at Newcastle, as long as they were not defrauded by corrupt agents.[139] There is even an instance of the commissioners agreeing to pay quarterers an extra shilling per man per day in order to induce them to receive two "extremely ill" men waiting to be admitted to a private-contract hospital.[140] Upon receipt of a letter in the summer of 1712 from Dover concerning "the Uneasing of the Towns People there on account of the Debt due for their office," the commissioners wrote the Lord Treasurer requesting money.[141] The letter to Harley recalled the commission's "promises [given] after Michaelmas last, upon the assurances we received from the Lord Treasurer of being duly supplied, makes the people very uneasy, whom we deal with."[142] Reference to the people of the ports as part of a plea for money was nothing new in the commission's correspondence with the Treasury. What is remarkable is the admission of a promise made by the commission to the people that the Lord Treasurer's inaction jeopardized. The commission might not always have liked working with ordinary people, but it could not work without them in good faith.

Indeed, the commissioners knew early on that their superiors wanted naval health care to be managed in a way that did not overly inconvenience the public. For example, the Admiralty ordered the commissioners to prepare accommodations for the sick men of the returning Vigo fleet away from the centres of Plymouth, Portsmouth, and Chatham "for preventing the spreading of the Distemper," which, being infectious "may been very prejudiciall to her Majesties Service, and very much hinder the Preparations against the next Yeare."[143] Similarly, in the presence of the privy council, the queen told the commissioners that, should local people ever be unwilling to quarter seamen with infectious diseases, "the commissioners might cause Empty houses or Barnes to be fitted up and furnished with bedds etc in the nature of hospitals hyreing nurses and other fit persons to attend them." Nonetheless, the queen went on to recommend that there be "no unnecessary expence therein so nothing should be wanting for the relief of those seamen who had service Her Majesty so well."[144] Herein the sovereign expressed a paradox at the heart of the preservative ethos underlying naval health care in the early-eighteenth century. On the one side, care had to be managed so that seamen were "carefully and diligently looked after, and that all possible caution bee taken for useing them well, in order to the effecting their speedy recovery."[145] Likewise, the navy could not afford to foster ill will among the people who received, lodged, and cared for its sick and wounded. But on the other hand, the Crown's financial capacity, like the nation's stock of able seamen, was limited. Saving men could not be allowed to ruin the navy's credit. As we have seen, at times it proved to be exceptionally difficult for the system of naval health care to preserve simultaneously the lives of seamen, public monies, and popular trust in the regime.

SECURING CARE AT PRIVATE-CONTRACT HOSPITALS

Between the spring and autumn of 1703, the fifth commission convinced the Admiralty that town quarterers, particularly landladies, were no longer adequate as care providers. Landladies presented moral dangers to effective care in the eyes of the commission. However, as we will see later in connection with Gosport's hospital, reducing the number of female care providers did not necessarily diminish the utter dependence of the sick and hurt service on good nurses. Ordered care still needed care workers.

The advent of naval hospitals run by private contractors was, as Kathleen Harland rightly argues, the most significant development in health care for seamen during Queen Anne's War.[146] As previous chapters have noted, the idea of naval hospitals was not new to the eighteenth century. Indeed, prior to 1670, Dr Whittaker and John Evelyn had suggested that the Royal Navy needed hospitals for its sick and injured seamen. Establishing private-contract naval hospitals at the turn of the eighteenth century could be seen as a good and necessary event in the prehistory of the permanent medical institutions constructed almost half a century later.

The three private-contract hospitals established from 1704 represented firstly a stratification of care sites in England into categories of greater – those with a hospital – and lesser – those with town quarters for seamen only. A hierarchy of care sites reflected the reality that some places regularly received the most sick and wounded seamen, and thus a higher demand for care space and care work. Secondly, the hospitals at Rochester, Gosport, Deal, and Plymouth centralized care space with a view to improving the quality of care work, while reducing the risk of men deserting the service. Hospitals were thought to be a superior means to preserve the navy's manpower and material resources, a contention that Harland sums up under the slogan "manning, money, and mercy."[147]

Given the difficulties confronting medical practitioners charged with healing seamen at the ports, a desire to centralize care space at a hospital makes sense. It is not hard to see a characteristically early modern drive for order underlying both the move to prioritize certain places as sites for care and to concentrate seamen in care to particular buildings.[148] Such a centralization of the spaces for care work was, from an administrative perspective, consistent with a broad trend in contemporary European armed forces to rationalize how they obtained necessary support services.[149] Often these sorts of changes had gendered consequences. Moves toward administrative specialization or bringing more systematic practices to administration could create new norms that tilted toward men.[150] For example, in the provision of food and drink, rationalization equalled the militarization of procurement, which between roughly 1650 and 1800 arguably propelled the marked decline in the number of women who joined armies on campaign.[151] In other cases, governments, concerned about the moral disorders that women associated with armed forces were seen to cause, tried to supress the number of female camp followers.[152] The introduction of hospital contractors – private individuals who ran care spaces as an enterprise on behalf of the navy – at the great ports drastically reduced the number of people with whom the commissioners had to engage at three coastal communities.[153] At Rochester, Deal, and Portsmouth, three male contractors replaced dozens of female care providers.

The commission for sick and wounded made two attempts to alter the framework of naval health care at major ports during 1703. In February, the commissioners first proposed converting a public house at Deal (called The Pelican) into a hospital. The Admiralty's response was to inquire if seamen could be kept at such a place "cheaper than in Quarters."[154] Days later, the commissioners contacted Dr Adair of Rochester "to send reasons for a hospital." Within a week, the commission determined to acquire a "particular account of the convenienceys" of a hospital at Rochester, along with a similar report from "all the officers hands."[155] Sometime later that month, the commissioners submitted a proposal for naval hospitals to the Admiralty, which in turn directed the Navy Board to study and comment upon it. The Navy Board's response to the proposal, dated 2 March, was negative.[156] The Admiralty then rejected the commission's proposal twice on financial grounds in June.[157]

Despite this outcome, the commissioners did not relinquish the hospital concept. Three months after the Admiralty's rejection, the commissioners accepted an external proposal for four hospitals to be undertaken by a former agent of the service, Rawlins Brownjohn. The ex-agent highlighted his personal experience with "complaints and ... the Grievances and Mischiefs [that] attend the sick and injured in ill quarters and publick houses" in port towns. Negligence at these sorts of town quarters had cost seamen's lives, while the proprietors' knavery robbed other sailors of their goods and pay, to their "great discouragement." Brownjohn proposed to acquire private houses to serve as hospitals and to supply them with "careful nurses and good provisions."[158] Two days later, the commissioners decided that their Instructions gave them the authority to begin negotiating with Brownjohn about his idea. They also prepared a list of the major problems, labelled "mischiefs," with care management and care providers at town quarters.[159]

Perhaps feeling emboldened by Brownjohn's rationale, and knowing that it is easier to ask for forgiveness than for permission, the commissioners evidently concluded an agreement with the former agent to provide quarters for sick and wounded seamen as a "Gentleman Undertaker"; then they proceeded to inform the Admiralty. However, Prince George and his advisors were still not in favour of a contract-hospital method for providing care at the great ports, with Brownjohn as the lead enterpriser.[160] At a late-October meeting of the commission, Brownjohn's plan was justified not as a remedy to medical and moral failures at town quarters but instead as a way to save men's lives. The plan for hospitals was intended, so the commissioners affirmed, "only to prevent the want of Quarters for such Seamen as could not be Entertained for want of Room in Town or were quartered in Staging Houses in the outports so that the Physicians and Surgeons times were so much taken up in walking from one house to another that the men could not be sufficiently attended."[161] Thus, the real problem with the existing method of procuring care space at the ports was that it wasted medical practitioners' time and energy. This argument is perhaps the one the commissioners emphasized as part of their presentation to the Admiralty on 10 November.[162] On that date, the commissioners convinced the Admiralty to order their "putting the sick and wounded into private houses," suggesting buildings dedicated to care, in the manner of a hospital.[163] Thus, the inconveniences of the town quarters, not the mischiefs, were to be remedied by putting sick men into hospitals. By mid-December, the commission had found and acquired the Admiralty's approval for hospital contractors at Rochester, Deal, and Portsmouth.[164]

The preservative ethos underpinned both the commissioners' proposals for, and post-hoc justifications of, the adoption of hospitals at select sites of naval health care. The privately contracted hospitals would, it was argued, save the Royal Navy men and money. The case had two components. The first focused on method, or how the hospitals allowed for better manpower management and more effective care. Hospitals saved lives and kept men for the navy. The second case centred around moral hazards, or who was providing care and under whose oversight. In this instance, the commissioners were concerned to show that hospitals would preserve men from self-interested and incompetent care workers or care providers. The methodological argument for hospital-based care appears more often in both prospective and retrospective justifications, and, as I suggested above, probably had more traction with the commissioner's superiors. The moral case, by contrast, was more pronounced when the commissioner had to defend its alteration of naval health care on shore against the protests of their social inferiors.

The commissioners' first proposal for contract hospitals, which must be inferred from the Navy Board's March 1703 report, highlighted the existing system's methodological and moral failings.[165] The commissioners had argued that hospitals would save money and bring more order to the delivery of care. The Navy Board's reaction was to dismiss the commissioners as naive for thinking that a standing capital charge, issued to serve a yet-unknown number of seamen, could save money in comparison to the present system. The commissioners had also complained about the decentralized nature of the town quartering system: at certain times, thousands of men were quartered at miles from each other, which was a barrier to effective care that a hospital would overcome. The commissioners evidently also thought that cases of fraud perpetrated by quarterers upon weakened seamen could be contained at hospitals. Similarly, there it would be harder for sick frauds – seamen only pretending to suffer – to escape the attention of medical practitioners at hospitals. Seamen would also be spared the depredations of bad nurses, the sort of care workers who gave patients the wrong food, neglected to clean their beds, or else did not administer the prescribed medicines. More generally, sick and wounded seamen who were lodged at public houses caused disruptions, gambled away their pay, and often relapsed "into fevers" because of drinking hard liquor to excess. In short, the commissioners thought that the town-quarter system of care incentivized care providers and care workers to defraud the navy of its treasure and deprive it of its sailors. In the view of the commission, the "many poor people [who] fell into the way of providing quarters for sick and wounded sailors, and make a livelihood of it," could no longer be trusted "to behave themselves otherwise in these matters."

The failure on financial grounds of the first proposal for hospitals probably encouraged the commissioners for sick and wounded to try a second, but differently oriented, attempt with Brownjohn's scheme.

94   Early Modern Naval Health Care in England

The first proposal had envisioned the navy splashing out "great sums of money" that could not be expected "while the Nation is at so vast a Charge in the present Warr." However, the commissioners understood that Brownjohn sought no investment in capital stock, and "no addition to the allowances, officers or salaries already established."[166] No mention was made of the quality of the people Brownjohn would employ at his hospitals. But the catalogue of eleven "Mischiefs" of the town quarters provided only negative evidence of the chaotic conditions and dishonesty the commissioners hoped Brownjohn's hospitals would eliminate. The former stemmed in large part from where the men were kept: in towns with insufficient accommodations; dispersed over large distances; in overcrowded beds, and with too many opportunities to escape, to fake their illness, and to infect the surrounding community.[167] The negligence of care and the defrauding of men were blamed on the malfeasance of the quarterers or landladies themselves.[168] The fact that many such people believed that it was in their and the navy's joint interest to provide care for the seamen did not move the commissioners from their commitment to hospitals, as events in the spring and summer of 1704 at Portsmouth demonstrated.

The commissioners preferred to trust female care workers employed as nurses at private-contract hospitals more than female care providers serving as landladies over care spaces. Moreover, the prospect of interacting with female care workers was more likely to have been distasteful to physicians than laymen. Dr Adams and Dr Morley belonged to a profession that was already associated with the feminine sphere, due to physic's focus on the body and its products. Employing private contractors to run naval hospitals placed greater social distance between the administrators of naval health care and the embodied nature of care work. Male contractors could play the role of intermediary between the commissioners and the largely (but not wholly) female care contingent upon which the operation of such hospitals depended. At the great ports, the members of the fifth commission for sick and wounded and their agents would interact with, and inspect the work of, a handful of male care entrepreneurs. Thus, the shift to private-contract hospitals from town quarters at three great ports elevated the status and enhanced the professional authority of physicians within a branch of the armed forces that had long valued the medical contributions of surgeons.

The preservative ethos underlying the commissioners' reformation of naval health care is also evident in three statements composed shortly before and just after the return of peace in 1713. While the method-ological advantages of hospitals for saving men and money featured in all three, only the first accented the moral hazards once posed by female care providers. One reason for the difference in emphasis could be that the first statement, written in 1711, looked back on the changes initiated eight years earlier. By contrast, the second and third were ele-ments of proposals for maintaining care for seamen under a retrenched peacetime establishment, one in which the commissioners presumed that the superiority of hospitals for saving lives and money would be taken as read.

In the summer of 1711, the commission restated its rationale for re-formed care management at the great ports in a report on the state of the sick and wounded service's debt submitted to Lord Treasurer Robert Harley. Under the report's second article, which concerned the £26,733 debt for six quarters (of the year) out of eight due to the con-tractors and quarterers, the commissioners recollected the "inconve-nient" practice at the war's outbreak of putting the sick and wounded into "Publick houses." The great dispersal of men into such places on shore meant that the physicians and surgeons "could not visit and ad-minister to [seamen] in due time as their occasions required." The com-missioners recounted "the ill accommodations most of those Houses afforded, and the carelessness and avarice of their Landladys, whereby great numbers of her Maj[jestie]s seamen perished." The resort to hos-pitals at the great ports "of Rochester, Deal, Portsmouth and Plymouth" had, by contrast, "provided fitting Receptacles and accommodation for the sick and hurt seamen that they might be all together, and due care taken of them in all respects."[169] The centralization of care at these ports afforded the navy greater efficiency, in that all the men were to-gether, while offering the men the care owed to them for their service. Trusting sick and wounded seamen to the landladies would have, in this view, served only the selfish interests of insouciant women, at great cost of men's lives. Care that had been overseen by women was, so the report asserted, by definition both ruthless and reckless.

Careless landladies did not, by contrast, feature in the commission-ers' 1712 "Observations" on the sick and wounded service at the home ports. In this document, the quartering of seamen on shore at private houses "having been found inconvenient," it was deemed proper to replace them with hospitals. Under the management of "able Persons," not only had "the lives and future service of many of Her Majesties subjects ... been preserved to the publick, but the expence has been considerably lessened."[170] Both the methodological and moral issues were distilled, in this retrospective rationale, into inconveniences that were superseded by competent contractors. The fact that the enterprising hospital contractors had been liable for "providing Bedds, Bedding, and other necessaries, more particularly at Gosport and Plymouth," thereby reducing the sick and wounded service's draw on the public fisc, was further proof that the 1703 reformation was a Good Thing.

The commission for sick and wounded was not alone in this judgment. In preparation for a major retrenchment, in which all officers of the service, except those at the great ports, were to be dismissed, the Admiralty agreed to the commissioner's proposal that it was "more advantageous to Her Majesties Service to place sick men into an hospital together, than to disperse them into Towne quarters."[171] In peacetime as in war, the best way to preserve the lives of seamen was to keep them as much as possible at one place. Dispersal meant disorder and disease leading to loss; centralized care saved money and men.

The commissioners' preservative ethos also animated its arrangements with contractors, and their instructions to officials working at the ports. The fact that this message was consistent whether the board communicated to inferiors or superiors is not insignificant. The commissioners were, it appears, of one mind in what they wanted the sick and wounded service to do, and expected everyone in the service to share their vision. Singularity of purpose very probably contributed to the service's greater effectiveness during Queen Anne's War, whatever one's feelings about the commissioners' unwillingness to trust female care providers with responsibility for overseeing spaces for care.

The single surviving contract between the commission and an undertaker puts preservation at the core of the hospital's function, while re-emphasizing how it would remedy the moral and managerial hazards of the town quarters. The foundation for the agreement for the care of sailors at Rochester between enterpriser Mr Sayer and the commissioners was the contractor's offer to look after them "for the Preservation of many of their lives, by Providing for them private Quarters, and other necessaries at your own Expence for the allowance of 12d per diem for the Dyett and Entertainment of each man, as hath been hitherto given in Town Quarters." The preamble concluded with a list of "all the Mischiefs that have been attended in the said Quarters," which Sayer had "engaged to the utmost of [his] power to prevent." Unsurprisingly, the mischiefs enumerated in the agreement were the same as the ones presented to the Admiralty in autumn 1703.[172]

A closer consideration of the Rochester hospital agreement's terms and Sayer's subsequent difficulties suggests that the commissioners were more interested in keeping men from deserting than saving money for the navy. The desire to preserve manpower was, and is, an enduring theme of warfare and medicine across time and space.[173]

The agreement stipulated that Sayer was responsible for finding and fitting up suitable accommodation "for not less than 800 men." The commissioners promised to reimburse him the cost of his initial capital outlay, should he be replaced by another contractor or should the Crown decide to run the hospital itself. But nothing in the agreement mentioned what Sayer could expect in relation to his investments in buildings and supplies if the Royal Navy suddenly no longer were to need care for its seamen. Presumably, the commissioners and Sayer expected that his quasi-monopoly over care at Rochester would generate sufficient income to cover his costs and eventually make the establishment profitable. The commissioners' agent at Rochester was to be instructed to quarter "all the sick and wounded seamen set on shore at the said Place" at the house provided by Sayer. The undertaker was to be paid the same amount per man per day as care providers – landlords or landladies – to provide the seamen with the "necessary and convenient accommodation Dyett etc as shall be fit for persons in their Condition as according to the Direction after the Physicians and Surgeons of the said Port." This meant that the hospital was not in fact lowering the cost of care, since the commissioners were to pay Sayer the same amount per man as it had when relying on town quarterers. The hospitals were not saving the Crown money but keeping men for its sea service.

Hospitals promised to preserve seamen's lives and the navy's manpower. The reiteration of the eleven "mischiefs of the town quarters" in the agreement with Sayer shows that, in the view of the commissioners, private-contract hospitals were supposed to keep seamen in naval service by healing them quickly and carefully in one and the same place, thus reducing the loss of manpower due to relapses of illness, excessive time in care, or desertion. The prioritization of keeping men over saving money was not unnoticed by higher authorities, although not favourably. In mid 1705, Lord Treasurer Godolphin demanded that the commissioners put together a plan "for the better and more frugal Management" of the sick and wounded service with a view to lowering its "Extraordinary Expence of the Public Money."[174] In the spring of 1706, the Admiralty requested an explanation from the commissioners for "the difference in charge between sending the sick and wounded for care to Sheerness," a community without a hospital, "and Rochester."[175] The commission replied that Sheerness "is so bad a place that many die who are put on shore there, which occasioned the establishment of the Hospital" at Rochester.[176] The quality of its town quarters and demanding landladies probably contributed to the commissioners' negative assessment of care for seamen at Sheerness. That said, there were also reasons to doubt the quality of care at Rochester. Three years earlier, a ticket agent and activist for seamen, John Tutchin, reported to the Admiralty on complaints "of the ill usage of such sick seamen as are put on shore" at Rochester.[177]

Rochester private-contract naval hospital, which the Crown had established "on purpose," was for the commissioners less about saving money and more about preserving manpower. The hospital did not, if a postwar account is accurate, generate much reward for its undertaker. Sayer, according to an estimate from a representative of his estate, had spent £1,500 for a house with room for four hundred men. It was claimed that he lost eventually £2,300 because of a dishonest steward.[178]

The commissioners for sick and wounded seamen justified their centralization of naval health care at certain ports as a practical and moral necessity. Hospital care at Rochester, Portsmouth, Deal, and Plymouth would save lives and money for the navy, and save men from female care providers the commissioners deemed sub-optimal. This perspective is clear from events that transpired within months of the opening of a hospital at Portsmouth. In the summer of 1704, a group of forty-seven sailors' widows and landladies from Portsmouth and the neighbouring community of Gosport submitted a petition to Queen Anne; it was endorsed by the mayor and two bailiffs. The petition was a protest against the recently erected hospital. In the petition, the women asserted that "between 300 and 400 families in Portsmouth depend on looking after sick and injured seamen." The hospital deprived them of the opportunity to care for sick and wounded seamen, and now these same families were suffering serious hardships. The petitioners asked that, instead of relying on a hospital, the queen's government allow Portsmouth's "poor widows" once again to "enjoy their ancient privilege of quartering your sick and wounded men, solemnly promising to take due care to nurse them well, which will add new life to the trade of the said towns."[179]

The official reply, sent to the Secretary of State, suggests that commissioners Adams and Morley saw landladies and widows as particularly culpable for the "mischiefs of the town quarter" system. The commissioners introduced their response by declaring that they had proposed centralizing care work at hospitals in order to prevent "such abuses as have been so apparently committed by these Petitioners." In other words, widows and landladies were notoriously culpable for the eleven chief problems of the quartering system, which the commissioners' reply proceeded to reiterate. For example, they claimed that widows and landladies charged with caring for sick and injured sailors replaced prescribed medicines with alcohol, and encouraged their patients into "disorderly ways of living more fatal and chargeable to them than their original distempers." Indeed, Doctors Adams and Morley asserted that the fundamental failings of the town quartering system arose from the "destructive genius of these Petitioners," working in tandem with the "licentiousness of the Seamen." Additionally, the commissioners rejected the petitioners' claim that they were starving from a lack of work. The commissioners declared that the sailors' widows had been offered employment as nurses at the hospital, which the women had "scornfully refused."[180] Clearly, in the minds of the medical professionals on the fifth commission for sick and wounded, independent female care providers were a proven source of disorder in what was by nature an unacceptably disorganized system. The ministry evidently agreed, and Portsmouth's private-contract hospital for sick and injured seamen remained in operation.

However, much to the commissioners' embarrassment, their strident condemnation of female care providers was shortly contradicted by naval officers. In late September 1704, Rear Admiral Dilkes and four ships' captains inspected the hospital at Portsmouth. They found 201 double, and 39 single beds, which they stated were "meanly and coarsely furnished." In their report to the Admiralty, the officers went on to criticize the hospital's location, next to a swamp that emitted bad odours when the tide was low. The hospital was also, they thought, situated too far from where the sick and injured could be landed conveniently. Most tellingly, the officers observed that "the number of women employed as nurses at the hospital is far too small." Consequently, the level of care available to the men "must be much inferior to what they have when disposed of into sick quarters."[181] The response of the Admiralty to Dilkes's report was to order the commissioners to put some of the men from the hospital into town quarters until a better location for the hospital could be found.[182] Evidently a more healthy location was found, and, by the end of 1705, not a single sick or injured sailor was in care in a private house in Portsmouth.[183] Nevertheless, the incident showed that private-contract hospitals were not necessarily better sites for care than private houses.

In response to the officers' report, the commissioners wrote to agents and contractors to "consult and propose to the Board what orders may be necessary to be observed by the seamen for their better Government and preventing of Disorders, that have frequently happened."[184] This request suggests that the commissioners acknowledged that their managerial reformation had not in fact solved the so-called mischiefs at town quarters that they had described to the Admiralty in September 1703.

The fifth commission for sick and wounded sponsored a partial centralization of the naval health-care service in England. Like similar processes undertaken elsewhere in early modern Europe, the centralization of care into private-contract hospitals at certain ports had wider social consequences.[185] The centralization of English naval health care after 1703 diminished women's opportunities to work as care providers. Centralization did not, however, reduce the navy's dependence on women willing to do care work.[186]

During Queen Anne's War, the navy needed and wanted to secure care space at important ports. It also wanted these spaces to offer good care. Thus, in a postwar plan for the "accommodation and Preservation" of seamen at Gosport and Portsmouth, the commissioners claimed that the proposed hospital contractor, Christopher Clark, would find suitable private houses with "good Bedds, Carefull Nurses, and Wholesome Provisions ... with Separate Lodgings for men in contagious Distempers."[187] In this view, a more centralized and rationalized system of naval health care worked well if it employed good, careful people.

THE CARERS IN AND OUT OF HOSPITALS

Onshore care for sick and wounded seamen was grounded on asymmetrical relationships between the navy – the consumer of care – and care providers. Generally, the navy demanded care for sailors that local people sold on credit. During Queen Anne's War, as during previous conflicts, care providers had almost no influence over the terms of payment, particularly when it occurred. Care providers could and did resist working with the navy when they thought and felt inadequately attended to, or were simply unable to do anything more for the seamen disgorged into their communities.

The introduction of private-contract hospitals after 1704 installed an additional asymmetry into England's naval health care system. The commissioners for sick and wounded restricted their interactions with landladies operating as care providers, while continuing to depend upon willing female care workers to heal sailors. The commissioners seem at times to have regarded their interactions with landladies as necessarily difficult, while at other times found relating to nurses a difficult necessity. The actions and decisions of the commissioners suggests that its members viewed female care workers as essential components of the system, but not entirely trustworthy. The administrators' lack of trust in women is most evident in their unwillingness to consider forming partnerships with female care enterprisers.

The commissioners for sick and wounded knew that in certain communities there were numbers of women who were keen to provide care for seamen. In December 1702, prior to promoting the hospital idea, the commissioners' physician at Gosport reported that the "landladies are desirous of entertaining the sick and wounded to be brought on shore and claime a Preference above their neighbours therein."[188] Less than two years later, probably many of the same people petitioned the queen against Gosport's new hospital for denying them their "antient privilege" of quartering seamen.[189] However, the commissioners had determined that willingness did not always correlate with trustworthiness, and so, at great ports such as Gosport, large numbers of seamen were made the responsibility of one contractor. However, seamen would have needed a similar number of nurses to look after them at the private-contract hospital. At places where town quarters were the only source of accommodation and provision, the fifth commission was, like its predecessors, compelled to take for granted the capacity of local people to care, if at times begrudgingly.

Local circumstances were often decisive for how the commissioners for sick and wounded interacted with care providers and those who represented their community's interests to the navy, as the case of care work along the mouth of the River Tyne shows. On at least two occasions in 1705 a local magistrate, and governor of Tynemouth castle, Colonel Villiers, represented to the commissioners that the town's inhabitants refused to receive any more seamen until they were paid their three years' worth of arrears. Villiers reported that when he had threatened to supress these *refuseniks'* licences to serve alcohol, they had asserted "that they had rather draw no drink then be obliged to take Sick Men into their Family, and not be paid for it." Evidently, the commissioners had responded that "these Ale Wifes should be paid in Course."[190] The agent at Newcastle, Nicholas Cockburne, apparently was not on good terms with either Villiers or the locals, which might explain why the governor wrote another plea for money on behalf of the "Poor Aile Wifes" who had previously quartered seamen on Villiers's warrant.[191] At no point in Villiers's correspondence with the Admiralty or the commissioners did he suggest that the women's resistance to quartering sailors was illegitimate. The commissioners had broken their trust with the people and needed to make things right if they hoped to preserve the lives of seamen set ashore in the northeast.

Unsurprisingly, where local care providers did not have a powerful advocate to present a grievance to the commissioners, their concerns were more likely to be brushed aside. For example, care providers at Sheerness, at the mouth of the River Medway, had an interest in looking after as many seamen as possible. The navy, for its part, wanted to transport as many men up river to the hospital at Rochester, while leaving only the most serious cases behind at Sheerness and nearby Queenborough. At the end of 1708, the agent at Sheerness, Mr Fairfax, reported that the landladies threatened to receive no more seamen unless he left behind "8 or 9 men at Queenborough well enough to go to Rochester." The commissioners reminded the agent that he should only leave the "very desperate cases" there, and "therefore the Landladys threats are not to be heeded." They went on to insinuate that Fairfax's predecessor lost his post in no small part for his inability to ignore "the Landladys clamour."[192] However, while the commissioners did not always enjoy dealing with landladies, they did not necessarily treat female care providers unfairly.[193] Agents of the commission were, for example, directed not to interfere with landladies' tickets for pay.[194] Nor was it a problem for the board to pay "£89 due to Sev[eral]l Quarterers" to Elizabeth Buck, "their Attorney."[195]

At the ports served by private-contract hospitals, the commissioners for sick and wounded were less dependent on the goodwill of female care providers than was the case during previous wars. However, care work undertaken mostly by women remained the system's foundation both within and without hospitals. As noted above, shortly after the opening of Portsmouth's naval hospital, ships' captains complained about its lack of nurses.[196]

During Queen Anne's War, the number of people involved in providing care space fell in comparison with previous conflicts. The shrinkage stemmed from medical and moral concerns expressed in word and deed by the commissioners for sick and wounded. Put baldly, the commissioners were willing to trust women to care for seamen's bodies, but were reluctant to entrust women to run care space and/or oversee care workers. Two phenomena bear out this conclusion. The first is evident from one of the few quantitative records of care providers surviving from this period. As mentioned above, an account of the seventy-six sick and injured seamen quartered at Rochester from August to December 1703 lists sixty-four quarterers, sixty-three of which bear a female name.[197] By contrast, an abstract of the sick and wounded service's accumulated debt as of April 1711 lists twenty-seven communities of care provision in England, of which only seven show a female care provider. Rochester, served by a naval hospital since 1704, is not one of them. Of the seven communities where women provided care on their own accord, in only two, Hull (50 per cent) and Woolwich (43 per cent), did women compose more than a third of the number of care providers.[198] Providing care space for seamen at coastal communities was a much more masculine enterprise during Queen Anne's War. And this seems to have been what the fifth commission for sick and wounded wanted.

The commissioners received and rejected at least two proposals from women to undertake care work in the manner of the hospital contractors. The first, from Mrs Beate Cole of Southampton, was reviewed by the local agent, Mr Levermore, and not recommended to the commissioners.[199] The second, from Margaret Hicks of Rochester, perhaps the same person as the second listed quarterer on the 1703 register, was submitted in the spring of 1713.[200] Hicks proposed to contract for the "Entertainment of Sick Men £10 per cent cheaper than what Mr Knaxton does now contract for." Commissioners Herbert and Adams justified rejecting Hicks's plan on the grounds that their existing contractor, Mr Knaxton, had lost money on the South Sea stock previously used to pay for his services. Additionally, the reduced demand for care meant "his Undertaking [is] scarce worth the while or charge he must be at." Besides, in their view Mrs Hicks's "conveniences are not such as will answer."[201] Evidently, the commissioners' long-stated commitment to save both lives and money had gendered limits that Margaret Hicks's probable experience in care provision, and her acknowledged thrift, could not overcome.

Naval health care underwent quantitative change during Queen Anne's War. It was more expensive than ever before, more reliant on paper-driven technologies of accountability, financially more secure than previously, and more centralized. Three private-contract hospitals were established at Portsmouth, Deal, and Rochester from 1704 at the behest of the fifth commission for sick and wounded seamen. The hospitals reduced the commissioners' dependence on women to provide care space at the great ports. These hospitals, and the existing naval hospital at Plymouth, were meant to save money and save men for the navy. In other words, hospitals would, in the minds of the commissioners, improve the quality of care work available to seamen on shore by putting it under the oversight of male contractors. However, naval health care at the beginning of the eighteenth century remained utterly dependent on women to provide care work, whether it happened at a hospital, at a pub, or in someone's house.

The contexts for care changed during Queen Anne's War, but its content did not. The system responsible for securing care for injured or sick seamen had become more complicated by 1714, but the basic work of attending to their needs – ensuring they had clean clothes and bedding, adequate diet, proper medicines – had not, and neither had the cohort of people who did almost all the work.

CHAPTER 5

Naval Health Care during the Early Georgian Era, 1715–1739

Although the scale of on shore naval health care was retrenched drastically following the Treaty of Utrecht, it continued to operate and perform relatively well over the following quarter-century.[1] During this period, naval officials strove to implement to a greater degree the preservative ethos of saving lives, saving money, and keeping seamen in the navy. Having secured care spaces through the establishment of private-contract hospitals at the great ports, the overseers of naval health care began to direct more attention toward the conditions of care in these spaces. Early-Georgian naval health care saw the beginning of efforts to make care on shore orderly, which meant the capacity to monitor accurately where and for how long sick or injured seamen were in recovery. Ordered care also involved providing sailors with clothes, clean single beds, adequate and appropriate food, and sufficient numbers of attentive care workers.

The fact that the system of naval health care continued uninterrupted past the end of Queen Anne's War is one of the most important aspects of its early modern development.[2] Paying for the care of sick and injured seamen became a standard state expense. For all but one of the parliamentary sessions between 1715 and 1738, there is a line for sick and hurt seamen in the Navy Board's annual estimate of the expense of the Royal Navy.[3] The estimate was presented either in the autumn (1720, 1721, and 1724) or in winter. Evidently the figures were first sent up from the commissioners for sick and hurt to the whole Navy Board.[4] The total sum submitted for December 1715, following more than a year of peace, was £8,051, of which £749 stemmed from the previous reign.[5] If this amount is taken as a baseline, we find that eleven of the following twenty-two years witnessed higher expense estimates, which presumably reflected at least in part higher actual spending on care, and eleven years of lower expense estimates. Unsurprisingly, the years of

106   Early Modern Naval Health Care in England

operations in the Baltic (1718–1721) and war with Spain in the West Indies and the western Mediterranean (1726–1727) make up part of the group that exceeded baseline spending.

The parliamentary estimates for the annual cost of naval health care from 1715 to 1738, nearly twenty years of peace, amount in total to roughly £175,150. By comparison, the cost of care for sick and injured seamen during the Nine Years' War, 1689 to 1697, totalled £185,334, which was £10,184 more.[6] These figures point toward how much money the long Georgian peace saved British taxpayers in the quarter-century after Queen Anne's War. Nonetheless, keeping up the sick and hurt service for seamen during a time of peace helped to preserve and even improve it, much as continuing the sea service itself sustained and benefited the fleet.[7]

Naval health care was not free from strife and problems between 1715 and 1739.[8] The private-contract hospitals at Deal and Gosport contracted in size and succumbed to corruption. The main sites for onshore care, Plymouth and Gosport, proved unable to manage a surge of sick and injured seamen in 1734 and 1735.[9] Nonetheless, the fact that the system continued to operate in the absence of a major maritime conflict is significant, for it demonstrated the navy's commitment to preserving the lives of its most valuable resource, absent a national emergency. Importantly, between 1715 and 1739, naval officials continued trust in the capacity of ordinary people to provide care space and perform care work for seamen, sometimes to a degree not seen since the late-seventeenth century.[10]

This chapter examines how naval health care was maintained and increasingly ordered during two and a half decades of peace. Ordered care meant accounting for both money and personnel. From 1730, the drive to provide care that was better ordered also involved regular visits to the ports to inspect the conditions of care. The greater attention to accounting for men, money, and the conditions of care during the long Georgian peace went a long way to preventing the system from experiencing a catastrophic collapse at the outset of the next major war.

A SYSTEM OF CARE PRESERVED FOR PEACETIME

The peacetime naval health care system emerged between 1713 and 1715.[11] The two-tiered scheme for onshore care that was established in 1703 remained. Agents for the sick and hurt commission were retained at Gosport and Plymouth. At those places, care took place at privately contracted hospitals or town quarters. Elsewhere in England, a surgeon agent might be employed periodically to look after seamen and find them quarters in town.

The responsibility for sick and hurt seamen fell to the Navy Board, as it had from 1699 to 1702. Two or three members of the Navy Board retained the title of commissioners for sick and hurt seamen: John Fawler (1715 to 1740); Richard Burton (1715 to 1727); Kendrick Edisbury (1716 to 1736); William Cleaveland (1727 to 1732); and Francis Gashry (1737 to 1741).[12] Neither Fawler nor Burton had any medical training, which meant that, for the first time since 1689, the commission for sick and hurt seamen did not include a medical professional. The commission's office moved from Westminster, where it had been since 1702, back to the old Registry office at Tower Hill, much closer to the Navy Office.[13]

The Instructions which framed naval health care after 1715 were designed for peacetime. Soon after their appointment, commissioners Fawler and Burton reviewed a set of documents "relating to the sick and wounded office when managed by two commissioners of the Navy" in 1699, including the "Instructions" of July 1698, which had been prepared by the Navy Board.[14] Burton and Fawler evidently "read and consider'd" the old instructions, then decided on changes to the regulations that made sense in peacetime. The Admiralty subsequently approved the annotated instructions.[15] After a further examination of the management of care during Queen Anne's War,[16] the two commissioners presented a proposal for a domestic and foreign naval health care establishment, which the Admiralty accepted on 27 May 1715.[17]

Saving money was a higher priority than stopping men from deserting the navy during peacetime. The Admiralty encouraged the commissioners to seek "consideration and directions" if at any time they found "the Publick Expence may be retrenched, either in the Discharging of any of the aforesaid Officers, or in any other Branch of the Business of their Office."[18] Fawler and Burton recommended a severely retrenched naval health care establishment.[19] Nonetheless, they argued that it was "absolutely necessary" to retain the private-contract hospitals at the great ports, plus a surgeon-agent at each of them.[20] Thus, the two-tiered system of naval health care constructed under the fifth commission for sick and wounded from 1703 survived postwar fiscal and administrative retrenchment.[21]

Despite the emphasis on thrift, at its core naval health care continued to be concerned with saving seamen's lives. Having secured the system's existence and a minimal number of sites for care in England, the commissioners intended to improve it by making it more visible and more ordered. These aims are evident, for example, in the instructions the commissioners' prepared for Oliver Birkby, appointed surgeon for Rochester in late spring 1715. Most (nine) of the directives concerned the surgeon-agent's interactions with seamen, primarily to restore them to health and to ensure that they did not become a burden on the system. Ensuring seamen were cared for and cured would involve a combination of regular visual inspections and the checking and registering of data onto forms. For instance, "all sick and hurt Officers, seamen and others set on shore" were to bring and to present "a printed Certificate according to the following form." The Rochester-based surgeon was to "take care" that all men were lodged at the town's hospital (run by contractor Thomas Knackston), and Birkby was to visit the men staying there "not less than once a day." Additionally, Birkby was to ensure that he "diligently and with [his] best skill and judgement administered physic and medicaments as necessary for their speedy recovery." Necessary and proper accommodation for men included finding supplies of "good and wholesome Dyett, Lodging Fire Candles Nursing." Birkby's duties including mustering the men in the hospital twice per week or more frequently "to the End that those that are recovered may be Discharged from the Hospital, and that such as have absented themselves may be timely Cheq'd and Discharged." Should the surgeon observe "any Men to be sent on Shore unnecessarily vizt such as in health," he was to inform the commissioners of the men and his commandeering officer's name immediately. At Rochester, saving money was not, in theory, to conflict with saving lives.

Paper-based records were important for monitoring care work on shore. The instructions for agent Birkby included the proper accounting forms for keeping track of the costs of care on a monthly and quarterly basis. The forms recorded sailors' names, their entry and discharge dates, and the number of days they spent in sick quarters. The agent was also to keep a Book of Names of all the quarterers who provided accommodation for seamen not staying at the hospital. The commissioners also encouraged the Rochester agent to relay data that could improve health care. They directed Birkby to "give information from time to time of any Matters that may be of Concernment for the better management of this Service."[22]

The commissioners did acknowledge that saving lives sometimes demanded spending more money, especially in cases where the care conditions were poor or seamen needed additional attention from care workers. For example, although Birkby was not allowed to pay people who quartered seamen more than 12d. per day per man, which had sometimes happened during the war, in the case of seamen with smallpox, quarterers could receive 6d. per day extra "to defray the Charge of Nurses for the first twelve days."[23] Similarly, Rochester naval hospital's contractor, Thomas Knackston, agreed that "the better accommodation and preservation of many of the lives of sick and hurt seamen" included the provision of separate beds, wholesome provisions, and "careful Nurses" for seamen.[24] Thus, seamen were well cared for, provided they had their own beds, good food, and help attending to their basic bodily needs. When and where these conditions did not obtain became a greater concern for naval officials between 1715 and 1739.

Despite being concerned to save money, and absent the high demand for care that characterized wartime, naval officials could be convinced to spend money if it meant improved care conditions. In the autumn of 1733, the commission for sick and wounded requested that officers of Plymouth's dockyard survey the condition of the naval hospital. The survey revealed that the hospital, located east of the town, was "in so ruinious a Condition that it is dangerous for [men] to lodge in any part of it." The surveyors estimated that a thorough repair of the hospital would cost £401.[25] A document listing the necessary repairs indicated a two-storey building, with two wards on its south side, three wards on the north side, and three wards above stairs. There appears also to have been a surgery, a nurses' room, a cook room, and a front hall.[26] In the report on the hospital subsequently submitted to the Admiralty, commissioners Fawler and Edisbury claimed that it could hold 165 men. They asserted that a thorough repair of "the house" was "a work absolutely necessary to be done."[27] The Admiralty then approved the commissioners' contracting "with some proper persons to perform the said work," and a contract was made with Sir Nicholas Trevanion, the resident commissioner at Plymouth dockyard, to effect the repairs.[28] This represented the largest expenditure on domestic naval health-care infrastructure for nearly two decades.

FINANCIAL ACCOUNTABILITY AND MANPOWER MANAGEMENT

Corruption was long understood to be a kind of disorder.[29] Several investigations into irregular financial dealings, including those of an allegedly fraudulent alehouse keeper and of the contractor of Rochester's naval hospital, testify to the danger that corruption and waste posed to the commissioners' vision of a well-ordered system of care for seamen. They also highlight the connection between financial accountability, or saving money, and keeping track of the number of men in care to preserve the navy's manpower.[30] For example, the allegations levied against Benjamin Dixie, a publican in St Botolph Aldgate, hinged upon his defrauding the commission for sick and wounded seamen during Queen Anne's War. Five former seamen and one sailor's widow testified in the autumn of 1717 that Dixie variously secured tickets for admission to St Bartholomew's Hospital from men who never entered the institution.[31] Dixie, who evidently operated the Cork and Bottle just east of the hospital in Little Britain, was also a quartermaster to the commission.[32] This probably means that his establishment lodged men who were waiting for admission to the hospital.[33] Dixie was accused of acquiring money from the commission for sick and wounded's officers "under the names of several persons by procuring people to personate the reall persons that were Intitled" to the money.[34] Similarly, in the autumn of 1727, the commission for sick and hurt was ordered by the Admiralty to investigate the conduct of Rochester hospital's contractor, who was apparently "receiving an Allowance for Men that are not actually Subsisted by them." The contractor evidently also extended the length of some men's stay by recording the death date of a deceased seaman at the hospital differently from his actual date of death, thereby increasing his charge for care.[35]

Accurate financial records could be decisive for investigations into corruption. In Dixie's case, the commissioners obtained an account from the Navy Board's ticket office of the "Persons mentioned in the Information" against the landlord,[36] and a report from the steward of St Bartholomew's Hospital.[37] This information, along with a search of the books from the fifth commission, evidently showed that none of the informants against Dixie were "entered in the books of the commission for sick and hurt seamen, nor the books for St Bartholomew's hospital." Ultimately, attorney general Edward Northey's January 1718 opinion on the merits of the case against Dixie was that "there is noe ground for a prosecution on any of the matters objected against" him.[38]

The commissioners responded to the actions of the Rochester hospital contractor by suggesting a new way of keeping track of the seamen. In the autumn of 1727, the Admiralty, led by the recently appointed Lord Torrington, directed the commissioners to come up with a way to reduce the possibility of fraud at the hospital. They suggested that, to stop the contractor from charging for the accommodation of non-existent patients, the clerks of cheque, not only at Rochester but at all the ports, should muster the sick and hurt men at hospitals and town quarters.[39] Although the Admiralty at first resisted this suggestion, from November 1727, clerks employed at naval dockyards were ordered to muster the sick and hurt twice per week, and to transmit their account of the numbers to the commissioners. At ports without dockyards, the local agent was to provide a weekly account for the commissioners of the number of men, their condition, and the circumstances at the town quarters.[40] These measures were explicitly intended to stop "the undertakers [contractors] for quartering the sick and hurt seamen there receiving any Allowance for Men who are not already subsisted by them."[41]

The practice of having clerks or agents muster seamen in care lasted two years. In December 1729, the Admiralty received a petition from the clerks at the dockyards, in which they outlined their difficulties fulfilling the order. The clerks reported that the distance from the yards to some of the hospitals was large, which made it "Laborious to go to them and return." The job could not "be done Especially in bad weather without the use of a Horse." Additionally, the work of mustering the men, "casting, Transcribing and sending to the Board their Muster books at the End of each Quarter" was "not only Extreamly troublesome but requires all imaginable Care." Lastly, the clerks "generally Muster in Person, which among contagious Distempers and Dying Persons renders their healths very precarious." Perhaps unsurprisingly, the clerks concluded their petition not by asking to be relieved of their duty but for "an Additional Clerk, and such an allowance for their Contingent Charges" as the Admiralty saw fit.[42]

Subsequently, both the commissioners for sick and hurt and the Navy Board recommended a return to the former practice of requiring surgeon-agents to muster sailors in care on shore. The commissioners suggested that surgeons, having no financial interest in extending seamen's stay at sick quarters, could be trusted to muster men and to ensure "that the Entries and Discharges of the men born" in the quarterers' books "were right and true."[43] The Navy Board argued that putting "persons of integrity" in the post of surgeon "would as effectively prevent undertakers receiving any allowance for men that were not actually subsisted by them," and that the clerks of cheque (senior dockyard officials responsible for finance and administration) could not be expected to do their regular duties carefully "even in time of peace" while spending two days each week counting seamen. Additionally, the

Navy Board pointed out that the navy could not afford to hire any more clerks, especially since the "Musterings of Seamen in Sick Quarters may undoubtedly with proper care be well performed by Surgeons or Agents as formerly."[44]

The Admiralty agreed to the recommendation to discharge the clerks from mustering sick and hurt seamen. Henceforth, the surgeons would perform the work of counting the men and providing a report of the number to the commissioners. The goal of the musters remained to "prevent any Fraud which may be attempted by Persons who receive and subsist the men in Quarters."[45]

Suspicions about a dishonest contractor at Rochester had necessitated new regulations intended to better preserve the navy's financial resources. The brief experiment with clerks and the mustering of seamen on shore failed because it placed too heavy a burden on their time and energy. However, the fact that it was tried at all demonstrates the navy's concern with saving money and preventing fraud in a period of retrenchment. It also highlights the fact that the navy had not abandoned all concern to maintain manpower, and the importance of naval health care in reaching this goal.

Naval health care on shore usually provided seamen with the opportunity to desert. Sick or hurt seamen, wrote Captain Philip Cavendish, made "nothing of going away from their Sick Quarters." Without some expedient to "prevent Desertion ... a Ship which has the misfortune of being sickly will soon be incapable of doing the Service."[46] Consequently, in an effort to reduce the level of desertion, early in the Nine Years' War, the Admiralty had ordered that ships' paymasters "putt a Query against each Mans Names that shall be sett on Shore for Cure, for the Stopping of his Wages" until he returned to his own or another ship.[47] By putting a Q (for Query) next to a sick or hurt seaman's name in the ship's pay book, the navy stopped his pay until he reboarded his or another ship. An entry in the Admiralty minutes from early May 1715 suggests that senior officers thought the policy was no longer needed; sick and injured seamen were to be discharged "on the pay books of ships at the end of the month."[48] The peacetime navy needed fewer men, so sick and hurt sailors set ashore for cure were deemed discharged after thirty days. Against the advice of the commissioners for sick and hurt, the Admiralty kept the practice in its General Instructions.[49] However, the "Draught Instructions" for ships pursuers, drawn up toward the end of 1726, did not mention a requirement to put a Q anywhere on the book "of all men that shall be set sick on shore."[50]

Toward the end of the decade, the Admiralty re-emphasized the policy of using the letter Q to stop the pay of seamen on shore for care. Probably the Qs were restored as part of a broader effort by Lord Torrington, First Lord of the Admiralty since mid-1727, to reduce the level of desertion through better regulation. The Qs feature briefly in Deputy Admiralty Secretary Thomas Corbett's papers about naval administrative practice prepared for Torrington.[51] On 22 April 1729, the Admiralty noted that the "directions about putting Qs on men who desert sick quarters" had been sent to ships' captains and the commissioners, and that "notice thereof [was] to be affixed at the several Hospitals."[52] The notices were to be set in "such Publick places in the Hospitals or Quarters" where the seamen would "best take notice that should they leave their Quarters, and abscond from his Majesties Service, they will not only forfeit their Wages, but subject themselves to be tried and punished as Deserters."[53] Putting Q against the names of "such as do not return to their Ships" from sick quarters was the ninth article of the first printed set of instructions and regulations relating to the naval service, approved by the privy council and released in early 1731.[54]

Manpower management remained a key component of naval health care during the 1730s. In 1731, the navy issued for the first time a set of *Regulations and Instructions*.[55] Six of the eleven articles under the heading "Rules to be observed in sending Sick or Hurt Seamen out of his Majesty's Ships for Cure" related to keeping track of where seamen were and stopping them from deserting the navy. For example, article two focused on the proper use of tickets authorizing the sending of seamen on shore for care, article five outlined the procedures to muster the men at hospitals or town quarters, articles six and seven directed captains to receive recovered men, "though the Ship be at a distant place from the Hospital, unless [the man] be unserviceable." Seamen who were restored to health were to be sent "to their own ships, but if they are full, to keep them, or spare them to other ships." Clearly, the rules and regulations relating to naval health care that were either introduced or reaffirmed under Lord Torrington aimed to make the process clear and thus less subject to loss. The same aspiration animated the efforts to assess more regularly the conditions of care on shore.

ASSESSING THE CONDITIONS OF CARE

The 1731 *Regulations* show what good care for seamen entailed. For example, seamen were not to be set ashore without clothes or bedding (article two). If men could not be set down with clothes, the purser was to provide for them "out of the Slop Clothes" (article three). Captains should "take care to send the sick men" with an officer, accompanied by the surgeons, and "carefully secured" in transport "from the Weather, and to land them at the nearest Place to the Hospital" (article four). Most significantly, the eleventh article ordered admirals, commanders-in-chief, and commissioners of the navy to visit the hospitals "frequently and see how men under Cure are treated," especially in connection to the attendances of the physician and the quality of the food. During these hospital visits, the senior officers and administrators were to "examine the Men and hear their Complaints," the "better to come to Knowledge of any Abuses" and "willful Mismanagement." In other words, naval officers had authority to review the conditions of care at the private-contract hospitals and town quarters. The quality of the medical care men received, and the quality of the food provided to them, were central to what the navy regarded as good care on shore.

The *Regulations* provide an insight into what good care for sick and injured seamen looked like to the navy by 1730, over seventy years after naval health care first emerged as a system. Good care meant clean clothes for seamen, appropriate medical treatment, and good food. It also meant ensuring that these goods and services were provided to the satisfaction of the seamen. Periodic visitations to hospitals by naval officers had occurred in the past, and captains had been ordered to muster sick and injured men on shore during the latter stages of Queen Anne's War.[56] The fact that the order to undertake regular visits "where Hospitals are established" was introduced very shortly after the Admiralty had ordered local surgeon-agents to muster the sick at hospitals, suggests that they were not entirely happy with the results of this directive. More pointedly, the order to visit hospitals shows that Torrington's Admiralty knew that conditions at the privately run establishments could deteriorate to a level at which seamen were ill-treated. The fifth commission for sick and wounded's goal of saving lives by centralizing care at hospitals was far from realized.

The conditions of care for seamen at several ports during the early Georgian era are partially visible thanks to the survival of a handful of inspection reports. They provide important insights into the qualities that officials believed constituted good care for seamen, and what conditions endangered it.

The centrality of good food for care is evident from the earliest surviving report about the conditions at Rochester, one of the so-called great ports with a private-contract hospital. Commissioner Kendrick Edisbury, appointed in 1717, inspected the hospital there and found everything in order. On 1 May 1717, Edisbury found forty-six seamen at the establishment. He judged the wards, sleeping arrangements, food, and the practice of care to be "all very good in their Kind." "The practice of the hospital" Edisbury reported, "is to give each Man a pound of flesh every Day and Dinner either of Beef, Mutton or Veal, besides which, they have for Breakfast, and Supper, Broth, Milkporridge, Bread & Cheese, as is most Suitable for them." The men, the commissioner noted, said that "they are well Supplyed both with Provisions and Medicins, and proper Care taken of them by the Nurses." Edisbury concluded that Surgeon Birkby and contractor Thomas Knackston were carrying on well with the "Care and Cure of the Sick and Wounded" at the port.[57] The quality of food also featured in Edisbury's report about the state of Gosport's hospital in the summer of 1729. He noted that while there he had "viewed the Beef, Mutton, Bread, Butter and Cheese provided for the sick men, which were all good in their kind." He claimed to have asked "the sick men whether they had good usage, and had everything necessary in their several conditions," which they "declared they had."[58]

The hospital at Rochester evidently continued to operate well into the 1720s. A letter from Admiralty secretary Burchett to the commissioners at the end of 1719 directed "care to be taken of sick Men in the Hospital at Chatham," which probably meant Rochester.[59] At some point in the 1720s, following the death of contractor Knackston, the commissioners entered into a new contract for managing the hospital with one Frederick Hills.[60] The final mention of conditions at Rochester recalls the issue that had most vexed the commissioners during Queen Anne's War. Secretary Burchett reported in the spring of 1724 that sick men in transport by boat to Rochester's hospital had died along the way. The Admiralty ordered that accommodation for sick men be "taken care of at Queenborough," just south of the mouth of the Medway, presumably in town quarters.[61] Once again, the hospital's location upriver was costing the navy at least some of its men.

The old problem of paying care providers on time re-emerged at Deal in the spring of 1734, when about three hundred men from Sir John Norris's fleet were set ashore sick.[62] Commissioner Edisbury was at the town to provide quarters for sailors "while the Hospital is full, and [men] cannot be Entertained in Town Quarters." He reported that as of 16 June, fifty-eight men were lodged at the hospital, 241 in quarters in town. In an echo of circumstances at Plymouth four decades earlier, Edisbury identified the problem at Deal as involving both a lack of money for care providers, whom he called "the Housekeepers," and a dishonest hospital contractor.[63] An inquiry into the situation had shown that "the Poorer sort, unless they had ready money to go to Market, cannot be supplied with the necessary Dyett" used to feed men in care. Additionally, the people who took in the sick and hurt seamen complained that they "were paid 5s. per week by our Contractor for receiving the men, although he receives from the Crown 7s. the established Allowance." Still, the people of Deal "choose to take five shillings rather than wait the arrival of payment." To encourage the town's people "to take in more seamen," Edisbury claimed to have "publicized ... That all such Housekeepers as are inclinable to take them in shall be paid at the End of each Month." Such an action would, he claimed, remove the objections made by the poorer sort that "cannot stay for their money to the end of the year."[64]

The result of Edisbury's efforts to convince the people of Deal to take his offer of money for care is unknown. However, Deal's private-contract hospital was not equipped to treat more than a few dozen seamen at one time. Significantly, Edisbury showed more willingness to have local residents look after sailors than his predecessors on the commission had during Queen Anne's War. There is nothing in Edisbury's report to suggest that he thought the problems at Deal required greater investment in the town's hospital. Good care for sailors at Deal could, in his view, happen at a hospital or at a private house.

Inspections showed that the quality of conditions of care at Gosport and Portsmouth evidently varied over time. As was the case at Rochester and Deal, the neighbouring towns had a hospital and a brace of town quarterers. Edisbury conducted an inspection in the early summer of 1729, during which time he had found "347 men in the Hospital" and private quarters, although how many were in each he did not indicate.[65] Although "26 men died in the past month" of those set sick ashore, Edisbury seemed satisfied with the conditions at the hospital. He found the food was "all good in their kind." The sick men did not have any complaints to report concerning their "good usage and necessary requirements." Nonetheless, Edisbury recommended that a physician be appointed to visit the men "for the Preservation of the Poor Men's lives" while Sir Charles Wager's squadron was off Spithead.[66] The Admiralty subsequently agreed to his suggestion, and appointed one Dr Brady as physician at the port.[67] Brady was re-appointed to look after seamen at Portsmouth in the late summer of 1734, as "great numbers of sick," many of them fevered, were set down at the town.[68] A later request for compensation from the Physician General James Lidderdale claimed that between seven hundred and nine hundred seamen of Admiral Norris's squadron were treated at the "Hospital and the Sick quarters."[69] If true, this was probably the highest number of sick and hurt men cared for in England since 1714.

The sudden surge in the demand for onshore care in 1734–35 also produced the one surviving example from the period of an officers' report on the conditions of care, almost certainly written in compliance with the printed *Instructions* of 1731. Unlike Edisbury's account five years previously, the officers' inspection of Gosport hospital revealed much about which to complain.

The November 1734 officers' reports on care conditions at Gosport complained about overcrowding, bad food, and inadequate nursing. Having visited the hospital, Vice-Admiral Philip Cavendish, Lieutenant Richard Hughes, and a Lieutenant Dilkie, noted that there were 380 men at the hospital, lying in beds with linens that went unchanged for a month or more. The agent, or deputy-contractor, had reportedly claimed that his contract with the navy did not include washing men's sheets. The food at the establishment seemed satisfactory to Hughes and Cavendish, if not a little bland. On muster days, the broth had leeks but no vegetables such as turnips, cabbages, or carrots, "nor even any sort of Greens." The pottage had no oatmeal or herbs. The beef was good, when boiled, as were the bread, beer, butter, and cheese. The officers were not impressed by the deployment of care workers. On average, there was at the hospital one nurse for every sixteen men. This ratio of nurses to patients was deemed insufficient to keep the place clean, itself a prerequisite for restoring the men's health.[70] The officers concluded that "the want of due regulation of diet and sufficient number of servants to keep the hospital sweet and clean does contribute greatly to their illness if not their death."[71] For his part, Lieutenant Dilkie reported similar complaints from patients about lacklustre broth, dirty and louse-infested bedding, and an unkempt hall. One seaman claimed he was still waiting to see a surgeon, another that the daily bread allowance was insufficient. Dilkie had nothing to say about the quantity of nurses but instead made a pointed remark about the quality of their care. The seamen said, he reported, "that the Nurses never sit up longer then Midnight, which will serve but one, the ill conveniency of this is that the Men that are sick and weak are obliged to get up by themselves in the Dark, was it not for the good nature of others that lay by them."[72] Thus, the hospital contractor allegedly did not care enough to provide more than the minimal necessities of nutrition and an inadequate number of nurses, almost exactly the same problems as had been reported of the first hospital contractor at the town in the autumn of 1704.[73]

The reports of 1734 show that centralizing care work for seamen at hospitals run by private contractors did not necessarily result in better care conditions or higher-quality care work. Seamen might still be neglected. The contractor could be motivated to spend as little as possible on provisions and care workers, so long as he could collect money from the navy. Indeed, at ports with hospitals, the navy was committed by contract principally to put men under the care of its hospital contractor. An untrustworthy or negligent contractor could seriously undermine the prospects for men's safe and speedy recovery to a much greater extent than one or two care workers looking after a handful of sailors. From the perspective of the mid-1730s, one could argue that the shift from a health care system in which care happened at many sick quarters, to a more centralized one that blended contract hospitals and housekeepers, had produced mixed results. One problem with this arrangement was that, absent regular inspections, the contractors could defraud the navy, costing it manpower, and seamen their health, if not also their lives.

Nonetheless, the choice to centralize care space at private-contract hospitals did, at least on one occasion, facilitate a more orderly approach to managing epidemic disease, and maintaining good relations between the navy and local people. In the spring of 1735, Plymouth's mayor, magistrates, and common councillors presented a petition to the Admiralty in which they complained about the dangers of the "sick men" in their midst. "Great numbers of seamen have been set ashore from the squad lyeing in Hamoze," many more than could possibly be "accommodated in the Hospitall near the Town." Consequently, the "government's contractor" had put seamen in "many private Lodgings." Given the prevalence of the "worst Sort of the small pox and malignant and spotted fevers" the seamen suffered, many parts of the town were infected, according to the petitioners, "to the great detriment of the Inhabitants, the spoiling of Markets, the Loss of many persons Lives."[74] The petition ended with a plea to remove the seamen from the town.

The Admiralty responded to the petition by ordering the commissioners to find proper ways to move the sick and hurt outside Plymouth, and to employ "at the Publick expence" at least one physician, Dr Seymour, to "put a stop to the Distempers occasioned by their being quartered there."[75] The commissioners and their local agent proceeded to cast serious doubt on the Plymouth petitioners' characterization of their agent's relationship with locals and his efforts to locate care space for seamen. The commissioners had, they claimed, ordered Plymouth's surgeon-agent, Mr Gortley, not to place any more seamen inside the town, and that "for the better Preservation of the Seamen's lives." However, the commissioners pointed out that, in their complaint, Plymouth's governors had not "given any Instances of the spreading of the Contagious Distempers and the loss of many person's lives." Additionally, they observed that "at Rochester and Portsmouth, the Town's People, when the Hospitals have been full, have Entertained double the number of sick men without the least complaint, and have thought it an Advantage to all the Trading People."[76]

A subsequent letter from agent Gortley suggested that the complaint from Plymouth's leaders was not about the dangers of contagion only. The petition was, said Gortley, "a Surprise to the Town in General" and was the cause of resentment among many "Hundreds of the best Traders and Gentlemen of the Town and Country." These sorts of people were, Gortley asserted, "sensible of the Advantages that accrue from the Ships of War, and entertaining the Sick Men." The agent claimed that smallpox was a problem at Plymouth "before the Ships came here, as well as fevers." The one man who had succumbed to smallpox had been "taken ill at his own house." To "prevent all manner of Reflection from the Town," he had not quartered any men with contagious diseases there. When the hospital had filled up, Gortley "drew out the recovered, and placed the [sick] in their Room." The contractor of Plymouth hospital and Gortley had, he admitted, rented "a small house at the extream end of the Town, where he [could] quarter 12 men, and was to be a Reservoir to make Room in the Hospital." This small house, although not yet used, "being nigh on an Alderman's house, he resents it." That man, Gortley was informed, was the driver behind the "Unnatural Petition." The agent concluded his letter by testifying that the residents of Plymouth hoped that the commissioners would quarter sick and hurt men there, "that they may evidence themselves to be, as they are, a Humane Merciful People"[77] – and, we might infer, people who understood providing care space and care work to sick and injured seamen as an economic opportunity for their households.

LOOKING BACK TO THE FUTURE

Significant characteristics of naval health care continued after its peacetime reconfiguration in 1715. Parliament funded care for sailors annually. Privately contracted hospitals operated at great ports such as Gosport and Plymouth. The commissioners for sick and wounded worried about and investigated corruption, sought to collect accurate information on men in care, and to stop them from deserting. In a word, they continued to aspire to save lives while saving money and keeping men in the navy.

Nonetheless, naval health care experienced important developments during the quarter-century interval between the War of the Spanish Succession and the War with Spain of 1739. These changes were quantitative in nature but qualitative in effects. Naval officials sought more accurate counts of the men at hospitals, both to prevent fraud and monitor desertion levels. The conditions of care at the hospitals were subjected to more regular inspections by various branches of the navy, including officers and, of course, the commissioners.[78] The goal of these assessments was to ensure that seamen were clothed and thus warm, well fed, well treated by physicians and surgeons, and well attended by a sufficient number of nurses. While the navy wanted seamen treated at hospitals in the first instance – at least at those ports where one existed – its officials were not averse to turning to local people to provide space for care when the demand required it. Although the sources do not state it directly, it was also always the case that local people, and women in particular, remained essential to naval health care as the main source of care workers. Care work within a hospital or privately operated town quarters underpinned the system in 1739 as it had at the end of Queen Anne's War.

Thanks to the early-Georgian navy's regulations and on-site reviews of care conditions, it was at least possible to aim for more ordered care on shore as war with Spain appeared probable. Thanks to the continuing reliability of local care providers and care workers, naval officials were confident in the capacity of their health care system when hostilities with Spain commenced. Events would ultimately vindicate that confidence, after first testing it as never before.

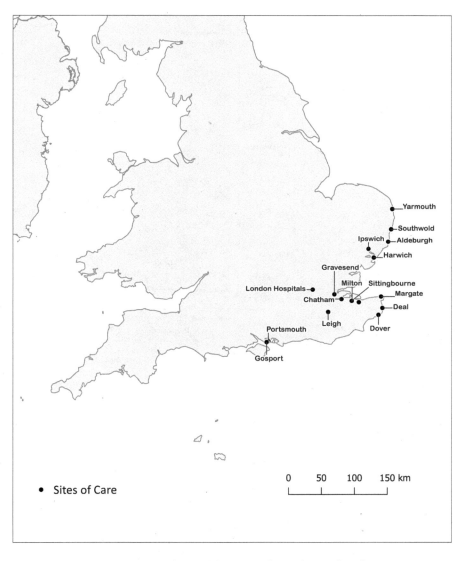

FIGURE 5.1 Sites of Care, Third Dutch War (1673).

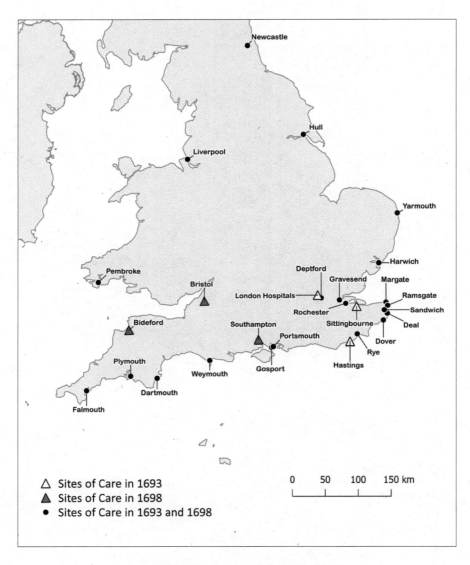

FIGURE 5.2 Sites of Care, King William's War.

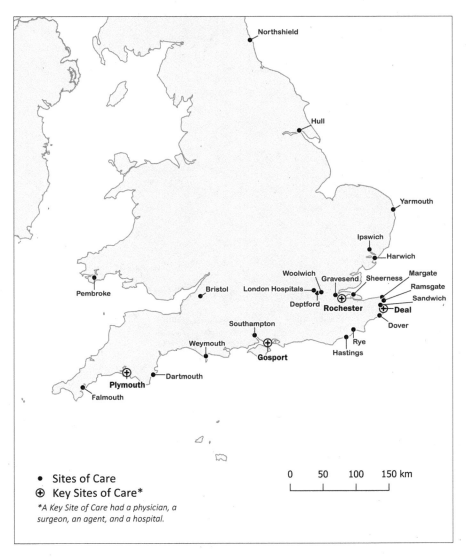

FIGURE 5.3 Sites of Care, Queen Anne's War (1712).

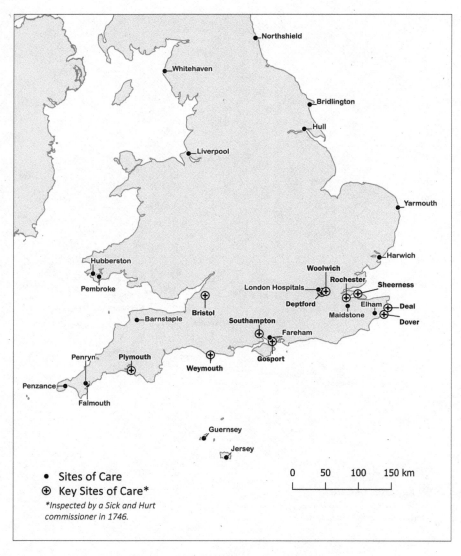

FIGURE 5.4 Sites of Care, War with France (1747).

CHAPTER 6

Failing and Succeeding to Provide Care during the War with Spain, 1739–1744

Histories of naval health care in England tend to portray onshore care during the early 1740s as exceedingly poor: "deteriorating," a "disaster," and "in crisis."[1] Such judgments are based on the numerous complaints from officials during a terrible typhus epidemic within the fleet, an outbreak that naval officials called the Great Sickness, lasting from late 1739 to early 1742.[2] This chapter takes a different view of care for seamen in the war against Spain.[3] In contrast to the performance of the Royal Navy at sea, which enjoyed a few signal successes very early in the conflict, but disappointed public expectations thereafter, the navy's system for care on shore failed to meet its own high standards initially, but later achieved a measure of effectiveness and stability.[4]

What mattered most to naval officials, both before and after the Great Sickness, was not where care happened but that it was properly ordered and so preserved seamen's lives. Ordered care demanded, first and foremost, careful people, most often women of coastal communities working as landladies and/or nurses. For example, in spring 1740 commissioners Fawler and Gashry fired off a letter to Dr Brady, the physician and victualler appointed for Portsmouth, demanding to know why the seamen there were "not better provided with nurses and servants which you are particularly enjoyned to do." They ordered the doctor henceforth to follow strictly his instructions about providing men with food and "as Physician to them also for their preservation." In case Brady had forgotten what those instructions were, the commissioners reminded him of the first three, including first that the men are "provided good beds, careful Nurses, wholesome provisions and all other necessary accommodations with separate Lodgings for men with contagious Distempers and a single bed to each man." Article 2 stipulated that the diet of men in care follow the surgeon's and physician's directions. Article 3 stated that at least one nurse attend every twenty men, every man to have clean sheets when first entered into sick quarters, new sheets monthly, their shirts washed with soap provided to them, and "a sufficient number of servants to keep the Hospital sweet and clean."[5] Good care for seamen meant keeping them separated according to disease, in distinct beds, and that the spaces in which they lay be kept free from dirt.[6]

Throughout the war, naval officials also expressed consistently their hope that the cost of health care for seamen would be constrained. If a way could be found to save money, the commissioners and the Admiralty were almost always willing to consider it. Thus, the Admiralty directed the commissioners to examine Captain Vincent's arrangements to provision the temporary sick quarters he set up on the Isle of Wight, and "give [their] opinion of savings to the government by this method."[7] The commissioners showed themselves keen to bring down costs, as when they negotiated the terms to reopen the hospital at Plymouth. A prospective contractor, Mr Cooper, was willing to accept the contract for supplying the food if he could claim the cost of bedding "considering the dearness of provisions." The commissioners replied that Cooper could buy the former contractor's bedding and cradles (standing bedsteads, used instead of hammocks for sick or wounded sailors), if they were altered to meet the commioners' standard, but he would not get more than the accepted rate of "1s. per man per day."[8] While the commissioners considered it a "Duty to propose any new Expence which shall appear to be for the good of the Service," they had "an equal Regard to the retrenching or avoiding any that may be unnecessary to it."[9]

Healing seamen as cost-effectively as possible meant little if they subsequently deserted or "Ran" from naval service. Keeping men in the navy was an ongoing challenge for the managers of naval health care, especially in wartime. Admiral Philip Cavendish complained to the Admiralty in the autumn of 1741 that "in one day I had an Account of Twenty or thirty of our best Seamen that went away from their sick quarters in a body, and many others go off as soon as they can crawl."[10] In one week during March 1743, thirty-two men ran away from Rochester's private-contract naval hospital.[11] Required to explain the sailors' action, the local agent expressed his frustration, considering "that they want for nothing" at his facility. Nonetheless, he found "they are often gone, which I have thought almost impossible for them to get out of their beds."[12] One reason to keep hospital ships off places such as Gosport was to stop men running away.[13] Health care had to include man management if it was to benefit the navy.

Care during the War with Spain 127

What follows shows how administrators, naval officers, and ordinary people struggled mightily and successfully to provide care space and adequate care for thousands of seamen between the autumn of 1739 and the spring of 1744. Quantitative records, which are relatively plentiful from this period, reveal the incredible scale of the demand for care during the Great Sickness, and the efforts undertaken to find care space. The commissioners for sick and hurt seamen found many ordinary people to provide space for care, a significant accomplishment given the scope of the demand. The commissioners also found town quarterers capable of offering seamen the kind of conditions on shore needed to preserve them for the navy. The system for care continued to rely on women to undertake necessary care work, albeit often without adequate regard or recognition. The commissioners' trust that ordinary people were up to the task of providing proper care conditions was vindicated in the scandalous conduct of Plymouth's hospital contractor. That trust was also demonstrated in the commissioners' equivocal support for a proposal to construct permanent naval hospitals in England.

THE BURDEN OF CARE DURING THE GREAT SICKNESS

During the war with Spain, the West Indies theatre saw the greatest number of sailors who needed medical attention. However, as in previous conflicts, most seaman received care at one of the chief ports along the southern coast of the British mainland.[14] Tabular records that landed in Sir Robert Walpole's papers provide unparalleled data on the number of men who received care, and where it was offered, during the Great Sickness. The figures suggest that the naval health care establishment faced an incredible challenge within months of the war's outbreak, particularly at Plymouth and Gosport. For example, a document representing the number of seamen in care on shore between August 1739 and August 1740 shows that Plymouth experienced a 200-per-cent rise in the demand for accommodation from April to June 1740, or from 656 to 2,003 men ashore, though that astonishing proportional and absolute increase did not surpass the leap at Gosport the previous autumn, where the number of seamen in care rose from 143 in August 1739 to 603 the following October. The same document also indicates that June 1740 saw the highest demand for care on the mainland, with over five thousand men on shore in either hospitals or sick quarters.[15] Another month-by-month tabulation of the number of seamen on shore at Gosport and Plymouth between January and August 1740 suggests that, over the five months from March to July, more than one thousand men were quartered at both ports. Another table shows that, from the start of the war to August 1740, nearly sixteen thousand sailors were cared for at mainland ports, of which 52.5 per cent were at Gosport (8,326) and 23.5 per cent (3,737) at Plymouth.[16] In other words, during an unprecedented naval health crisis, three out of every four sick or injured sailors were treated either at Gosport or at Plymouth.

An even more sobering numerical sketch of the Great Sickness's operational consequences is evident from an abstract of seamen sent "to Hospitals or Hospital Ships" between July 1739 and November 1740. Parliament ordered this reckoning from the commissioners, along with figures for the number of men who had recovered, or died, or deserted.[17] The abstract sent up to the members claimed that over 26,500 seamen ended up in either a hospital or hospital ship during the war's first sixteen months. For eleven of those months, more than one hundred men died every thirty days, and more than one thousand were in care on shore. In nine months, more than one hundred deserted the navy. During six of those months, all three totals were achieved.[18] In sum, 2,360 seamen died and 2,143 deserted over the report period. Unquestionably, the Royal Navy faced a massive mortality and manpower crisis in 1739 and 1740, on an unprecedented scale. The Great Sickness and its aftermath could not but critically impair the navy's capacity to engage in decisive action in the war's early phases.[19]

Officers and naval administrators grasped at explanations for the rampant sickness. In mid-June 1740, from his vantage point off Gosport and Portsmouth, Admiral Philip Cavendish observed that the fever ripping through the fleet was "no more Epidemical ... than Ships Fevers used to be." He did concede, however, that "where Men are kept in so much Filth and nastiness, and so badly attended it is not to be wondered at, that so many have Dyed."[20] The same month, the Admiralty deliberated over the "great and unusual Sickness that has raged in the Fleet for several Months past, and in different parts of the World has been a very great hindrance to the Operations" at sea. They surmised, "the same may have arisen from the Fleet being supplied with bad and unwholesome Provisions," and ordered the Victualling Board to investigate its contractors for fraud and its supplies for spoilage. The Board subsequently reported that its provisions were "sweet, sound, and in all respects as good and wholesome, as We have ever known." They concluded that spoiled food was not the problem, but "rather that it may have arisen from the general unhealthiness of the late extraordinary and uncommon Seasons, and other causes that do not fall under our Inspection."[21] In blaming the weather of the recent months – one of the coldest winters on record – the Victualling Board was not far off the mark.[22] The movement of many people onto ships after spending months crowding together indoors to keep warm would have provided lice that were bearing typhus bacteria, living on unwashed clothes, ideal conditions to proliferate.[23]

The following year was also deemed, in retrospect, "very sickly" by the commissioners for sick and hurt.[24] Then, gradually, during the first half of 1742, they sensed that the Great Sickness was over.[25] As the winter of 1742 closed, the commissioners perceived signs that the number of men needing care on shore was falling. The Gosport agent, Mr Butler, reported "so great [a] decrease of the Sick at Gosport, as will admit a discharge of some of the assistant surgeons."[26] The news from Plymouth a few days later was that the "Number of men are decreased."[27] However, at the same time at Port Mahon, almost one thousand lodged at the hospital.[28] Still, on the mainland the decrease in number turned into a decline. Two assistant surgeons at Gosport lost their positions in September 1742 because of falling demand for care.[29] The next spring, more junior staff at Gosport and Plymouth lost their posts because of "the small number of sick": an assistant surgeon, a quartermaster, and labourers (people who prepared medicines at a dispensary).[30] The Great Sickness was over.[31]

The war with Spain witnessed more inquiries into the number of seamen in care on shore, and how many were lost to death, desertion, or disability – the latter condition recorded as "discharged." The Navy Board required a weekly account of the number of seamen marked "R" (for Run) from Gosport's contract hospital from June 1741.[32] By the spring of 1743, the Admiralty, under First Lord Daniel Finch, Earl of Winchilsea, ordered quarterly statements of the total number of men who had deserted.[33] While it may be the case that systematic numerical investigations represented a "new vision" taking form among senior naval officials, their traces point to a qualitative conclusion about the naval health care system.[34] For the most part, the established mix of contract hospitals and town quarters offered adequate care capacity for the navy's sick and injured sailors.

Nonetheless, at the start of the Great Sickness, the conditions in which seamen were supposed to heal at Gosport and Plymouth provoked serious complaints about overcrowding and filth. These two ports, along with Rochester and Deal, hosted private-contract naval hospitals to which sick and injured seamen were sent in the first instance. Seamen were to be lodged in town quarters when the hospitals were full. Given the exceptionally high demand for accommodation and care work during the Great Sickness, it is difficult to imagine a scenario in which the sudden arrival of hundreds of fevered seamen would not have resulted in a hygienic nightmare, especially for officers keen on cleanliness. Landladies and nurses concerned about contagion lingering in bed linens might have preferred to destroy dirty bedsheets rather than wash them.[35]

Reports about the number of men on shore and the number Run, submitted at first sporadically but eventually at regular intervals, combined with offhand references in other kinds of correspondence between officials at ports and the commissioners in London, suggest that finding sufficient space for care was sometimes extremely difficult, especially in the summer of 1740. However, the main complaints emanating from Gosport and Plymouth centred on the conditions in which care occurred, not if and where it could happen. The "if and where" questions of care on shore had troubled, sometimes profoundly, the fourth and fifth commissioners for sick and hurt during the wars of King William and Queen Anne. By contrast, there was almost never a shortage of people willing and able to quarter sick and hurt seamen during the Great Sickness. The fact that officials complained mostly about the conditions of care at the chief ports, not the lack of it, is indeed a sign that the naval health care system did in part overcome the extraordinary epidemical challenge of 1739 to 1742. Thus, the people at the ports who offered to care for seamen prevented a health care crisis from turning into an unmitigated catastrophe.

Data collected at Gosport supports a more positive appraisal of the role of local people in the performance of naval health care in the war's early phase. Ordinary women and men served as indispensable auxiliaries to the navy's sick and wounded service on shore. Of the 818 men receiving care there in the third week of April 1740, 461 were in town quarters.[36] Upon the arrival of Sir Chaloner Ogle's squadron on 8 July, the commissioners subsequently ordered the town's surgeon-agent, Sir James Barclay, "to provide good and convenient quarters for such numbers of sick men as the hospital at Forton (Gosport) and *Blenheim* hospital ship at Portsmouth will not contain."[37] Barclay later reported that 720 of Ogle's men had been quartered ashore, including many at the nearby town of Fareham, "where the people are ready to receive many sick, but the uncertainty of the service continuing makes them unwilling to buy Bedding."[38] Barclay's observation might give some insight into why some naval officers found the sick quarters so repulsive: care providers, uncertain as to how long they would be quartering seamen, did not bother to procure additional beds or bed linen, nor offer the time and expense necessary to keep what they did have clean.

By the following February, the number of sick sailors at Gosport had "very considerably decreased."[39] Four months later, the hospital held just under three hundred men, well within its capacity of 350.[40] The arrival of around one thousand sick or injured seamen in August 1741 presented yet another massive challenge at Gosport. The town's hospital, ordinarily the preferred site for care, could in no way accommodate so many sailors. While Admiral Cavendish again complained to the Admiralty about the lack of space at Gosport, the commissioners for sick and hurt were not overly concerned about the situation.[41] Gosport hospital and quarters together could hold, they claimed, "upwards of 1,600 men;" the latest account from their agent showed "but 1,069 on shore." Once local people got paid for quartering seamen before 30 June 1741, the commissioners believed, any lack of space at Gosport would be overcome.[42] Over the course of the next two weeks, Commissioner Hills found room for two hundred men at Portsmouth, and buildings capable of holding another one hundred.[43] Cavendish eventually acknowledged the "great Pains" taken by Hills "procuring Quarters for our sick people that remain on board."[44]

Gosport, Portsmouth, and other coastal communities, however, did not have unlimited capacity to care for seamen. A breaking point appears to have been reached at the beginning of June 1740, which saw the highest number of seamen, 5,039, on shore.[45] One captain's actions provide a strong indication that the system for care on shore faced total collapse in early-summer 1740. Captain Vincent of the *St Albans* took matters into his own hands and found accommodation for some of his sick "upon the Isle of Wight in a Barn, which [he] hired for that purpose."[46] When the number of men needing care increased, Vincent acquired access to another building, into which he put men "with the worst degree of malignant fever."[47] In June 1740, the contractor at Plymouth, Humphrey Buttall, reported that about five hundred sick men from Admiral Balchen's squadron were "already taken care of to his satisfaction." The contractor had no doubt that "in a few days" he could "provide for all."[48] By the end of July 1740, a total of 730 men were in care at St Helen's on the Isle of Wight.[49] Clearly, without many ordinary people willing to provide care for sick and injured seamen, on whom officials such as Buttall could rely, naval health care on shore would have collapsed completely during the Great Sickness.

As we will see below, Buttall's ability to procure space for care at Plymouth was not always matched by attention to the quality of care performed within it. Obviously, it was hugely important that sick and injured seamen received good treatment ashore. And good treatment meant clean beds and bedding, and the ability to discriminate between different diseases. Nonetheless, the fact that the qualitative aspect of naval health care did not perform well during the early phase of the Great Sickness does not mean that the system itself was in crisis, let alone doomed to fail. One important reason that the blended arrangement of private hospitals and town quarters remained a viable option for the Royal Navy in the aftermath of the extraordinary challenge from 1739 to 1742 was the good relations that existed between its agents at the ports and their local partners in the provision of care space and care work.

ORDINARY PEOPLE AND THE PROVISION OF CARE FOR SEAMEN

In contrast to their predecessors on the fifth commission for sick and hurt during Queen Anne's War, the commissioners serving during the war with Spain strove to build care capacity for seamen by establishing and maintaining good relations with care providers in coastal communities. The commissioners and their agents did not always find enough people at the ports who were willing to take in or look after sailors, usually because the demand for space was extremely high or represented too great a financial risk. However, there is almost no record of resistance from local people to caring for seamen. This fact does not prove, of course, the genuine absence of hostility to helping the navy restore sailors to health. Yet the almost total lack of complaints within the sources from residents of ports, coupled with clear signs of the commissioners' attempts to build trust and goodwill with people who might give care, represents a marked departure from the stance taken by naval officials during Queen Anne's War. The commissioners for sick and hurt during King George's war with Spain treated local people as vital auxiliaries in the provision of care for seamen at home.

Prompt payment and conscientious officials, including hospital contractors, fostered good relations between naval officials and local people, even in the middle of the horrendous conditions of 1740 and 1741. Initially, the commissioners regarded five months as a reasonable, if not always attainable, period to settle their accounts with the quarterers of seamen. "All persons" who had any charge on the board's account from 1 January to 31 December 1739 were to be paid at the navy's pay office after 29 May 1740.[50] By mid-1741, care providers from Rochester and Deal could expect payment once a quarter.[51] Naval officials knew that delays in paying the people diminished their willingness to host seamen. In early May 1740, the physician at Portsmouth reported his "great difficulty" accommodating seamen – which should not have been very surprising, given that the sick and hurt service was nearly eighteen months behind in its payments. In response to this situation, the commissioners proposed immediately sending £800 to the contractor toward reducing the amount outstanding, "so housekeepers [would be] more willing to receive sick seamen."[52] Payments or even notifications of them sometimes encouraged local people to quarter seamen. In September 1740, Gosport's surgeon-agent, Sir James Barclay, claimed, "since the publication for payment, the Quarterers are very ready to take in Sick Seamen, even more than they can conveniently lodge."[53]

The commissioners and the Admiralty were not impressed by agents, such as Barclay, who dithered sending in the records of payments owed to people. The quarterers used the fact of arrears as a reason "why they are not able to provide better" for seamen.[54] At one point the commissioners brusquely reminded Barclay that, if he had been more conscientious, he "would have had his money and the Quarterers also had been paid, for want of which the Poor People may have been obliged to sell their Ticketts, which 'tis to be feared does ultimately affect the poor people quartered with them."[55] Justifiably impatient local care providers contributed less to the recovery of sick seamen.

Naval officials granted requests put to them by local people for the sake of staying on good terms. Gosport quarterers petitioned the Admiralty in the summer of 1741 to allow payments to take place at nearby Portsmouth rather than in London. This change would allow local people to collect payment from the navy, instead of via an intermediary such as a ticket agent, who usually would discount the ticket's full value.[56] The commissioners agreed with the idea, reminding the Admiralty that, in fact, it had been the "Practice in the late war with

France."[57] Restoring the former method of paying at the ports would reduce the problems arising from the current one. The reform would encourage "housekeepers to Entertain the Sick and Wounded People ... when Occasion shall require, but really better Enable, and very likely dispose them to use such People with more Care and Tendering than otherwise they may do."[58] The Admiralty agreed to the reversion, and by the end of August 1741, the commissioners had confidence that their agent at Gosport, Mr Porter, would not lack quarters for sick and injured sailors.[59] They even encouraged the agent to "inculcate on their minds that they will be paid quarterly."[60] A week later, agent Porter claimed, "Payment of the Quarters has much encouraged the People to take in the sick."[61] Local people's enthusiasm seems to have been real and enduring. Early the following January, the commissioners proposed retiring the *Blenheim* hospital ship to the Admiralty. One reason they gave was "the late regular payments" for sick quarters at and around Gosport "produced so good effect that some hundreds of men can now be provided for more than could before." Indeed, the commissioners suggested that putting more seamen into town quarters would in fact "contribute much more to their recovery."[62] A stronger statement of trust between naval officials and ordinary people is hard to imagine.

The reversion to the old method of paying people at the ports benefited both naval officials and local people and, in turn, evidently improved conditions for the care of sick and injured sailors. The pursuit of mutual advantage grounded, in theory at least, relationships between the British state and its many business partners.[63] However, not all partnerships between the state and local providers were between substantive equals. Hospital contractors had a qualitatively different relationship with the navy than quarterers. Despite the commissioners' preference for the type of care offered in Gosport's town quarters to the *Blenheim*, generally they preferred seamen to get care at the local hospital, reserving town quarters for circumstances when the hospital was full.[64] Nonetheless, the conditions for care provided at the pubs and houses of ordinary people could sometimes be preferable to the navy's own facilities.

At Plymouth, the commissioners for sick and hurt likewise strove to stay on good terms with local people. Unfortunately, the actions of their agents made this at times more difficult than at Portsmouth. For example, one of the complaints raised against the Plymouth hospital contractor, Humphrey Buttall, was his mistreatment of quarterers. In

July 1740, after receiving a report from Captain Hildesley about the conditions for care, the commissioners wrote "to [Buttall] to tell him, that if We find that any Complaint of the badness of Quarters is occasioned by his not giving the full price allowed by the government," they would immediately end his contract.[65] Buttall's contract was eventually terminated, but not, as will be discussed below, chiefly because of his defrauding the people who quartered sick men.

Regular, if not timely, payments were key to keeping ordinary care providers willing and ready to serve sick and hurt seamen. In this area of interaction, the navy succeeded despite the enormous challenges of the 1740–42 epidemics. At no time during the war with Spain did the commissioners report on the desperate plight of unpaid landladies or other local traders as part of a request for money. While it might have been the case that a rhetoric of local catastrophe had less purchase with the Treasury than four decades earlier,[66] it is more probable that it was never used because things at ports were better. As noted above, by the midpoint of 1741, the commissioners committed themselves to paying the people at the ports four times per year.[67] The Treasury issued the money needed for these payments from within two to three months of the request, but often within the same month. The funds to pay for sick quarters and hospital accommodations were sourced from diverse streams of public revenue: reserves (the sinking fund), the land tax, levies on consumption (the malt duty), and lotteries.[68] The fiscal instruments of the British state had no trouble paying for both war-making and care-taking operations during the early 1740s.[69]

Payment for care generally did not go into arrears. For example, on 6 August 1740, the Treasury issued £18,700 from the sinking fund to clear the cost for sick and hurt seamen to 30 June.[70] At the end of the same year, the surgeon-agent for Plymouth reminded the commissioners that the quarterers would "expect to be paid in December agreeable to the publication made some time since," suggesting that they expected the navy to keep its promises.[71] The commissioners usually did not disappoint. Commissioner Gashry, for example, oversaw payments owing on half a years' sick-quarters cost ending 31 December 1740, amounting to £2,640, on 23 February 1741.[72] Sometimes the people at the ports waited longer for payment, although not always because money was not available. Sir James Barclay's inability to organize and clear his account books delayed the payments at Gosport several times. Thus, the Midsummer 1740 quarterers costs were paid over several issues the following year.[73] Perhaps because everyone involved recognized that

1740 had been an exceptional year, there was more patience over the delay of payments, despite Barclay's tardiness. Nonetheless, without a consistent flow of money from London down to the ports to pay the people who cared for the seamen, no measure of patience could have prevented naval health care from collapsing utterly.

Money was not a problem confronting the managers of naval health care during or after the Great Sickness. Given the struggles previous administrators and agents faced in the 1690s and 1710s, this reality represents a remarkable advance. The financial base of care for sailors during the war with Spain never once buckled or bent.[74]

The Great Sickness of 1739 to 1742 did not ultimately break the existing naval health care system. The remarkable fact to emerge from all the interactions that underpinned the huge numbers of men and money tabulated for the Admiralty and parliament during and after the epidemic is that dirty beds and crowded conditions were the chief complaints. Considering the many thousands of men taken in at Gosport and Plymouth, albeit in conditions that they (and certainly modern historians) probably deemed suboptimal, it is a wonder that more did not go wrong.

The capacity of coastal communities to care for thousands deserves comment if not commendation, considering the continental scope of the mortality crisis of the early 1740s.[75] Likewise, the effectiveness of the commissioners for sick and hurt warrants mention: at no point during the war with Spain did the board hold more than three members. For half of 1740, the height of the Great Sickness, only two men, Fawler (in his post since 1717!) and Gashry oversaw the naval health care administration. Only in July 1740, with Fawler's exit and the entry of William Bell and Nathaniel Hills, was the commission's complement brought up to three, where it would remain for the next three and a half years.[76] By contrast, five men served on the commission during Queen Anne's War, under much less trying circumstances. Bell, Hills, and, from March 1741, Charles Allix, did not always do well, but neither was their performance, given the unprecedented challenges they faced, anywhere near to poor.

ORDINARY PEOPLE PRESERVING SEAMEN
THROUGH ORDERED CARE

Ordered care was not beyond the capacity of private-contract hospitals or town quarterers, even during the Great Sickness. Depending

Care during the War with Spain

137

upon who was asked, the care conditions for sick and hurt seamen at both Portsmouth and Gosport from the late autumn of 1739 to the early winter of 1740 was either precarious or satisfactory. In November 1739, Admiral Cavendish reported that the hospital and quarters there were full. The one surgeon-agent, Sir James Barclay, and his one mate "of the Hospital at Gosport" could in no way "give the requisite attendance on the Sick Men sent ashore."[77] However, two months after Cavendish's observation, Admiral Balchen visited the sick quarters at Gosport, then holding about four hundred men, "and was much surprised, after what I had heard, I had not one complaint." The hospital, he learned, was "in very good order."[78]

Nevertheless, shortly after Balchen's visitation, Barclay appeared to have lost control of the situation at Gosport. Overwhelmed by the demand for care spaces, the surgeon let conditions within them deteriorate to unhealthy levels. In late April, Cavendish described the "ill condition of the sick" at the town, prompting the placement of a hospital ship in Portsmouth's harbour.[79] Overcrowding in sick quarters concerned the admiral the most. "I cannot say that the putting so many sick men in one house and one bed proceeds from any fraud in the Contractor," he wrote, "but think it's rather from the want of Room."[80] Another officer, Captain Crawford, worried about the proximity of men's beds, which were "Shifted but once a Month (One Nurse to Twenty Men)." He also noted that men in sick quarters had opportunities to walk about town, "Selling their Clothes and getting Drunk with Drams etc." All this would be, he thought, "a great Hindrance to their Recoverys."[81] Similarly, the dockyard commissioner, Richard Hughes, observed rooms for seamen at Gosport that were "very Dirty, Offensive, low, small, and much crowded." At some places, "two Men lying in One Bed, in some Three, the Bedding was very Slutish."[82] Confined and dirty spaces, combined with easy access to alcohol, threatened to make seamen sicker.

Properly ordered care demanded sufficient space and adequate numbers of informed care workers. Learning of Cavendish's complaint, commissioners Fawler and Gashry scolded Barclay, an experienced ship's surgeon, for his apparent failure to provide the men with "convenient Quarters when the Hospital is full, also good wholesome Dyett, Lodging, Fire, Candle, Nursing and other Accommodations." Likewise, the commissioners expressed disappointment that Barclay evidently failed to give care providers "Directions for keeping Quartering Houses Clean," since he knew that "Cleanliness is a great means towards the Recovery of the Men." Instead, the commissioners had news about "twenty or thirty [men] crammed into a little alehouse, and two or three in a Bed of different Distempers ... and no Nurses or servants to take care of them." Had care workers been provided, the quarters would have been kept clean and "several Mens lives might have been saved."[83] Under Barclay's supervision, it appeared that care at Gosport town quarters actually endangered the lives of sick and injured seamen.

Barclay consistently denied the substance of the complaints about disorderly conditions at Gosport town quarters and its hospital. Very ill seamen got, he claimed, single beds. He did not ram men into "little Alehouses," but "into Publick Houses ... fitted like Country Inns, [which] have higher and better Rooms than the private houses."[84] Barclay subsequently acknowledged that "the greatest number in any One room are four Beds and that but in one Mrs Nortons in Middle Street where the ceiling is about 10 foot ... the Room well-lighted and a sufficient distance betwixt the Beds."[85] The surgeon likewise rejected the charge that the sick lacked nursing care, "there being in all great Houses at least Three besides the landlady."[86] Barclay explained that the apparent gap between the reality of conditions at Gosport and the officers' representations of them were caused by the latter's self-interest. At the base of officers' descriptions of dirty and crowded town quarters, Barclay asserted, lay their ambition "for building a Royall Hospital."[87] Some officers seemed to want to use an extraordinary situation to push for a new method of naval health care.[88]

The complaints about the lack of space and inadequate conditions at Gosport had two immediate consequences.[89] The first was temporary and practical: Captain Vincent made his own arrangements for care on the Isle of Wight. There, so he claimed, fewer seamen died than did in town quarters or Gosport's private-contract hospital.[90] The second effect was more theoretical: in early June 1740, the Admiralty issued its first set of regulations prescribing the necessary conditions for preserving the lives of seamen in care.

The ten "Rules and Instructions, for the better Management" of "Lodging, Dieting, and attending the Sick and Hurt Seamen" put cleanliness and sobriety at the centre of rightly ordered care. Proper care conditions maintained the boundary between purity and danger and clean and unclean, and sorted the sick according to the danger of their diseases.[91] Hospital wards and rooms in town quarters were "to be kept Clean, and not crowded." Bedding likewise should be "kept

Clean and often Aired," and the sheets cleaned and/or changed every three weeks. Agents and surgeons should avoid mixing men who had "contagious Distempers" with those who did not. The sick should be kept separate from the healthy. The "unjustifiable practice" of putting two men in the same bed was to end immediately. Additionally, dangerous substances were to be kept out of sick quarters. Pubs that sold strong liquors should not host sick seamen. Nurses and other care workers were to have "strict Directions" not to bring spirits into hospitals or town quarters, "it being a Practice of pernicious consequence to the Health of the Seamen." The penultimate rule stipulated that "a Sufficient Number of Nurses" attend seamen on shore. However, officials were directed to pay attention to quality as well as quantity when recruiting nurses, since "many of these Women are nasty Drunkards, Negligent, and unfit for the Office."[92] While not always deployed charitably, the image of the intoxicated nurse in the pre-Nightingale era was not socially constructed only.[93]

The revised general instructions for the commissioners of sick and hurt set out in February 1742 recapitulated the centrality of cleanliness and careful nurses to orderly care.[94] The fourth to seventh articles of the Instructions conveyed the essence of the June 1740 Regulations. Overcrowded spaces were to be avoided (#4); where possible, one man was to be laid in one bed with clean bedding (#5); men with different diseases were to be kept in separate rooms (#6); and men were not to be quartered where strong liquor was sold (#7). The Instructions also focused on the conduct of the people most responsible for keeping conditions clean and orderly. Article six also stipulated that for every ten men in care there was to be "one proper Nurse." The next article set out what should happen to a nurse who acted improperly, for example, "should she bring liquor to seamen, the nurse should be immediately expelled" and "never to be restored." The recognition that "failing to stop the entry of liquor" into care spaces often produced "the worst Consequences to the People themselves, of great hindrance to the service, and of considerable unnecessary expence to the Crown," justified this harsh sanction.[95] Proper nurses were necessary for orderly care. Improper nurses undermined the preservative ethos at the heart of naval health care.

Throughout the war with Spain, both the old and new commissioners worked to prevent the conditions of shore care from deteriorating as they had at Plymouth and Gosport in 1740.[96] One area of particular concern was keeping men with different diseases, such as "Malignant

Fevers and Small Pox," separate from others.[97] In March 1742, the commissioners succeeded in convincing the surgeon at Gosport to secure distinct wards at the hospital for "Itchy people."[98] The Admiralty, for unstated reasons, subsequently overturned this arrangement by ordering men with that particular skin condition to stay on the *Blenheim* until cured.[99] Unsurprisingly, the desire to sort sick people according to ailment was not limited to naval officials. At the end of 1742, the commissioners investigated a petition from one Edward Burton, who asked that "his Brother now Sick at Woolwich may be moved to his House at Deptford." Burton claimed that "his Brother lay in a little dirty Room without any Sheets, and was almost suffocated with the Stench of the Buckett of a Man who had the Flux." The agent at Woolwich was instructed always "to put Men of different Distempers in different Rooms, according to his Instructions."[100] Orderly care required care workers to classify seamen according to their diseases.

Sailors themselves sometimes acted in ways that undermined orderly care. Near the end of the summer of 1740, the surgeon-agent at Plymouth reported on the "Riotous Behaviour upon Recovery" of the seamen at the hospital, which "destroys all order." Commissioners Fawler and Gashry thought that the answer to the problem was to get the men back on ship as quickly as possible.[101] However, officers might not always act in the interest of orderly care on shore. Discipline at sea did not translate directly to land. Consequently, officers could not command seamen ashore, and might even encourage them in their disorders.[102] Indeed, Commissioner Hills warned his colleagues that the "irregularities" encouraged at Plymouth hospital by Captains Hildesley and Rycaul might mean that "no Contractor will keep it long."[103] The fact that Portchester castle had walls made it briefly attractive to the commissioners as a hospital, since "the people could not have it in their power, as have now, to Straggle about and commit such disorders as they often do, to the occasioning of Relapses and extraordinary expence to the Crown."[104]

The inability of some seamen to moderate themselves while in care undermined the aim of restoring them to active duty at minimal cost. Yet the system was not equipped or purposed to preserve discipline among seamen.[105] Reporting from Plymouth in the spring of 1741, surgeon Wyatt acknowledged that sailors often remained at the hospital for a long time because of "the Obstinacy of their Distempers," and sometimes due to "their own Irregularity."[106] The commissioners refused for good reasons to allow their agent at Lisbon to give wine to sailors at his hospital, "since the People can have no Title to anything but what is proper to their Condition, but likewise very dangerous to them, as it might tempt them to Excess, and Occasion Relapse."[107] In the autumn of 1743, Wyatt put a guard at the hospital for Royal Marines, "their having been frequently mutinous, often dissatisfied with their Diet without Cause, their abusing the Nurses and often himself, and also licentious Behaviour and unbridled Lust they often add the Pox or other Distempers to the Diseases they already labour under."[108] In this case, both the surgeon and nurses evidently endured alcohol-fuelled misbehaviour from men in care. In other cases, the female care workers' actions or inaction gave cause for concern. Men in sick quarters expected their bedding to be washed regularly, which normally nurses did. Unwashed bedding, as we have seen several times above, provoked complaints from officers and seamen.[109] This fact might explain the pessimism expressed by the commissioners about the nurses of the *Blenheim* looking after the seamen's beds. "Due care is hardly taken to change the peoples Bedding as they are wet or fouled," the board admitted. If the ship's surgeon, Mr Beers, did not investigate the matter of cleaning beds himself, "other people hardly will, and especially the Nurses."[110] The implication that nurses on the hospital ship were the least likely to attend to the cleanliness of bedding points to a paradox that the next and final section of the chapter will examine.

Orderly care as envisioned in the naval health care system's normative guidelines, and the commissioners' particular directives, assumed the presence and performance of proper nurses – ideally one to every ten seamen receiving treatment.[111] But however necessary female care workers were to naval health care, they both represented and enacted dangerous disorders that risked upending all the time and treasure spent on preserving men for the Royal Navy.

THE NECESSARY AND PROBLEMATIC CARE WORKERS

Female care providers and care workers made up the corporeal base of naval health care during the war with Spain. Officers and administrators recognized that seamen could not be healed and returned to active service unless many women provided sick quarters and/or worked as nurses. This recognition was grounded on the fact that sick quarters overseen by women often provided good care, and that hospitals, both real and envisioned, relied on many nurses to function. However, naval officials understood that female care workers could also pose a threat

142   Early Modern Naval Health Care in England

to seamen's health. On at least one occasion, the managers of naval health care found a way to sustain its preservative ethos by shifting the cost of care over from a contractor to nurses. While care work performed by nurses was unquestionably important to the navy's sick and hurt service, nurses themselves were seldom a priority.

Women could and did provide proper spaces for care during the first phase of the Great Sickness. A 1740 survey of the hospitals and sick quarters in and around Gosport offers data about the participation of landladies in naval health care to an extent unavailable for any conflict after the Second Dutch War.[112] Evidently prepared for Admiral Cavendish and presented to the Admiralty in May, the survey shows the overwhelming predominance of female care providers as of 30 April.[113] Of the 113 named quarterers at Gosport, 102 were women.[114] Together, these women lodged and provided for 818 seamen. The hospital near Gosport held 350 men in fifteen wards, each one served by one or two nurses. According to the survey, four complaints from sailors stemmed from sick quarters, of which one did not concern its interior condition.[115] The other three seamen's complaints concerned bedding, which was either "extremely dirty" (Mary Cousins, hosting seven men), or lacking sheets (Mary Debney, hosting thirteen), or one bed sitting in a store cellar (Joan Winwod, hosting fifteen). Significantly, no complaints were observed at any of the largest sick quarters, including those of Catherine Norton, quartering twenty-five seamen, Ann Hayes with twenty-six, Mary Wyley with twenty, Elizabeth Hayes's pub, holding thirty, Mary Russ with twenty-six in her pub, and Mary Bone with twenty. At Fareham, all seven quarterers were women, and all had at least two men per bed, whose conditions were similar "as those at Gosport." By contrast, the complaints coming out from Gosport's hospital ranged from the quality of the broth, lack of beer, thin milk porridge, insufficient attention to a seaman with a wounded leg, and beds not changed after removing a dead body. During the early phases of the Great Sickness, seamen at Gosport were better off in private quarters run by women than at the navy's own hospital.

The survey's data suggest that seamen in quarters were in more crowded conditions than might have been the case at the hospital, but that, in April 1740, a lack of space for seamen was not reason to complain. It is unclear whether the condition of beds for sailors, their cleanliness, was more of a concern for officers than for seamen themselves. Certainly, unclean beds featured in the reports submitted by Cavendish and his captains.[116] Given the number of men lodged in sick quarters, it would have been very difficult to keep their beds and cradles as clean as could be expected on board ship. People hosting fewer men could have kept their spaces cleaner. Unsurprisingly, one Mary Moss of Gosport's Middle Street, for example, offered the one man staying with her bedding that was "very Clean and in decent Order." However, considering the unprecedented nature of the demand for care space at Gosport in the first six months of 1740, it is no wonder that Sir James Barclay, the surgeon-agent, prioritized finding and keeping places with high capacity over ensuring that those places were kept clean. Barclay claimed that "two men lye in one Bed when We were strained, some of the Houses endeavored to have three in one Bed, which I remedied as soon as I could." It was fortunate for him and the Royal Navy that the women of Gosport and environs provided space for the sick and hurt that most of them seem to have thought was good enough.

Both local agents and the commissioners acknowledged that the availability of sufficient care workers was essential for good care wherever it happened. Thus, around the time of Cavendish's survey of sick quarters, Barclay reported to the commissioners that "as to the Nurses ... the Landladys allow a sufficient number." He noted, "in one of the Houses, which is the best Quarters in Town and has above 20, there are three Nurses, besides the woman of the House, and in proportion, to the numbers in each House they have Nurses."[117] About a month later, the contractor for Plymouth's hospital affirmed that he always employed nurses at a ratio of "one to Ten" seamen, "with a Reserve of one or two if to be had."[118] This ratio of carers to patients, if indeed true, met the guideline established by the Admiralty's subsequent Instructions.[119] By contrast, the ratio of nurses to patients on the *Blenheim* hospital ship the following spring sat at one to sixteen.[120] Most other statements that mentioned the necessary number of nurses for a hospital settled on one to roughly every fourteen men.[121]

The correspondence back and forth between agents, naval officers, and the commissioners for sick and hurt seamen suggests that officials recognized, not always explicitly, that naval health care depended on nurses to function. A crisis such as the typhus epidemic, the so-called Great Sickness, obviously demanded more nurses than normal. However, more nurses at work did not necessarily mean sailors received better care.

The navy wanted nurses to provide proper care, and complained when they did not. For example, Captain Vincent visited Gosport hospital during the epidemic's early phase and found it very unsanitary.

144 Early Modern Naval Health Care in England

He recommended "frequent and necessary changes of wholesome, dry, clean bedding and linen, together with a more just distribution and regulation in having more careful women as nurses to keep the sick neat and free from vermin."[122] Four weeks later, Admiral Cavendish, unconvinced about the quality of care at the sick quarters of Gosport, pleaded with the Admiralty to order the sick and hurt seamen into the *Blenheim* hospital ship. At both the hospital and town quarters, Cavendish declared, seamen lay "two in a Bed for the most part, and what they call Nurses to attend them, are Rotten whores that ply about there houses, where they force from the poor sick men a Will, and then destroy them with Ginn."[123] Cavendish's letter suggests his deep distrust in the motives of local care workers toward their patients. It also indicates the identity of those who decided what constituted proper care work: naval officials. For example, a proposal from Russell Revell for the contract of Port Mahon's hospital included an article in which he promised to "procure such a Number of Nurses as the physician and surgeon shall judge proper, the said Nurses to be sober and diligent and approved by him."[124] Women might be expected to work as nurses, but they could not, so naval officials sometimes believed, be expected always to work up to official standards.

Naval officials did show a degree of paternalistic concern for and trust in those women working as nurses, particularly at hospitals. While still the contractor for Plymouth hospital, Buttall denounced the action of his chief critic, Captain Hildesley, for endangering the safety of nurses. The officer had, so Buttall declared, encouraged his seamen to such insubordination "that soon after the Nurses were beat, and in the Evening, one of them used in a most barbarous and shameful manner."[125] The hospital subsequently provided separate cabins for its nurses, possibly to enhance their privacy and security.[126] Nurses were also entrusted with a degree of authority over their male charges. Evidently, hospital nurses had keys to the wards' doors. They unlocked the doors at night, so that nurses could enter and administer medicines. This practice, which also occurred at Greenwich Naval Hospital, apparently scandalized a Spanish surgeon.[127]

Unfortunately, not all nurses were trusted to serve sailors so reliably and carefully. The nurses of the *Blenheim* hospital ship, its surgeon alleged, "made use of the Bedding and Sheets put on board for the Sick." The commissioners told him to charge the cost of the materials to their wages.[128] At times, the commissioners sounded resigned to the problem of intoxicated nurses. Writing to the agent at Gosport, they admitted that "as to the Nurses getting Drunk, [we] don't know of any method intirely to prevent it, but when they are found so are turned out."[129] This admonition implied that the agent would not have trouble finding replacements. However, from the view of naval officials, a ready supply of female labour did not necessarily provide care workers of the requisite quality.

Naval health care needed female care workers to operate, but its managers usually made them a priority only when they were in short supply or acted in ways that threatened orderly care. At times, down-playing the importance of nursing could even support the preservative ethos. In the spring of 1741, the commissioners managed to convince an entrepreneur to include bedding in the operating cost for Gibraltar's naval hospital by lowering the amount allocated for nurses and assis-tants. The rate charged for each nurse per day was reduced from 1s. 3d. to 1s. 2d.[130] It was not a large sum, but significant for showing where the board's priorities lay in this instance: good beds for seamen and tighter belts for nurses.

Nurses did not have any say in questions of their pay, their working conditions, and hours of work. The navy's archive sheds next to no light on what they thought about caring for sick and injured seamen. One very indirect testimony comes from a minor complaint arising in the summer of 1743. A Devon justice of the peace, John Fowell, notified an officer of the Royal Marines about one George Williams, recently "cured of the Itch" and discharged from Plymouth hospital. While en route to his regiment at Winchester, Williams died in Fowell's parish of South Brent. Fowell claimed that his estate, lying along the road to Exeter, was "frequently troubled with poor unhappy Soldiers and Sailors whose misfortune it is to put into the Hospital from whence they are often discharged as cured when in fact they are worse than when put in."[131] In their reply to Fowler's complaint, Plymouth's phy-sician, Thomas Vincent, and surgeon, William Wyatt, stated that the hospital's assistant surgeon and "Sarah Clark the Nurse, together with the Chief Nurse, Assert and are ready to make Oath that George Wil-liams ... never was in Salivation nor treated for his Cure of the Itch."[132] A nurse's word was not ignored when it could preserve the reputation of naval health care on shore.

The managers of the Royal Navy's sick and hurt service were nearsighted in relation to nurses: in general, they saw nurses (and landladies) when their actions created problems that compelled com-missioners or their agents to look closely at conditions in hospital

146   Early Modern Naval Health Care in England

wards or private dwellings. This moral and managerial blind spot has not been the focus of previous histories of naval health care in the war with Spain. Instead, historians have highlighted the ways officials at ports bungled their response to the Great Sickness. In this they have taken their lead from officers such as Admiral Cavendish and Captain Vincent, appalled by what they saw in the hospitals and town quarters: the crowded conditions, subpar provisions, dirty beds, and disorderly care workers. However, considering the nature of the challenge facing naval health care in England from late 1739 to mid-1742, the officers', and historians', negative view of its performance should be modified. Things could have been much worse. Nonetheless, the case of Plymouth hospital for seamen does convey a sense of how bad conditions could get during an unprecedented period of epidemic illness.

PLYMOUTH'S PROBLEMATIC PRIVATE HOSPITAL CONTRACTOR

The scandal over care conditions at Plymouth in the early phase of the Great Sickness provided negative evidence of what ordered care was meant to do. The case unfolded in three acts. Local investigations seemed to resolve the first two phases, while the third and final one involved an inspection by a London-based administrator. The key players included the hospital contractor, Humphrey Buttall, several ships' captains, the Admiralty, officials from Plymouth's naval dockyard, the commission for sick and hurt, plus dozens of unnamed nurses and hundreds of seamen.

The drama began when the Admiralty received a complaint from Captain Firth of the *Ruby* about "the miserable condition of the sick Men in the [Plymouth] Hospital, and that the Hospital was in a very nasty condition."[133] The allegation of "Scandalous proceedings of the Contractor and Surgeon" at Plymouth then reached the commissioners, who ordered the dockyard commissioner, Philip Vanborough, to investigate. The commissioners also demanded an explanation "as to what is complained of" from surgeon Gortley and contractor Buttall.[134] In his reply to the accusations, Gortley emphasized the hospital's cleanliness and his actions to ensure it. "I have caused," he claimed, "several Nurses to be turned off (dismissed) and endeavoured to get better in their Room, and given them strict Charge myself, as well as the contractor, to keep the Men clean and wholesome."[135] The hospital contractor likewise stressed his concern to employ good nurses at his facility. "If

Nurses have been bad," he conceded, "it has given me pains, which I always Redressed in the best manner I could by turning them of[f], and getting others in their room ... notwithstanding a Complaint may come from that Quarter, and as it is almost unavoidable." Buttall assured the commissioners that "I have sufficient numbers of them [on] purpose that the sick may not want for help, and that the wards might be kept clean and wholesome." In case the commissioners had forgotten that the challenges Buttall and his coworkers faced were unusual, he noted that he had "never had a quantity of seamen before save in 1734."[136] Commissioner Vanborough of Plymouth naval dockyard confirmed the gist of Gortley and Buttall's accounts. "The chief part of the Complaint," Vanborough acknowledged, "has been occasioned by the Difficulty of procuring proper Nurses, nine of which have died within these two months, and several have been discharged for Ill Behaviours." Vanborough suggested that normally the contractor employed one nurse to ten seamen. He concluded that the hospital was not "so bad as the Complaint sets forth," although he promised that "they will be kept closer to their business in the future."[137] The commissioners accepted these three explanations, thanking Vanborough in particular "for his Care and Trouble in Visiting the Hospital," and his desire to prevent more complaints.[138]

Six weeks later, the complaints at Plymouth resumed, with another Captain, Hildesley of the *Grafton*, reporting on "the miserable Condition of the Sick Men" there. Again, the Admiralty ordered the commissioners to make inquiries.[139] The following day, the commissioners notified the Admiralty that Gortley had resigned "on account of his present infirmities." In light of the "great number of sick now ashore at Plymouth," the commissioners recommended hiring one Mr Wyatt as his replacement.[140] Two days later, they asked surgeon Wyatt, their locally based physician, Dr Seymour, and Commissioner Vanborough, to make another "strict enquiry" into the allegations of the "Shocking Situation" at Plymouth.[141] Within a week, Dr Seymour reported that seamen at Plymouth "have been as carefully attended as in any Hospital in Europe."[142] Wyatt, a former ship's surgeon, wrote that the hospital and town quarters were the best that could be hoped for given the short notice and high demand; the *Grafton* alone had put 383 men ashore. He denied that seamen were mistreated at the hospital or kept there after they had recovered to defraud the navy.

Wyatt's letter implied that the trouble at Plymouth stemmed mainly from the actions of captains and their men. For example, while the surgeon did concede that "many [seamen] have been discharged sooner than I thought they should, and I fear may have relapsed," he qualified this admission by claiming that "it is always done by the express order of their Officers." Similarly, Wyatt claimed that, "when the Number of Sick and Hurt was greatly reduced, with more space in the Hospital and good Sick Quarters in Town," he had attempted to remove men belonging to the *Grafton*, then quartered at Oreston, to Plymouth, "that they might be more immediately under our Care."[143] A few men had been transferred to the hospital, only to be "ordered by Captain Hildesley to Oreston again." The captain evidently believed that "more lives would be saved if they were Lodged at Sick Quarters." Wyatt asserted that "though those who are most dangerously ill are always put into the Hospital, yet few in proportion have died there than in Sick Quarters." Wyatt also alleged that Hildesley had visited the "old Hospital" on 17 July in order to "redress irregularities and represent willful mismanagements." This evidently included telling his men staying at the hospital that "the Physicians, [Wyatt], and others concerned were their Servants, as our Bread was owing to them, they were our Masters." Consequently, Wyatt claimed, order at the hospital broke down. In particular, "the Nurses are abused, beat, and forced to leave their Wards; they have been frequently changed, the new Ones are forced to fly from the Violence of these Rioters, who get Drunk, come in at all hours of the Night, threaten the Lives of the Nurses, and most inhumanely disturb the rest of the other poor sick creatures." In sum, according to Wyatt's account, the captain's visit to Plymouth's naval hospital "introduced more confusion, Riot, and Disorder, than Contributed to rectify abuses."[144]

Wyatt's report succeeded in convincing the commissioners for sick and hurt that Hildesley's complaint about conditions at Plymouth were "without Foundation."[145] The report also confirmed what his predecessor, Gortley, and the hospital contractor previously stated about the importance of nurses for the work of hospital. The surgeon's rebuttal to Hildesley's complaint likewise reminded officials of the necessity of order for hospitals to do their work properly. Officers and seamen could choose to flout the rules of the hospital, thereby making conditions for its key workers – nurses – insufferable. Those receiving care also had a responsibility to act in ways that helped toward healing. However, Wyatt's July 1740 report was not the last word on the state of care at Plymouth during the Great Sickness.

Less than three weeks after the commissioners declared the case at Plymouth closed, the Admiralty received a complaint from a Captain Rycaul about "the Badness of the Mens Lodging, the want of Care, and the Impropriety of their Dyett." Hildesley also was back with a complaint about "the ill Treatment of the Seamen in the Hospital and Quarters," which he evidently equated with "Fraud and Murder." Commissioner Hills, himself a former ship's surgeon, resolved to go down to Plymouth "to come to the Truth of the matter."[146] Before the month ended, Rycaul sent in another account of "many and Gross abuses alledged to have been committed by the officers of the Sick and Hurt seamen" at Plymouth, "both in the Hospital and Town Quarters." The commissioners responded to this latest accusation by terminating its contract for the hospital with Buttall and placing all responsibility for quartering seamen with Wyatt.[147] The Admiralty ordered Hills to journey to Plymouth and Portsmouth to inspect the hospital and town quarters there "and rectify whatever he finds amiss."[148]

Hills arrived at Plymouth on 12 September. His investigation there lasted until 12 October. He then moved on and spent several weeks assessing the situation at Portsmouth. His final report about the conditions for care at Plymouth the previous spring and summer reached the Admiralty on 18 November.[149] The report did not vindicate the former contractor and contained a harsh judgment against the former surgeon-agent, Mr Gortley. Consequently, Buttall lost his contract to run Plymouth's hospital for seamen. Parts of the hospital were subsequently evacuated, while the "old Hospital," probably the original King's Hospital, got whitewashed.[150]

Buttall had breached his contractual obligations, so Hills judged, by failing to attend adequately to the need for good order within the hospital. This failure left unchecked the spread of dirt, inadequate food, and disorderly relations between nurses and seamen. The contractor did not "keep the Hospital supplied with proper Bedding, for such as [Hills] found there, were both very old, dirty, and out of Repair, the Sheets were in as bad a Condition." Seamen slept on mats that "were foul and very full of Flees, Bugs, and Lice." Food served at the hospital "had often been very bad, and the Beer Sower & and not fit to drink." Buttall employed one nurse in a hospital ward with fifteen to twenty men each, plus one woman "to see they did their duty, and that the Peoples Victualls were properly dressed." Hills found it a "great Indecency" that "these Nurses lay in the Wards among the people,"

150   Early Modern Naval Health Care in England

so he gave the nurses "a little Ward to themselves." The commissioner learned that "some Nurses, it seems, had fallen into a way of Exchanging the people's Provisions for Geneva,[151] & bringing it to them in the Hospital, but that as soon as this was discovered, these Nurses were expelled." To better "preserve good order in the Hospital," Hills had directed the surgeon Wyatt to put one of his assistants in each ward throughout the night.[152]

In his reply to Hills's report, Buttall claimed, true to form, that conditions at the hospital were not unusually dirty, and that he did in fact care about cleanliness. For example, Buttall pointed out that "Matts will unavoidably Harbour Flees and Lice." At any time that "it was known that a matt was foul, or unfit, it was always taken out and a new one put in its room." And in order "that the men might be kept clean in every part of their Bedding, as well as carefully attended," Buttall had employed at the hospital not "onely one nurse to about twenty men as by my Instructions, but one Nurse to about ten, or less."[153] Buttall did not, however, attempt to refute Hills's observation that nurses were sleeping with seamen in their wards, and bringing in gin. Indeed, hiring more nurses for the hospital than his Instructions required might have understandably, although unintentionally, produced those outcomes.

Buttall also breached the trust of local people, Hills contended, by not paying them what they were owed. Instead of the standard seven shillings per man per week, Buttall "quartered the other people in houses of the Town, at the Rate of Fifteen pence (1s. 3d.) per man a Week," roughly five times fewer. From this small amount of money, local people "were obliged to find the Men, not only in Lodging Washing & Attendance, but in Firing, Candle Water gruel & Milk Porridge, others in only some of these Articles." However, "the people declared" to Hills that "they seldom had their Bellys full, & particularly not enough of Bread." To prevent future complaints about care at Plymouth, Hills had publicly promised that all who lodged and provided sailors "with every thing necessary & fitting to people in their Condition, shall have the Kings full Allowance of twelve pence p man a day, and be constantly paid it at the end of every Quarter." Hills confidently predicted that "the poor Men who shall have Occasion to be put to them for the future, will meet with much better Treatment than has been practiced at that port for some time past."[154]

Buttall disagreed entirely with Hills's characterization of the contractor's treatment and provisioning of care providers and seamen. In the contractor's view, his dealings with local people enabled him to find more space in which to quarter sick and injured seamen. Buttall admitted that he had quartered the men in town at 15d. per week, but that "as the men, were well taken care of, and in good quarters, I did my duty." Indeed, he claimed that "instead of being onely able to Quarter 200. And those with difficulty at first, I could and did in less than a month's time Quarter 800 with Pleasure." All the seamen staying in sick quarters, Buttall insisted, "had a pound of Bread, and a pound of good Beefe, Mutton, veale, or lamb a day, without any manner of Doubt."[155] After a decade of working as contractor at Plymouth, Buttall insisted that he had always "treated the sick men with as much Humanity as twas possible for any one, and never had the least complaints against me till the late unjust ones."[156]

The commissioners did not dispute Buttall's long-standing concern for the seaman; the problem was how he manifested that concern. Buttall was too much his own operator. Inadequate oversight of the contractor allowed disorder to prevail at both the hospital and the town quarters.[157] The former surgeon-agent, Mr Gortley, was "very deficient of his Duty, not only as Surgeon but as a Cheque upon the Contractor." Had Gortley done as he ought to have done, the "Contractor could never have committed the Fraud ... in the Victualling, and Lodging of the Poor People set sick on shore."[158] Nothing in Hills's report or the commissioners' concluding summation suggests any consideration of mitigating factors, such as the fact that, during an unprecedented epidemic, the surgeon-agent might have worried about things other than the close oversight of Plymouth's hospital contractor. Likewise, the commissioners might have, in their deliberations, considered the severe difficulties facing any contractor hoping to find sufficient quarters, adequate food, proper nurses, and ways to keep men clean, amid an exceptional demand for space and care. In their eyes, Buttall proved inadequate to the role, however much he cared about seamen's health. In other words, the system of naval health care did not fail in a crisis, one of its private partners failed the system.

The scandal over the conditions of care at Plymouth hospital and town quarters concerned matters not unique to the war with Spain: overcrowding, lack of cleanliness, inadequate nursing, and disorder. However, one of its consequences was truly unprecedented. For a while, care in the community took priority over care at the hospital. This shift from centralized to dispersed care was consistent with an

152   Early Modern Naval Health Care in England

increased reliance upon and trust in the capacity of local people to offer good care to sick and hurt seamen in co-operation with the local administrators of naval health care.

In the late spring of 1741, the commissioners wrote to the Admiralty to explain why "none of the Sick Men put on shore at Plymouth are sent to the Hospital." In reply, the commissioners recalled the complaints that led to Buttall's dismissal as contractor, "the Cradles, Bedding and Nurses." The cradles and bedding that Buttall supplied "must have made very painful Lodgings for poor People who stood in need of Ease and Comfort." The contractor paid nurses "generally but two Shillings a Week," and dismissed them "as the Number of Men decreased." With such employment terms as those, only "the most indigent, and perhaps the most unfit Women in the World," would agree to serve at the hospital. Uncomfortable beds and careless nurses discouraged seamen from joining the navy. Consequently, the commissioners were prepared to do whatever was necessary "for the Preservation of the Lives of those who become Sick or Wounded." However, not having found anyone of business willing to provide adequate bedding and nursing, the commissioners decided to leave the hospital unused.[159] Moreover, the commissioners knew that "there were Town Quarters for between Four and five Hundred Men, where, in the general, We believe them to be better accommodated than they would be in the Hospital so lodged & so nursed as they were in the former Contract."[160]

During the second season of the Great Sickness, the commissioners trusted Plymouth's people to give better care to seamen in homes and pubs than at a hospital. This high level of trust in the capacity of ordinary folk to provide good care is all the more remarkable given the fact that, at the same time, the commissioners, the Navy Board, and the Admiralty were building an argument calling for the construction of three permanent royal hospitals for seamen.[161] On the ground, however, the provision of naval health care at Plymouth in spring 1741 looked more like what had existed under Charles II than William III.

The scandal of care at Plymouth in 1740 revealed old and new truths about early modern naval health care. First, it relied on good people, or at least people acting honourably. Second, the care provided at hospitals was not necessarily or always better than care in town quarters. Finally, the commissioners' response to the scandal shows a pragmatic flexibility in the face of changing circumstances. They were committed to finding space where good care would be offered by conscientious people, not to a particular place for care, such as a hospital.

Care during the War with Spain

The problems at Plymouth were personal. Humphrey Buttall, the contractor, did not provide satisfactory conditions for seamen's recovery in 1740, despite over a decade of experience. The surgeon, Gortley, failed to oversee the contractor's performance. In Buttall's case, we see a tension between normative expectations and unprecedented or unexpected realities. During a once-in-a-century epidemic, Buttall and Gortley's efforts to secure adequate care conditions did not satisfy the expectations of some seamen, officers, administrators, and local people. Part of the reason for the troubles Buttall and Gortley had was that they could not always know, especially in unprecedented or changing circumstances, whose expectations about care on shore – seamen's, officers', landladies', commissioners' – should take precedence. Naval health care's multiple goals produced another layer of problems for local agents: the system aimed to save both lives and money. Naval health care was always also about managing manpower. The final section of this chapter concerns a failed attempt to further centralize care to keep seamen in the navy.

THE BID FOR NEW HOSPITALS AND
THE PRESERVATIVE ETHOS

In the summer of 1741, the Admiralty, in conjunction with the commissioners for sick and hurt, submitted to the Lords Justices a proposal for permanent naval hospitals.[162] The proposal failed for reasons that are not clear.[163] Nonetheless, re-examining the process leading up to and surrounding the 1741 naval-hospitals scheme sheds important light on the relative significance of the key components of the preservative ethos as expressed by the naval officials during an extraordinary care crisis. Nonetheless, the rationales for the hospitals did not reflect the whole sphere of thinking about their benefits for seamen and the navy. For some, including the Admiralty, permanent Royal Navy hospitals were the most cost-effective means to fix a system for care in need of serious repair. For others, especially commissioners Bell, Hills, and Allix, royal hospitals could be a way to improve an already ordered system.

The Admiralty got the idea of constructing three permanent hospitals on shore for seamen, at Chatham, Portsmouth, and Plymouth, from the Navy Board in the spring of 1740.[164] Within a week, the Navy Board began an investigation, at the Admiralty's behest, into the method of treating sick and injured men, both at the existing hospitals and at town quarters, and "an Estimate of the Expence of Establishing

154   Early Modern Naval Health Care in England

the necessary number of Hospitals, and of the saving (if any) that may be seen to the Crown." The goal was better care for the men at less cost overall.[165] The investigation passed over to the commissioners. Given the extraordinary demand for care over the following four months, it is not surprising that their report about hospitals did not reach the Navy Board until the autumn.[166]

Stalled over the winter, the drive toward royal hospitals resumed a year after the idea for them first reached the Admiralty. The Admiralty directed the commissioners to consider "an establishment of an Hospital on a new Foot, capable of entertaining 1000 sick men." The cost of such an institution was to be compared to treating a similar number of seamen under the present method, and the cost of employing the requisite number of people "for the said Hospital in times of peace."[167] About a week later, the Admiralty ordered a comparison between the costs of naval health care during Queen Anne's time with the present.[168] By the beginning of April 1741, the Admiralty had approved in principle two 750-bed hospitals at Queenborough and Plymouth, and a fifteen-hundred-bed hospital at Portsmouth.[169] The commissioners then prepared detailed estimates of the costs of staffing and operating them, while the Navy Board undertook an estimate of the construction cost.[170] The total cost for the three structures amounted to £103,832, or £77,600 if they were built with three storeys instead of two.[171] On the same day that it submitted the proposal to the Lords Justices, 17 July, the Admiralty directed the commissioners to answer several questions related to the number of seamen in care since the war's outbreak. The reason for this additional request was "in order to enable them to explain the Advantages that will arise from the Erection of Hospitals at the Publick, and putting the Care of the Sick Seamen under proper Officers and Servants."[172] The commissioners' reflection on the public benefits of permanent hospitals arrived in less than a week.

The Admiralty's 17 July proposal on hospitals, and the commissioners' subsequent statement on the advantages of such facilities, convey common ambitions, overlapping concerns, and importantly divergent priorities.[173] The differences stemmed from contrasting appraisals of the present condition of naval health care at home.

The Admiralty's proposal began with an enumeration of the deficiencies of sick care at town quarters in terms that the fifth commission for sick and hurt under Queen Anne would have recognized. "Hired places and Houses" scattered up and down coastal communities made it difficult for medical officers to attend seamen. "None but Indigent

Care during the War with Spain 155

People receive" the sick and injured into their dwellings. There the men got improper food, shared beds, and bad treatment that caused death, "or if they Recover, to run away." The conditions of sick quarters were, the Admiralty insisted, "the principal cause of the Disaffection of the seamen to His Majesties Service." By contrast, seamen cared for at royal hospitals would be "treated with the Proper care and Tenderness," and provided with enough space "to walk or refresh their Spirits." Thus, the men could recover without "resorting to Publick houses, to intoxicate themselves with strong liquors and relapse." At the same time, the hospital would "prevent their deserting, and secure them" for the navy once healed. All these benefits to the seamen and the public, so the Admiralty argued, would come at an annual saving, when compared to the present system for care, of £3,450.[174]

The commissioners, for their part, agreed that permanent hospitals were warranted by the "Great Savings in point of Expence" to the Treasury. However, they articulated three more important reasons for the government to take the path to hospitals. First, great numbers of lives would be saved. Second, the "Ease with which People, when recovered of their Illnesses ... Desert His Majesty's Service" would lessen. Third, hospitals would persuade seamen "that whenever it happens to be their Misfortune to be Sick or Hurt," they could expect to get "all proper Tenderness and Care." Nothing else could "be a greater Motive to Peoples Voluntarily Entering into that service and continuing in it with Cheerfulness."[175] The commissioners made no mention of saving seamen from the inconveniences of dirty town quarters. And no wonder. Well-run sick quarters could sometimes do a better job of care than a poorly run hospital. About a month previously, they told the Admiralty that Plymouth's people had space "for between Four and five Hundred Men, where, in the general, We believe them to be better accommodated than they would be in the Hospital so lodged & so nursed as they were in the former Contract."[176]

The two rationales for royal navy hospitals emphasized distinct elements of the preservative ethos. The Admiralty suggested that care at permanent hospitals would offer better care at a lower cost, thereby saving lives and money. The commissioners' statement implied that permanent naval hospitals would cost less to operate than contract hospitals and quarters, and reduce manpower loss through desertion. At the same time, the Admiralty acknowledged that bad treatment at private quarters could induce seamen to break faith and desert the service. While not focussing on the problems care in the community posed to healing seamen, the commissioners likewise recognized that better treatment at hospitals could dissuade sailors from leaving. The commissioners did not claim, in contrast to the Admiralty, that disorder was an inherent problem among town quarters, or that quarterers were less than trustworthy as care providers. Thus, while the Admiralty presented the Lords Justices with a portrait of domestic onshore care that was endangered by delinquent local providers, and a system in need of major overhaul, the commissioners asserted that the existing establishment could be improved significantly by building hospitals. In other words, a revised model for onshore care would benefit the public by making the current system a bit better.

The commissioners' statement of the public benefits of hospitals suggests that, for them, where care happened mattered less than that it happened in good order. So long as the commissioners were convinced that most men got proper treatment, at a private contract hospital or town quarters, a significant transformation of the present system was not necessary. This outlook goes a long – if not all – the way to explaining why the failure of the hospital proposal to gain traction did not generate a renewed effort to convince either the Admiralty or the king in 1742 or 1743.[177] Other factors would have included the formation of a new Admiralty with a new outlook in March 1742 after Walpole's fall, and the diminishing of the Great Sickness a few months thereafter. A commission whose members seemed satisfied with a functioning, if sometimes creaky, system of care, not complacency or laziness or failure to see the trajectory of medical history, accounts for the continuance of the blended hospital and town-quarter model on the mainland throughout the rest of the war with Spain.

A permanent naval hospital was one of several possible solutions to local care conditions. For example, when the commissioners learned in early 1742 that Plymouth's surgeon, Mr Wyatt, did not "keep the Houses fitted up by Mr Cooper (the contractor) for the reception of sick and wounded seamen filled preferable to the private Quarters," their stated concern was Cooper's contractual rights. The board did not wonder at Wyatt's action on account of the inherent problems of town quarters.[178] Similarly, in mid-1743, the commissioners learned that Gosport's agent put "People into private Quarters, when there was room enough in the Hospital." They told Butler that they understood that he did not act "with any sinister view," but nonetheless "contrary to the Directions he is under."[179] The commissioners had good reason to correct but not sanction Butler, since Commissioner Hills had recently visited Gosport's sick quarters and "found them all in good order."[180]

The Admiralty's assessment of the "inconveniences" of town quarters chimed with some of what really was the case at a few ports at the height of the Great Sickness. But the commissioners' statement of the benefits of hospital care, written at approximately the same time, implied that all was not terrible at all the ports all the time. Care in the community did not always carry the dangers of disorder and dirt and drunkenness.

Naval health care at both Plymouth and Portsmouth underperformed for much of 1740. In response, the Navy Board, the Admiralty, and the commissioners for sick and hurt seamen proposed that the Crown construct three permanent royal hospitals for seamen. Nonetheless, at the very same time, the commissioners reaffirmed their trust in the ability of local people to provide adequately ordered care for seamen. That confidence was grounded in the system's financial viability, thanks to the effectiveness of the fiscal-naval state's financial capacity, and to a supply of conscientious local care providers and care workers. Even in the depths of the crisis for care spaces of spring 1740, naval officials set out the parameters for ordered care conditions on shore. The fact that, during the war with Spain, officials mostly worried about where and how well care would be performed, rather than how it could be paid for, is a sign of the system's strength and its improvement over the first four decades of the eighteenth century.

Over the period from mid-1742 to early 1744, the mixed system of privately contracted hospitals and town quarterers appeared to work well enough. At the beginning of April 1744, as Britain prepared to make war again on France, there was little on the horizon to suggest the necessity of changing the mode of propulsion moving naval health care toward its trident-shaped goal of saving lives, saving money, and keeping men.

CHAPTER 7

Disorders and Due Care for Seamen during the War against France, 1744–1748

Early-modern naval health care achieved peak performance during King George II's first war against France. At the same time, the Royal Navy initiated the most significant reform to its system for onshore care since the turn of the eighteenth century: the construction, at public expence, of Haslar hospital for seamen. Historians of naval health care tend to interpret the decision to build a permanent naval hospital to be the consequence of long-standing problems. For example, Coulter and Lloyd claim that the failings of the private-contract and town-quartering system were "obvious" from the early-eighteenth century, and by 1740 it was so "out of date" that "something new was needed."[1] Crimmin and Harland likewise suggest that the existing establishment for naval health care ashore could not meet the demands of war against France.[2] Indeed, the establishment of Haslar naval hospital was, these scholars argue, a logical and pragmatic reaction to the disaster of onshore care during the previous war's Great Sickness.[3] Thus, the successful application to build a permanent hospital, submitted to the privy council in the autumn of 1744, recapitulated and redeemed the failed application of three years earlier.[4]

This chapter argues, by contrast, that Haslar naval hospital owes its origin to an Admiralty-driven attempt to increase the level of discipline it could expect from sailors in care and care workers.[5] Reports of drunken disorder at Forton contract hospital served as the key rationale for constructing enclosed, navy-run spaces for care, the largest state investment in England's health care infrastructure since the Reformation. At the same time as this investment took concrete shape on the field at Haslar, care on the ground saw sustained success. The late 1740s witnessed peak care for sick and injured sailors, which itself was a continuation of the steady improvement already in place after the crisis period of 1739 to 1742. Regular visits to contract hospitals and town quarters by one of the commissioners for sick and wounded seamen, a

Disorders and Due Care during the War against France 159

practice that started in 1729, contributed to better care on shore.[6] The records of the sick and hurt service suggest that, by the later 1740s, private hospital contractors and sick quarterers could expect an annual inspection of the conditions for care from Commissioner Nathaniel Hills. As we will see below, Hills not only assessed the conditions in which men received care, and how well they were treated, he could order changes to the conditions if he deemed them necessary. Hills's reports about conditions at coastal communities, also called the "out ports," show how well naval health care performed, and indeed improved, over the course of the 1740s.

Historians' assessments of the war against France, often treated as part of the wider War of the Austrian Succession, vary according to their relative emphasis on historical continuity or rupture. Scholars who take a broader view, either chronologically or thematically, tend to portray the war as part of a longer set of eighteenth-century interstate and transoceanic competitions,[7] in which either overseas territories,[8] or European frontiers, proved decisive for the combatants' war plans and the conflict's outcome.[9] Other historians argue that the war represented the start of a new and more serious round of conflict involving France that was crucial for determining the balance between the great European powers and imperial geopolitics down to 1815.[10] Similarly, historians of the Royal Navy have pointed to the importance of the birth of a new approach to warfare at sea, later known as the Western Squadron, during the conflict. The squadron's capacity to patrol the Atlantic approach to the English Channel while also watching France's west coast ports proved instrumental both to securing command of the ocean and to preventing a seaborne invasion of mainland Britain.[11] A recent history of the Georgian Royal Navy's political culture also accents novelty during the war with France. Early in the war, so this interpretation argues, a new disciplinary regime, which owed its inspiration to Authoritarian Whigs' top-down centralizing vision for the British Empire, assumed control over the Admiralty.[12] Thus, the war's significance for different historians lies in part in their capacity to link developments within it either to an existing pattern, such as geopolitical competition, or to the emergence of a new one, such as contending political visions of the nature of the British imperium.

This chapter first examines efforts by naval officials during the war to address long-standing challenges to care for seamen, manpower management, and disordered care conditions. We will see that the commissioners for sick and hurt demonstrated a confident command of their

160   Early Modern Naval Health Care in England

and their subordinates' capacity to deal with these challenges compe-
tently. The chapter also highlights signs of naval health care's singu-
lar success during the war with France. This accomplishment emerged
from the potent combination of financial stability and due care from
the people at the ports. The capacity of ordinary people and the private
contract hospitals to provide proper care for seamen throws greater
light on the contingent origin of Haslar hospital, and the deliberate
exaggeration of the danger of drink and disorder at Forton, which the
popular consumption of gin had given great social and moral prom-
inence in the 1740s. To re-emphasize the unique circumstances of
Haslar's founding, the chapter concludes by foregrounding the conscientious labour of women as care providers and care workers.

CHALLENGES TO ORDERED CARE ON SHORE

Desertion of seamen from sick quarters or private-contract hospitals,
either individually or en masse, continued to vex naval officials.[13] Between 1 October 1744 and 30 September 1745, 1,645 sailors deserted
(ran) from the hospitals in England.[14] Perhaps even more to the Admiralty's frustration, they learned in late-November 1744 that certain
ships' captains sent men from their complements on shore whom they
did not like, not because they were very sick. In order to stem the flow
of so-called sick frauds to sick quarters, and to mitigate manpower
losses, the Admiralty ordered the commissioners to direct their medical officers to inspect seamen physically prior to their entering sick
quarters.[15] It is not clear whether this directive was ever implemented.
The fading of the Earl of Winchilsea's leadership over the Admiralty
could account for part of the reason the directive might have died on
the commissioners' desk. Alternatively, the commissioners might have
simply ignored the directive because they possessed sufficient confidence in their capacity to manage the reception of sick men on shore
without overburdening their surgeons and physicians with more work.

The commissioners asserted their and their local agents' competence
and good-faith management of naval manpower to their superiors on
the Admiralty. In the autumn of 1744, the former received a report from
one of its regulating captains that alleged mismanagement of care on
shore.[16] The captain claimed that seamen discharged as "unserviceable"
from one of the two London hospitals were first admitted based upon
what appeared wrongly diagnosed diseases or "some times when they

had no Distemper at all." The captain had examined a man put ashore as fevered who, in fact, had "no such condition" but instead had "the Tendon of his Kneepan divided by the Cut of a Cutlass, whereby he is unserviceable." In another case, a ticket showed rheumatism, "tho' his Disorder is the Palsey," while four other men similarly diagnosed as rheumatic had "no manner of Visible Ailments, and look as Healthy as any Man in England."[17]

The commissioners' response to the allegation rejected its implication of incompetence and lack of integrity on the part of their officials. If the disease stated on the ticket did not match the seamen's actual condition, "it must be by men's Mistake," not from an attempt to misrepresent the diagnosis. The commissioners reminded the Admiralty that sicknesses often stemmed from injuries; for example, a hurt kneecap could cause a fever. Concerning the allegation that some sailors might not appear sick because they were in fact well, and therefore sick frauds, the commissioners urged the Admiralty toward realism and forbearance. "As long as we have a Navy," the commissioners noted, seamen with various diseases will be set ashore. Everyone familiar with the "Nature of Diseases" knew that rheumatisms affected people in ways not evident to the eye, "though very painful to the Patient." Consequently, "there is great Room for Imposture in these Cases ... and there will be Imposters in spite of all the Skill of the Faculty, till they have acquired the Art of making as good a Judgement at heart, of what passes within, as without the body." In other words, in most cases an experienced official could be trusted to tell a fraudulent case from a real one.[18] In the end, the commissioners assured the Admiralty that "the Regulations which we and our Officers are already under, if duly attended to, will sufficiently answer all the necessary Purposes" of addressing the issues raised by the regulating captain.[19] The existing system of diagnosing seamen, while subject to some abuses, did not require any regulatory fixes.

The commissioners' confidence in the face of challenges manifests itself in their capacity to defend their agents and their practices from criticism. In November 1744, the Admiralty, still under the Earl of Winchilsea, demanded an explanation of an inconsistency in the weekly account of the number of men on shore sick at Gosport. The report indicated the total men mustered on one day as sixty-six, while at two other musters only twenty-four. The report likewise showed that only eleven seamen had "Run" from the town quarters."[20] The commissioners replied that "when so many People are sick on shore at that Place as are now, the Agent cannot muster in one day, Those in the Hospital and Those in Town Quarters." The seamen lodged at different places got counted on different days. Additionally, "no Man is made Run, either from a Ship or Sick Quarters" until he was recorded absent from three musters in a row. Thus, the differences between the three accounts stemmed from the dates of the musters: the one submitted on 8 November related to a muster taken on 3 November, the day before a large group of seamen departed Gosport without leave.[21] Thus, the agent had done nothing wrong, and the existing method of keeping track of men in care continued without revision.

As things transpired, the agent at Gosport whom the commissioners defended in mid-November 1744 was John Butler, dismissed the following spring for his misdeeds in quartering seamen.[22] And Butler was by no means the only official to fall under a cloud of suspicion for his conduct. The surgeon at Portsmouth, Richard Porter, nearly lost his post, after over twenty years of service, because he and his wife were found to have discounted quartering tickets sometime in 1741. Fortunately for Porter, the commissioners managed to convince the Duke of Bedford's Admiralty that the long-serving surgeon's mistake was not so egregious as to be unforgiveable.[23] A few years later, the commissioners showed a similar measure of loyalty to an official who himself seemed to lack that quality. Toward the end of 1746, the records at Plymouth's contract hospital prompted the commissioners to investigate their agent, Mr Morshead. In particular, the hospital's books showed that some men marked "dead" on one date were marked "Run" on a later date. The navy would then be "unjustly charged" with the cost of the men's quarters from the day of admission until the day of desertion. Called upon to explain himself, Morshead blamed the accounting irregularities on "the Assistant Surgeon or Nurses." Despite a finding that the agent was guilty "of a very great neglect of duty," by not following the proper method of mustering the seamen, Morshead suffered a fine of only £10, while keeping his post. The fact that Morshead appeared "unaccustomed to the method of muster in the Navy" mitigated his circumstances.[24] Even though allegations of inconsistent record-keeping appeared almost annually, the commissioners maintained the same method of tracking men in care.

Later in the conflict, a senior officer criticized the established practice of sending men from ports such as Gosport to London for cure. Again, the commissioners' reaction shows their high confidence in the

Disorders and Due Care during the War against France 163

existing methods of the naval health care system, given the perennial challenge of manpower loss from desertion.

Despite the commissioners' commitment to the existing methods for keeping track of seamen, in early 1747, the port admiral at Portsmouth, James Steuart, argued that significant reform was necessary. "We are in utmost need of Seamen," Steuart claimed, such that "too much care can not be taken to preserve and keep those already Engaged to the Service." The admiral pointed out that seven or eight men deserted weekly from the hospital at Gosport. He also took aim at the rule of sending chronically sick men from the outports to one of the London hospitals "for completing their Cures." While acknowledging that this rule aimed "to lessen the Expence of the Sick and Hurt Seamen to the Government," he speculated that "many of them by some contrivance or other, procure Certificates of their being rendered unserviceable," and so secured a discharge from the navy. An even greater number of sailors "when they get cured never return to their Ships, so that by the Mens thus being sent to the London Hospitals, we certainly lose a great many of them which in all probability would not be the Case were they kept in the Hospitals here." Steuart suggested that the medical officials working at the contract hospitals were "properly qualified to administer Physick and Surgery to every sort of Patient," just as well as those employed at the London hospitals. Thus, to reduce the loss of seamen en route from Gosport to London, Steuart proposed that the commissioners for sick and hurt direct Gosport's medical officers "not to send Seamen to the Hospitals in London without directions from the Commander in Chief," meaning himself. "I am persuaded," he affirmed, "the preserving Men to the Service by this Method will prove less Expensive to the Government than it is at in raising Men" to replace those who deserted after travelling to the capital.[25]

Within a week of receiving Steuart's letter, the Admiralty ordered the commissioners, in view of the "great numbers of men" lost to the navy, not to permit the transfer of sick or injured seamen from Gosport to one of the London hospitals "without acquainting the Commander in chief therewith, & receiving his Concurrence."[26] Thus, based on one senior officer's opinion, the Admiralty modified significantly a long-established practice of caring for seamen with serious ailments.[27]

The commissioners complied with the Admiralty's directive, but not without clearly stating their opinion that it was based on false premises and would damage the effectiveness of naval health care. Seamen were not, in fact, sent to London's hospitals to save the Crown money, despite what Admiral Steuart believed. The commissioners also pointed out that Steuart was wrong if he thought the directive would reduce desertions. Whether sailors healed while staying at Gosport or St Bartholomew's Hospital, they might choose thereafter to "enter themselves into the Merchant Service." Moreover, neither the private-contract hospitals "nor Hospital ships at the Ports are exempt from Desertion." As to the port admiral's claim that keeping men at the contract hospitals cost the navy less than finding replacements, the commissioners argued that the uncollected pay from deserters made up for the expense of pressing men.[28] About two weeks after their reply to the Admiralty concerning keeping men at the outports, the commissioners informed the senior board that Nathaniel Hills had reported from Chatham of "the Difficulties attending our Surgeons at that Place in procuring Directions from the Commander in Chief" at that place. The surgeon had claimed it was "very inconvenient as well as expensive" to send seamen to the commander at the Nore (an anchorage near the south-centre of the last narrowing of the Thames estuary) for his opinion on whether he thought them in need of further care at a London hospital, or else men incapable of additional naval service.[29] The Admiralty eventually allowed the surgeon-agent at Chatham to seek the opinion of the dockyard's commodore "concerning such men" from nearby Rochester hospital.[30]

Once again, the commissioners asserted the practical effectiveness of the existing system and its methods to deal with a persistent challenge to naval health care – in this case, the loss of men in care to desertion. The fact that the Admiralty altered, albeit slightly, their original modification of previously existing procedures was at least a tacit admission that the revised method was not an unmitigated improvement on the old one.

The strongest statement of confidence in the capacity of naval health care to address its challenges emerged early in the Duke of Bedford's oversight of the Admiralty. In the spring of 1745, the Admiralty directed the commissioners to "state the practice now in use relating to Sick Men put Sick on Shore." In particular, the senior board wanted to know what day of the month ships' captains recorded seamen as set ashore or discharged, and with which mark or designation. They also wanted to know when captains entered recovered men back into their ships' pay books, and what "Agents of the Hospital do when [sailors] are longer Sick than a Month?" Finally, what implications did the

Disorders and Due Care during the War against France   165

established recording methods on ships and at the hospitals have for seamen's pay?[31] In short, the Admiralty wanted information about the effectiveness of the current method of tracking when seamen went into and exited care on shore.

The commissioners replied the same day to the Admiralty's questions about putting men "Sick on shore from His Majesty's Ships and Vessels."[32] While not failing to acknowledge gaps between the ideal and the actual, the overall thrust of the reply highlighted the effectiveness of existing procedures. For example, as a rule, captains did discharge seamen if their stay on shore exceeded a month, signifying this kind of discharge on the pay books with the mark "Dsq (discharge query)."[33] However, "if the Condition of any of those People be such, as in reality to require a longer stay on shore than a Month, they ought not to be discharged at the end of that time, but continued in the Hospital or Quarters, till fit to return to their Duty." The commissioners truthfully acknowledged that "this Rule has sometimes been broken … by sending men on board before they have been well enough for it." The reasons for the rule breach included "the Surgeon's getting a second 6s. 8d. for cure, or for preserving to the Man the Currency of his Wages, and sometimes upon both Accounts." The sailors so "improperly discharged to their Ships" from sick quarters, the commissioners averred, "are generally again sent on shore, in a very few days." When this occurred and came to the commissioners' attention, which they suggested was not often, "proper Notice has been taken of it to our Officers." Captains and agents on shore did not always follow the rules, but the commissioners discovered the truth eventually and made the necessary adjustments.

The commissioners went on to explain the procedure by which seamen who remained in care more than thirty days moved from their ship's pay book to the hospital's book and then back into a pay book upon recovery. Essentially, a sailor on shore more than thirty days lost his pay from the period between his leaving sick quarters and his re-entering a ship's service.[34] In overseas colonial and foreign ports, however, a seaman's pay continued to run "how so ever long People are under Cure on shore." The commissioners regarded this "Indulgence" toward sailors recovering their health abroad "very reasonable," since they had "few Temptations to be long at an Hospital than is necessary for their Cure." The sick and hurt service could not afford a similarly relaxed approach to sailors receiving treatment at home, since "great

Inconvenience" and "unnecessary Expence" would follow the suspension of the "Dsq."[35] After all, sailors employed "in the Channel have many more Calls and Temptations to feign Diseases to get into Sick Quarters, than the Others."[36] Thus, the long-standing system of tracking the whereabouts of seamen in cure, which included elements first introduced in the early 1690s, continued to work reasonably well in the commissioners' considered opinion. The fact that the rules applied differently according to local circumstances showed the system's resilience and its capacity to adapt.

During the war against France, naval officers demonstrated increased concern over the conduct of seamen once they were lodged at either a hospital or at sick quarters. Excessive alcohol consumption by seamen while ostensibly in recovery fostered disorderly conduct that damaged property and their health. For example, the contractor of Deal's hospital complained in the spring of 1746 about "the Irregularity of the sick men, and the Damages they do him by breaking windows." However, the town's surgeon-agent assured the commissioners that "he found it out of his Power to keep them in Order."[37] That autumn, Commissioner Hills reported another complaint of disorder at Forton Hospital, this one concerning two drunken men and one nurse "coming in the Night before Twelve and One o' Clock." The threesome "disturbed the whole Ward, and threatened to turn some of them [sailors] out of their Beds." Hills had immediately discharged the men "for drunkenness and Abusing the Sick People." The nurse "was directly turned out of the Hospital," never to be employed again.[38] Then, early the next year, Admiral Steuart lamented the "want of a proper hospital" for seamen at Gosport. Sick and injured men quartered there had "access to all kinds of Debauchery, whereby many are destroyed and others tempted to desert."[39] Indeed, the danger that drink posed to men in care helped justify the postwar restoration of Plymouth's old royal hospital – used as a prison during the war against France – into a site for the "Entertainment of Sick and Hurt Seamen." Rather than relying on a wall to keep sailors separate from "spirituous liquors," the commissioners put their faith in the "Distance of the Place from the Town."[40]

Despite their seriousness and frequency, these cases of disorder did not point to broader or systematic problems with onshore care during the second half of the 1740s. For the most part, the commissioners for sick and hurt managed to minimize or mitigate the threat that excessive alcohol consumption or dishonest officials posed to ordered

Disorders and Due Care during the War against France 167

care. This success will become evident in the following section. Before demonstrating the predominance of proper care for servicemen on shore, it is necessary to examine for one final time naval health care's financial base.

PAYING FOR PEAK PERFORMANCE OF CARE

The Royal Navy's early modern naval-health-care establishment achieved its peak level of performance during the war against France, thanks in large part to the state's financial strength, the conscientious work of officials managing care on shore, and the labour of ordinary people providing and giving care, particularly women. As in previous conflicts, the care establishment was concentrated at London, Portsmouth, and Plymouth. The latter two towns functioned as care hubs, each holding a contract naval hospital, a salaried physician, a surgeon, and an agent. A further twenty-three to twenty-five coastal or fluvial communities in England were served by surgeon-agents who were paid 6s. 8d. per man for cure.[41] At all places except Gosport and Plymouth, hospital contractors and providers of town quarters received "12d. per man" for "Quarters Diet Nursing etc."[42] Of the seventy-two officials employed for the sick and hurt service in the summer of 1745, twelve oversaw the custody of prisoners.[43] From the second half of 1747 to the cessation of hostilities, taking care of prisoners formed the bulk of the commissioners' work, with nine additional communities hosting prisoners in 1748 than the year prior.[44]

The scale and scope of care and custody demanded by the war with France did not overburden the Royal Navy, nor coastal communities. The commissioners' minutes and correspondence never suggest that the sick and hurt service could not pay its costs, whether at home or overseas.[45] Parliamentary and political records suggest that the Royal Navy had little trouble managing its healing and carceral obligations.[46] Experienced as a portion of the Royal Navy's annual debt, the sick and hurt service, which included managing prisoners, never got close to 2 per cent. Indeed, in 1747, the year in which the charge of the sick and wounded office was at its highest during the conflict, the navy spent 98.5 per cent of its money on other expenses, such as wages, supplies, and victualling.[47] What mattered most, of course, was parliament's willingness to fund care for seamen. At least some members understood their responsibility for the cost of care, as is evident from the occasional request for an account of the number of sailors put ashore "into the Hospitals of the Kingdom," and the assent to fund the contribution of what became Haslar naval hospital.[48]

The strong financial base underpinning the navy allowed the Admiralty on several occasions during the war to propose or accept additional expenditures on care for seamen, especially if the money went to keeping them in the service. For example, in the spring of 1744, the Admiralty (Winchilsea's) queried the commissioners on the cost of transporting, feeding, and treating) seamen at London's hospitals.[49] The commissioners enumerated the so-called subsistence costs borne by the Crown in sending seamen to either St Bartholomew's or St Thomas's hospitals, and included a proposal to supress the 2d.-per-diem allowance permitted to sailors for food while they were staying in hospital. The reason for the suggestion was that the allowance sometimes undermined ordered care: "according to our Information, that Money is generally Expended in Spirituous Liquors, and thereby serves only to retard the people's Cure, and make many of them so disorderly as to occasion their Expulsion." Henceforth, the commissioners recommended "all Charges should be defrayed by the Crown, and That in consideration of the very scanty ... Allowance such people have upon the day of their admission into the hospitals, They be allowed six pence per man for that Day by this Office."[50] The Admiralty agreed to the proposal for the reasons offered by the commissioners.[51] Nearly two years later, the commissioners again managed to convince the Admiralty (Bedford's) to spend more money, in this instance the travel costs of men discharged from the London hospitals as unserviceable. The commissioners mentioned discharged men from "Scotland, Ireland or the remote parts of England." The junior board claimed that helping destitute ex-seamen return home was proper, "not only in point of Humanity, but Encouragement to the Service; that such Expence be defrayed by this Office."[52]

An examination of reports about care conditions for seamen at coastal communities suggests that ordered care prevailed at most places much of the time. Proper and orderly care provided by officials and local people characterized the conditions in which most sick and hurt seamen recovered their health until hostilities ended in the summer of 1748. The qualifying adverb "most" is significant, since it would be inaccurate to present the conditions for care of sick and hurt men as flawless: peak performance was by no means perfection. It bears mentioning, in addition to the below-examined complaints about care on shore, that in late

Disorders and Due Care during the War against France 169

1744 the commissioners had to reassure the Admiralty concerning the provision of medical care at Gosport's hospital. Medical officers at the port had reported that "Mr Stevens who constantly resides at Forton Hospital is very capable of what may be necessary to the present relief either in Physik or Surgery, of such People as may have occasion for it, either in the Night, or any other time of Our Absence."[53] A year later, the commissioners determined, after undertaking an investigation, that their surgeon-agent at Yarmouth, Mr Brown, "has not fully discharged his Duty to the Sick People who have been put under his Care." Although the commissioners recommended Brown's dismissal, they did point out that the captain who first brought a complaint against the surgeon – one Captain Shirley of the sloop *Hawk* – had left a fevered man on Yarmouth beach "about nine of the Clock in the Morning, and left [him] there ... till above four Afternoon." At that point, another group of sick men from another ship and "those who had the Care of them took Compassion on the poor Wretch, and carried him to Quarters with their own, where he soon grew delirious, and continued so till he died." Not only was Captain Shirley's conduct "barbarous, cruel and Unchristian," but also "contrary to the 4th Article of the Captains' Instructions."[54] Although officials employed in the sick and hurt service did occasionally fail to attend adequately to the men in their care, officers and seamen themselves could act in ways that undermined the provision of good care on shore.

Despite these and the previously discussed complaints, the system of naval health care performed, according to its own managers, at a high level over the second half of the war against France. In no previous conflict do so many reports of conditions for seamen at coastal communities survive. No set of records gives so many indications that sailors could expect due care and attention at private-contract hospitals and town quarters in Kent and along the south coast. For the first time since the navy began to administer health care for seamen through its own agency, its system – for the most part – gave them good care.

Care for seamen in Kent, as reported by Nathaniel Hills in the spring of 1746, occurred either at a private-contract hospital or in sick quarters. The commissioners visited five places to inspect their hospitals and/or sick quarters, including Woolwich, Deptford, Sheerness, and Deal. These communities ranked among the smallest centres for cure and recovery in England. Deptford had fourteen sick quarters, Woolwich had ten, and Sheerness had five. Deal had thirteen sick quarters and a private-contract hospital. Hills's report showed space for at least seventy-eight seamen at Deal's hospital, plus another forty-eight in the town's sick quarters. The three other communities had room for forty-two men. Significantly, in Deal, Woolwich, and Sheerness, over half the sick quarters were run by women: seven of thirteen at Deal; six of ten at Woolwich; three of five at Sheerness.[55]

Hills's report indicated that Kent's sick quarters and Deal's private-contract hospital offered decent care for sick and injured seamen, although not without areas for improvement. The surgeon-agent at Deptford acknowledged that, although a high percentage of "houses made use of for Quarters, were Publick Houses," and that at first "he was not able to get everything in order he could desire," nonetheless he was doing "as much as Possibly he could, and hoped soon to bring it about." Despite this admission, Hills ranked the overall conditions at Deptford as good. At Woolwich, by contrast, no pubs served as sick quarters, although some of the cradles in which men lay there were too small. The quarters "in General," Hills noted, "appeared in other respects to be Good and in Order."[56] Likewise, Deal's hospital "in general appeared in good order." Its wards held seventy-eight cradles, a few "not the proper distance apart." The contractor, Mr Underdown, had prepared a structure with room for 150 men that would soon replace this facility. Hills did point out that the Deal hospital contractor "complained much of the Irregularity of the sick men, and the Damage they do him by breaking Windows etc." However, the town's surgeon assured Hills that "he found it out of his Power to keep them in Order."[57] Evidently, property damage caused by a few disorderly patients sometimes could be consonant with generally good conditions for sick and hurt seamen.

While at Dover, Commissioner Hills found the conditions in the infirmary for French prisoners "very bad." The nurses employed at the infirmary told the commissioner that it was "impossible" to keep the place clean. Elsewhere, the conditions in which prisoners stayed were "extremly nasty." By contrast, the town's sick quarters for seamen were satisfactory and, according to the patients, "pretty good."[58] Similarly, the sick sailors at Rochester's town quarters "assured us they were taken due care of in every respect," and "were well attended by the Nurses." The town's private-contract hospital "appeared to be in good order," but did have a problem with fleas. Hills suggested as a remedy that the staff undertake frequent airing of the bedding, cleaning the floors with wet sand, and burning brimstone in wards as a form of fumigation.[59] Conditions at Sheerness as Hills reported them were good

Disorders and Due Care during the War against France 171

to excellent. "The Town Quarters were in Order and pretty good, but some of the beds had Matted and some boarded bottoms, which the Quarterers promised to alter." Hills found the hospital in the town in good order. He claimed that seamen at both sick quarters and Sheerness hospital had been "intirely satisfied with their Treatment, and the care taken of them by the surgeon and their Nurses, Particularly two on Recovery from bad Cases." Those two men, one of whom suffered from a serious skull injury and the other one a fistula, "assured [Hills] that had they been the Surgeons near Relations, he could not have treated them with more care and Tenderness."[60] The fact that Hills did not supress his discovery about the "nastiness" of Dover's infirmary for French prisoners lends credibility to the contrasting and glowing account of the work of the surgeon and nurses at Sheerness.

Hills returned to inspect the hospitals and sick quarters in Kent in the spring of 1747. Once again, he reported a mostly satisfactory situation. Good order characterized the town quarters at Woolwich and Deptford, Hills reported, with "the Men well taken Care of, and no Complaints of any kind." Some quarterers complained that the requirement to "make their Beds single" resulted in fewer married seamen lodging with them.[61] The men at Rochester's hospital had no complaints about their treatment, Hills noted. Their bed- and body-linen was "washed and shifted as often as appointed," their cradles properly spaced apart, and "the Wards clean." Upon hearing from the hospital's Matron that "some of the men had been disorderly by coming in at 11 or 12 o'clock at night, disturbing the Wards, and abusing the servants, for not letting them have Victuals and Drink at those unseasonable hours," Hills ordered the surgeon, Mr Hawes, "constantly and immediately [to] Discharge any Drunken or disorderly Fellows." Additionally, if it was found that any nurses had "connived at these abuses," the surgeon should inform the contractor and "insist on their immediately being dismissed from ever attending as Nurses again." Otherwise, the men there "were well treated in every respect."[62] At Sheerness, Hills heard "no Complaints." Here again, the men in care assured the commissioners that "they were well attended by the Surgeon and Nurses."[63]

At the hospitals and sick quarters along the south coast of England, Hills's reports indicated that care conditions appeared good to very good during the latter stages of the war against France. For example, the commissioner found that, at Fareham's hospital, he "met no complaints," and he was assured by every ward that "they were well attended by the Surgeons and Nurses." The wards were "kept very Clean, and the

Cradles at a proper distance from each other."[64] Similarly, all Gosport's sick quarters in the summer of 1746 appeared "Neat and Clean" to Hills the day of his visit. He also made a point to note that, "as this was the day appointed to begin the Pay, I presume they did not expect me, so hope they are always so."[65] At Forton Hospital, Hills heard patients "in every Ward" claim "their Provisions were all very good." Despite learning about another complaint about drunken sailors and nurses disturbing the peace of a ward during the night, the men told him "the Nurses in general take great Care of them." However, Hills did dismiss the two sailors and one nurse who had caused the nighttime ruckus. His concluding statement on the hospital reads like a realistic appraisal of what the sick and hurt service and its officials could expect of the conduct of seamen ashore. It is also an indirect refutation of the Winchilsea Admiralty's reaction to the drunken disorder there just over two years earlier. "The Whole Hospital at present," Hills's judged, "appeared to me to be as well conducted as it possibly can, considering the Men cannot be confined within the Gates, but some of them will get out, Drink, and thereby retard their cures."[66] While there is no reason to think that the commissioners did not regret this reality, they probably also doubted that confining the seamen to a walled hospital would diminish their urge to consume alcohol while in care.

Hills likewise found good food and good care for seamen on board the *Blenheim* hospital ship, at Southampton's sick quarters, at Weymouth's hospital for prisoners, and at Plymouth's Mill Hospital for prisoners during the spring of 1746.[67] Plymouth's Cockside and Saltram hospitals for seamen treated men well "in every respect," with "no complaints of any kind." The sick quarters at Plymouth, Hills reported, were "exceedingly good." Similarly, Bristol's Catch hospital for seamen, a "very convenient and Airy Place," half a mile from the nearest pub, was "kept very neat and clean," and its patients were "well contented with their Treatment." Moreover, "good care is taken of them by the Nurses, and the surgeon visits them everyday."[68]

Conditions for seamen needing care along the south coast and western ports did not deteriorate by Hills's next visit in the spring of 1747. The commissioner attended Forton Hospital "where [he] heard no Complaints whatever, the Hospital Neat and Clean, and everybody attending their Duty as they ought." Significantly, on this visit to Gosport Hills drew up a list of all the town quarterers as of 4 April. He graded the quality of the quarters from "indifferent" to "pretty good" to "good" and finally to "very good." Of the thirty-five listed sick

Disorders and Due Care during the War against France   173

quarters in the town, thirty-one were run by a woman. And of those thirty-one quarters, Hills ranked twenty-nine as either good or very good.[69] Clearly, care for sick and injured seamen at Gosport during the war with France depended heavily upon willing female care providers, the vast majority of whom offered conditions conducive to healing. Over two years later, Hills again visited Gosport's Forton Hospital, at which patients claimed they received daily visits from the surgeon, appropriate and adequate food and drink, and "that the Nurses gave due attendance." Those few men then staying in the town quarters likewise had "no Complaints."[70]

The visitation reports on the state of care for seamen in the nation's outports during the latter stages of the war against France suggest that naval health care performed well. It is possible that Hills, and his colleagues on the commission for sick and hurt, exaggerated the positive aspects of care at the hospitals and sick quarters. They might have had more incentive to promote the notion that, for the most part, care on shore happened in due order to an Admiralty keen to establish a new mode of externalized, authoritarian discipline upon the Royal Navy.[71] As will be discussed below, the commissioners' more relaxed approach to excess alcohol consumption at Gosport's private hospital in the summer of 1744 played a role in the decision to phase it out of operation. Thus, it is plausible to think that from early 1745, the commissioners might have wanted to minimize further executive interventions into the shape of care on shore. However, other instances examined in this chapter indicate that the Admiralty had ways of hearing about problems in the provision of care, or at least allegations of them. Had the Admiralty thought it reasonable to do so, they could have directed officers to visit the outports to confirm or refute Hills's reports. As we will see, Vice-Admiral William Martin performed an inspection at Gosport hospital around the same time as Hills's visitation in July 1744. Indeed, an officers' inspection of sick quarters was a practice dating back to the period immediately after the decision to contract with a hospital provider at Plymouth in 1703.[72] Admiral Steuart's complaints about Gosport also remind us that officers who distrusted care provided in spaces outside the navy's authority could be motivated to portray conditions on shore in a very negative light. Thus, the Admiralty and its subordinates had both motive and means to reject Hills's mostly sunny accounts of care for seamen at the ports from 1746 to 1749. But they did not. Thus, we have good grounds for thinking that naval health care on shore for seamen during the war with France performed well.

174 Early Modern Naval Health Care in England

Nonetheless, one report of disorderly seamen and nurses provoked a massive change in the structure of naval health care at Gosport.

DRINK, DISORDER, AND THE CONTINGENT ORIGIN OF HASLAR ROYAL NAVY HOSPITAL

A finely grained account of the process leading to the advent of the first permanent purpose-built facility to treat sick and injured seamen in England reveals several salient and largely overlooked factors at work in Haslar's emergence. First, the 1744 proposal for a permanent naval hospital, unlike its 1741 predecessor, did not arise in reaction to a set of challenges that could be apprehended as evidence that the existing mixed system for care – private-contract hospitals and town quarters – was not capable of providing ordered care. Rather, the proposal stemmed from the Admiralty's reaction to an account of disorderly seamen and nurses at Gosport's Forton contract hospital. Second, the situation at Forton was linked to the broader social problem of excessive plebeian consumption of spirituous liquors. Third, the Admiralty's response to disorderly seamen and nurses at Gosport, expressed as concern over the implications of intoxication for seamen's health and the potential loss of naval manpower, propelled the proposal up to the privy council. Unlike their predecessors of 1703, the commissioners for sick and wounded did not initiate the drive to reform the management of onshore care via a new institution.

The Admiralty's proposed solution to disorderly conduct at Forton Hospital – a permanent naval hospital – aligned well with the long-standing medical view that disordered conditions were the chief enemy of health. Consequently, disordered care conditions that threatened the health and even the "bare life" of seamen were also inextricably obstacles to victory at sea.[73] Both goals, seamen's health and victory, required the appropriate application of constraint, emerging from within a person (self-discipline) and emanating down from responsible authorities (imputed discipline).[74] Unquestionably, the Admiralty's desire to ensure that care happened in an ordered context derived from the need to retain the productive capacity of sailors (their labour power) in order to have a reasonable hope of contributing to the outcome of the war against France. Thus, the Admiralty was concerned about both the health of its "People" and their ability to serve, upon which the navy's capacity for force projection crucially relied.[75]

The process leading to Gosport's permanent naval hospital began in the late spring of 1744 with the arrival of Sir Charles Hardy's squadron. In response to an Admiralty query concerning the "Great Number" of seamen on shore at Gosport, the commissioners for sick and hurt reported on 20 June that "there was no greater Number than ordinary" in care. They assured the Admiralty that nothing "epidemical or extraordinary had been discovered in the Diseases of the people set on shore from that Squadron." Four ships (the *Cornwall*, *Duke*, *Princess Royal*, and *Sandwich*) of the eight-vessel squadron were "most sickly." The "most prevailing Distempers" among them included "continual and intermitting Fevers, Fluxes, Scurvys and Rheumatisms." The commissioners went on to suggest that the situation at the port was not bad. "For of 1337 men" reportedly on shore and in the *Blenheim* hospital ship, "only 391 were very ill, 346 were not dangerously ill, and 600 were on Recovery."[76] Nothing in the tone or content of the commissioner's letter indicated that the situation at Gosport in late June 1744 was anything other than well under control.

On the twelfth day of the following month, the commissioners sent Nathaniel Hills to visit the hospitals and sick quarters at Gosport and Plymouth.[77] Along with a routine inspection of care conditions at the two ports, the commissioners wanted Hills to conduct an inquiry into complaints that certain of their agents were discounting quartering tickets and putting seamen into sick quarters "though the Hospital is not full."[78] Both of these actions, if true, contravened the standing instructions of the sick and hurt service, dating back to 1740.[79] Within days of Hills's departure, the commissioners learned from their Portsmouth-based surgeon (Richard Porter) that the decreasing number of sick there allowed him to forgo the help of one of his assistants.[80] The situation at nearby Gosport would almost certainly have to have been the same for Porter to release one of his subordinates. Thus, conditions for sick and hurt at Gosport and Portsmouth in the summer of 1744 were not close to approximating the situation of summer 1740, during which time seamen were dispersed up and down the area into very crowded quarters. Moreover, upon visiting Forton Hospital on 19 July, Hills reported that he "found no complaints except the Bedding in some particulars falling short of the Sample."[81] Thus, conditions at Gosport's private-contract hospital seemed in relatively good order.

However, some time after Hills's departure for Gosport, the commissioners had received a compliant from the port, which they then directed him to investigate while he was still visiting the town. The complaint evidently related to "the people's being Drunk" while at Forton.[82] Ominously, two days earlier the commissioners learned from their agent at Sheerness, Mr Hicks, that seaman Peter Stannadel had perpetrated serious damage to the sick quarters there after returning from a night out "a little in drink."[83] The commissioners proposed that the Admiralty make an example of Stannadel, not only out of justice to Hicks but also "for the Good of the Service, as it may tend very much to keep other people in the Order necessary to the most speedy recovery of their health."[84] Drunken disorder in sick quarters threatened to undermine the foundations of care for sick and injured seamen.

Hills visited Gosport's hospital for seamen on 24 July 1744 and sent up his report the same day. In the report, he proposed a "Method for remedying" what he called "an Evil," namely, "the Abuses of the People being Drunk."[85] Whatever that method might have been, the commissioners' meeting minutes do not indicate that they decided to forward it to the Admiralty. This fact is significant, for on the very day of Hill's visit to Forton, Vice-Admiral William Martin likewise submitted a report of his visit to the same place to Admiral Sir John Balchen. Martin's report was subsequently forwarded to the Admiralty. Its account of the disorder there would be decisive for the emergence of Haslar Hospital.

Vice-Admiral Martin's report arose in response to complaints about the abuse of alcohol at Forton Hospital. The senior officer found that the "houses about the Hospital and adjoyning to it are a nest of gin shops who retail Spirituous Liquors to the sick open both Day and Night." The gate of the hospital, Martin claimed, likewise remained open "at all hours." The only person residing at the hospital who might be expected to "inspect frequently into the Wards to prevent disorders" was its contractor, "who is afraid to speak" to the seamen. Martin stated, "the Nurses and the Men deny that there is any spirit brought into the Wards, but it appears by other credible Witnesses that they often drink there, which Liquors must be brought in by the Nurses or such Men as are capable of going abroad, or both, they being under no restraint." Consequently, nurses and seamen were "often times Drinking and Dancing the whole Night long on the Green without the Hospital, the Contractor not daring to intermeddle." One way to prevent such disorders, Martin wrote, would be to revoke the liquor licences of the nearby gin shops. Nevertheless, the most effective solution, he suggested, demanded "a Place Walled in and Officers to reside within the Hospital." Those officers could monitor the men's movement in and out of the facility, while the wall would keep seamen inside. It would also keep out masters of merchant marine vessels who wanted to encourage sailors to desert the naval service.[86] Keeping seamen for the navy would mean locking them down at a naval hospital.

Over the next several days, the Admiralty received two more reports that touched on the situation at Gosport. The first relayed the findings of Hills's visit in June 1744, concerning allegations of irregular and fraudulent activities perpetrated by the commission for sick and hurt's agent, John Butler. No mention of the abuse of drink at Forton Hospital appeared in Hills's finding.[87] The second was the quarterly account of how many men "have Run from the Hospitals of England between the 1st April 1744 and 30th June following." From a national total of 288 seamen Run, 211 (73 per cent) deserted the navy from Gosport during the second quarter of the year.[88]

By the end of July 1744, the Admiralty knew of at least three problems besetting care for seamen at Gosport: an allegedly fraudulent agent; drunken disorderliness at the hospital; and a significant loss of manpower. How would they react?

For six weeks, no response emerged from the Admiralty office. Then on 14 September, the commissioners received word to attend the Admiralty at noon. Upon arriving at the Admiralty Office, the "Lordships respited the matter of attendance."[89] However, the minutes of the Admiralty's meeting that day note their consideration of a letter from Sir John Balchen, enclosing one from William Martin, giving "an account of the Irregularity and drunkenness among the Sick men on shore at Sick Quarters at Gosport." They then resolved to send a memo to the king, "proposing to erect hospitals at Chatham, Portsmouth, and Plymouth for the reception of Sick Men set ashore."[90]

The autumn 1744 proposal to build royal naval hospitals did not arise as a logical or necessary reaction to the crisis of the Great Sickness three years earlier. Neither was the fact that France and not Spain was the nation's chief enemy after March 1744 the crucial factor.[91] Martin's report of disorder at Forton private-contract hospital fit well into the political establishment's anxiety over the social, economic, and hygienic consequences of excessive gin consumption. The popular abuse of spirits such as gin generated profound public concern over much of the 1730s and 1740s.[92] Public figures argued that gin posed a threat to individuals, their families, public welfare, and even national security. For example, in early 1743, Lord Hervey told the House of Commons that "getting drunk with gin" destroyed not only the "health and vigor"

178 Early Modern Naval Health Care in England

of persons, but also "the state, because it prevails most among our most necessary and useful sort of people." By this Hervey meant "our poor labourers" who are "the support of our trade, our manufactures, our riches, nay, and our luxury too." The vice that was gin would likewise, he noted, "destroy our soldiers; it will destroy our seamen."[93] Hervey's fear found concrete expression in William Martin's report of the nest of gin retailers surrounding Forton Hospital.

The Admiralty's proposal to construct royal hospitals for sailors brilliantly deployed the previous July's sensational account of drunken disorder at Gosport's privately contracted hospital as proof of the existing system of naval health care's fatal flaws. It began with a reminder of the previous memo, sent up in the autumn of 1741, proposing three royal hospitals. The next sentence implied that the previous proposal's failure, and the present "want of hospitals," compromised seriously the navy's performance. The Admiralty claimed to feel it was their duty, considering the navy's great suffering "from the loss of Seamen, either by Death or Desertion," to renew the application for naval hospitals. To concretize the painful manpower losses, the memo noted the frequent complaints of "great Disorders and Irregularities committed at the place where the Sick Men are lodged near Gosport," and directed the privy council to William Martin's finding "such a scene of Drunkenness" as expressed in his enclosed report. The proposal then turned again to the problems inherent in the whole system, which damaged the navy's workforce. "The Want of Royal Hospitals," the Admiralty asserted, "is the reason that Lodging, Diet and Nursing of Sick Men is performed by contract, a method liable to abuses that are often fatal to the health of seamen." The existing system for care failed sailors not only in its essential requirements, but also in not providing a structure in which seamen could overcome their lack of self-discipline. The memo asked the king and council to consider "the Folly of the Poor Men" who intoxicated themselves with strong liquors while in the "height of their Distempers." They argued that the "great number that are swept away by such Intemperateness, and the Desertions of Great Numbers who recover" demanded a response from the government, a response emerging out of "Compassion to them and the Interest of Your Majesty's service." Building a hospital was, the Admiralty proposed, a medical, moral, and naval necessity.

The proposal concluded with a pragmatic concession: should the king think the expense of erecting three hospitals too extravagant, the Admiralty suggested "putting up one at Portsmouth" to house fifteen hundred men, at a cost of £38,000 spread out over four to five years. The charge of construction would be saved through reduced expenditures on maintenance and cure for seamen.[94]

The privy council received and read the proposal on 18 September. They directed a committee to study it and "a former memorial" about royal hospitals for sailors.[95] That committee included the Lord Chancellor, the Duke of Newcastle, Lord Carteret, Henry Pelham, and the Earl of Winchilsea, First Lord of the Admiralty: in other words, the core of the Carteret ministry. They evidently considered the proposal and Martin's report of conditions at Forton Hospital, then agreed to report their opinion "that the present method of taking care of Sick Seamen is attended with many and great Inconveniences." A royal hospital built at Portsmouth would constitute a "real service in preserving the Health of the Seamen."[96] On 7 November 1744, the king registered his acceptance of the committee's advice.[97] The Royal Navy would get a permanent hospital for sick and injured sailors.

The Admiralty under the Earl of Winchilsea pitched what was a problem in the conduct among some seamen and nurses as evidence of problematic widespread disorder within onshore care, for which a permanent naval hospital was the solution. Notably, the proposal for a permanent naval hospital did not emerge from the agency responsible for the administration of care for seamen. The commissioners for sick and hurt had not appeared especially concerned about the state of care in either the hospital or the sick quarters at Gosport in their correspondence with the Admiralty in June and July 1744. Moreover, the fact that the commissioners appear not to have sent up to the Admiralty Nathaniel Hills's plan to deal with the abuse of spirituous liquor at Forton Hospital would be consistent with a more relaxed appraisal of conditions for sick and injured men at the largest site for care in the land. The commissioners did not oppose the idea that permanent naval hospitals could serve as a mode to improve care, but neither did they think that such institutions were necessary for helping seamen recover their health, return to active service, and thus contribute to the success of the Royal Navy.[98] Town quarters, so the commissioners thought, could and did act as appropriate supplements to private hospitals when the latter became full.[99] This sort of equivocal support for the claim that royal hospitals were the only solution to the problem of diseased, disorderly, and deserting seamen might well have been known among the Admiralty, and could explain why they postponed their meeting with the commissioners on 14 September 1744. Perhaps the Admiralty also concluded that Vice-Admiral Martin's report gave them all the evidence they needed to persuade the privy council to save the sailors from their intemperate love of gin.

The Admiralty's proposal for a hospital at Portsmouth whose walls would hinder seamen's quest for gin obviously intended to limit their freedom and direct their conduct in preauthorized ways. Although this intent is regrettable from a certain modern understanding of person-hood, that the Admiralty would hold it should come as no surprise.[100] Naval officers as officers had more interest in preserving sailors as healthy units of labour power than in permitting self-directed be-haviour and flourishing as autonomous individuals.[101] It is very improb-able that anyone in Winchilsea's Admiralty gave a moment's thought to the way their institution might sustain modes of self-actualization among members of its largely coerced workforce.[102] The conviction that seamen needed to be constrained by their superiors from making decisions that could ruin their personal health – that is, imputed dis-cipline – reflected the traditional understanding of discipline and its connection to health, which, like justice, had both externally and in-ternally directed determinants.[103] Disordered environments, marred by dirt, foul air, overcrowding, and unwashed body and bed linens, did not promote recovery from sickness or injury. The Admiralty and naval administrators had responsibility over these external determinants of health. To ignore their responsibility would be to undermine their au-thority.[104] Likewise, the intemperate consumption of food and drink, especially powerful intoxicants, was unhealthy, and tended to lead to disorder.[105] Therefore, an attempt to construct an external setting that would make it easier to govern the personal conduct of sick and hurt men with a view to fostering their recovery, while no doubt paternalis-tic and diminishing of individual freedom, made eminent sense to an authority tasked with finding the manpower needed to advance the national interest.

The Admiralty's aim to constrain sick and injured seamen within a walled enclosure to promote their health connects to other efforts by contemporary European governments to bolster the health of their subjects, increasingly viewed as biological entities. This kind of biopol-itics, to use a term from scholarship focused on the history of European state formation and governmental power, made sense, given the fact that excessive gin consumption truly did ruin the health of already-weakened seamen. Incapacitated and dead sailors were obviously of no use to the navy.[106]

Gender was another crucial factor in the decision to build Haslar. Martin's report from Gosport mentioned nurses smuggling liquor and dancing with their patients. Concerns about inadequately supervised female labourers as a cause of disorder mapped closely onto broader fears of unreason that were often unfairly gendered female.[107] However, it was also the case that nurses were known on occasion to supply seamen in care with alcohol. The seventh article of the general instructions for the commissioners for sick and hurt required the immediate dismissal of a nurse found to have brought liquor to men under their care.[108] Whether that happened at Gosport in the summer of 1744 was a matter of whose testimony from those working and recovering at Forton Hospital that Vice-Admiral Martin had trusted – and evidently, he chose to believe unnamed witnesses instead of the nurses themselves.[109] Martin's distrust of the hospital's nurses went a long way toward shaping his sense of who was to blame for the disorders there, and what needed to happen to fix them. In a walled-off Royal Navy hospital, both nurses and sailors would be subject to closer supervision, and there would be fewer opportunities for smuggling, deserting, and cavorting. The royal hospital was thus in part an answer to a perceived systemic labour problem at contract hospitals: the untrustworthiness of some of their female care workers in the provision of ordered care.

The decision to build Haslar Hospital represented a contingent application of the preservative ethos, albeit one that was pitched to the king as morally and medically (if not historically) necessary to save naval health care. Moreover, concern for ordered care that preserved seamen's lives and their labour for the navy, while also constraining costs, existed independently of any broader debates over the nature of discipline and authority within the navy or the British Empire.[110] This is evident from the fact that, in the waning days of the Winchilsea Admiralty, it possessed sufficient gumption to recapitulate (in a somewhat sensationalized form) the proposal for naval hospitals first tabled in the terminal phase of Sir Charles Wager's board. Naval discipline during the mid-eighteenth century was not necessarily a partisan question, at least in connection to the sort of discipline required to guide sailors back to health without losing them to the merchant marine or debilitating intoxicants.[111]

Finally, without a strong fiscal base and financially powerful constituencies, the Admiralty's proposal for a large permanent hospital would never have been realized. The fact that the Carteret ministry could contemplate, in the middle of an enormously expensive war, splashing out tens of thousands of pounds for a massive building whose rationale could vanish within months should peace result from a surprise defeat or diplomatic revolution, is yet another testament to the awesome capacity of Georgian Britain's fiscal state.[112] That state could spend money on war and development, or both at once, thanks to a powerful blend of taxing and borrowing prowess.[113] What proved crucial for Britain's fiscal strength was its method for regulating public debt, which by 1744 was over half a century old. As Professor Kocka trenchantly observes, that debt was ultimately the responsibility of parliament and politically enfranchised population groups with significant financial power.[114] So long as the members of that institution and those groups saw fit to fund the Royal Navy, Britain could afford a war state that cared for its seamen at a comparatively high level.

The final section of this chapter sheds light on the extent to which, from 1744 to 1748, high-performance naval health care depended upon female labour.

WOMEN WORKING TO PRESERVE THE SAILORS

To a significant extent, naval health care on shore relied on women to provide or to give care to sick and injured seamen. As we noted above, in the spring of 1746, the majority of quarterers in three communities in Kent, Woolwich, Deal, and Sheerness, were women.[115] Of the thirty-five sick quarters at Gosport that Commissioner Hills visited in the spring of 1747, women ran thirty-one, of which the overwhelming majority – twenty-nine – gave "good" to "very good" care.[116] Nurses formed the bulk of the workforce at hospitals for seamen. For example, Fareham's hospital employed up to twelve nurses, twice the number of surgeons. Hills's report suggests that the contractor hired more or fewer nurses "in proportion to those of the Number of Sick."[117] In the future, Haslar naval hospital would continue to depend heavily on nurses. The Navy Board envisioned a facility with room for fifteen hundred seamen needing 105 nurses, roughly one for every twelve men in care.[118] The future of care work in the navy's permanent hospital would remain largely female.

In word and deed, the administrators of the naval-health-care system demonstrated their awareness of the service's dependence on women's labour. The commissioners' papers testify to attempts to treat female quarterers and nurses fairly. For example, in the autumn of 1744, the commissioners helped the widow of Deal's former hospital contractor

Disorders and Due Care during the War against France   183

to negotiate the transfer of property to his successor.[119] A few years later, the commissioners ordered the same contractor, Mr Underdown, to stop discounting sick quarterers tickets, "being of the Opinion it may be attended with bad Consequences to the Service, especially as his Servant had menaced one of the Quarterers if she did not do it."[120] Naval officials occasionally disagreed amongst themselves over what constituted fairness in dealings with female quarterers. In the autumn of 1747, the Admiralty ordered the commissioners to pay one Jane Norris of Deal two guineas for caring for two seamen, after the commissioners had refused to pay her one. Evidently, the junior board believed Norris had been too generous in provisioning the men in her charge, a belief that the Admiralty refuted.[121]

Although constraining costs formed a crucial component of managing care for seamen on shore, there were times when the commissioners for sick and hurt found it reasonable to spend more money on care workers. As noted above, nurses employed at Haslar Hospital would receive lodging. Soon after the facility began to receive patients, the commissioners recommended that its nurses get tables to store medicines and cradles for sleeping.[122] In the spring of 1746, the commissioners convinced the Admiralty to victual nurses working on its hospital ships "on the same Foot, in point of Diet, with the Sick People under their care." This action would, they argued, "be a great Ease to them, an Encouragement to their doing their duty cheerfully about the sick, and also prevent their being under any sort of Necessity to make an ill Use of what is allowed to their Men."[123] However, a few weeks later, the commissioners recommended the surgeon of the *Britannia* hospital ship ensure that its nurses not use bedding allotted to seamen.[124]

Nurses could expect treatment from the navy that was similar but not equal to that accorded the seamen in their care, at least on hospital ships. This differentiated treatment probably stemmed in part from women's diminished status in eighteenth-century England in relation to men. However, men in care were not always able to assert their de jure superiority over female care givers. Sick and injured sailors were truly vulnerable people, especially in relation to those charged with restoring their bodies to health. The commissioners for sick and hurt seemed aware of the reality of the dynamic disparity between the cared-for and the carer in their rationale for providing food to nurses on hospital ships. Victualling the nurses would, the commissioners stated, reduce nurses' temptation to misuse "what is allowed to their Men, which cannot but be very much in their Power."[125] Shifting and

184   Early Modern Naval Health Care in England

unequal power relations crosscut relations between nurses and seamen in care at multiple levels.

Plebeian solidarity occasionally overcame gendered inequality in sick quarters. As we have seen, more than once did seamen and nurses combine to produce alcohol-fuelled mini "orders of misrule" at contract hospitals and town quarters. In such cases, naval officials tended to judge both nurses and sailors on the same terms. Both the two seamen and the one nurse whose drunken revelry disturbed patients of one ward at Forton Hospital one night in spring 1746 lost their employment.[126] In cases where it appeared that a nurse (or nurses) bore sole responsibility for bringing liquor into sick quarters, to the detriment of orderly care, the nurse could expect dismissal. For example, Jane Pearce lost her place on the *Enterprise* for "selling a Bottle of Brandy to a sick man," who, when Commissioner Hills saw him, "was dangerously ill of a Fever." Hills later suggested assigning two nurses to each ward of the ship, who would bear sole responsibility for any liquor found in the ward. In cases when liquor was discovered, both nurses should be, Hills believed, "immediately Discharged, whether one or both be concerned in it."[127]

Official regulations, and the reports of officials suggest that some nurses fostered drinking among the men in their care. However, what portion of nurses engaged in the practice of supplying men "with spirituous liquors," and with what frequency, are unknowable. The sources point to instances when officials or the commissioners saw the effects of excessive alcohol consumption in sick quarters, which might represent only a tiny sample of the real number. The motivations for nurses providing men with spirits are similarly unknowable. Some seamen in sick quarters no doubt asked for it, not the least because alcohol was an elementary analgesic. Alcoholic beverages such as beer or ale also formed part of seamen's basic provisions; their daily consumption was what Phil Withington calls immanently intoxicating.[128] Depending on the seaman's condition and stature, a nurse might not have felt that she could refuse a request for a consciousness-altering drink. Indeed, some nurses might have believed that supplying intoxicating spirits to men in desperate conditions was itself an act of compassion. Whatever the reasons, the link between nurses and the immoderate consumption of intoxicants by men in care was not unique to the war with France.[129]

Nurses working at contract hospitals and hospital ships, and women providing town quarters for seamen, held sway over the conditions of care sufficient to disorder them severely. Men provided with spirits

Disorders and Due Care during the War against France   185

by nurses could destroy property, disturb their weaker fellows, and damage their own health. Nurses at times could join with seamen in producing disturbances within sick quarters. At the same time, sick quarters could not operate without nurses. Female care providers and care givers ensured that seamen ate what they needed, took their medicines, were supplied with clean clothes and clean bedding, and recovered in clean, airy rooms. No doubt, many sailors upon their arrival into sick quarters depended utterly on their caregivers to recover their health. By extension, the Royal Navy, ever in need of manpower, relied on care work to keep its ships supplied with labourers. The quality of care for sick and injured men determined in part the performance of the navy during the war against France.

Fortunately, most female quarterers and most nurses provided very good care. Most of what Commissioner Hills discovered during his visits to coastal communities to inquire about sick quarters run by women, and about nurses working at hospitals, suggests that they were conscientious toward sailors. At Fareham hospital in May 1747, the seamen claimed that nurses there gave them "due attendance."[130] Gosport hospital's nurses took "great Care of their Patients." The men assured Hills that "they do not want for attendance." Some caregivers demonstrated solidarity with each other and their patients. Hills expressed concern about the high ratio of seamen to nurses at the *Blenheim* hospital ship – 20 to 1 – but claimed that when any of the nurses became ill, "one of the Nurses from another Ward, whose Patients do not want Attendance in the Night, assists and sits up with those who do."[131] The following year, Hills likewise reported that nurses on the hospital ships gave due attendance to seamen.[132] Similarly, the private quarters at Plymouth in the spring of 1746 were reportedly "exceedingly good." The men lodged in the houses told Hills "great Care was taken of them by everybody concerned."[133] Good care did not diminish with the return of peace. Seamen at Gosport hospital in the summer of 1749 related that "the Nurses gave due attendance, and they wanted for nothing necessary for their different Distempers, either to eat or to drink."[134]

During Georgian Britain's first war against France, women constituted most of the people who provided sick quarters to sick and injured seamen. Most care workers in quarters and hospitals were women. Their labour was unquestionably a key factor in the success of naval health care on shore after 1744. It is thus more than a little paradoxical that a single report alleging the misbehaviour of a very few nurses at Forton

Hospital in July 1744 occasioned a significant reform of care conditions at Gosport. That report itself relied on the testimony of witnesses who contradicted what the hospital's nurses themselves claimed about their role in the incidence of drunken disorder at Forton. Because William Martin refused to believe the nurses, the Admiralty could use his report to portray naval health care in crisis and in need of serious transformation. Had the Admiralty not received Martin's report, had they Hills's reports of conditions at the outports and the due attendance provided by most nurses only, Haslar Hospital might have remained a dream until much later in the eighteenth century.

Most of the forgoing shows that, in fact, disorder did not characterize the bulk of naval health care on shore in the late 1740s. The system for care reached its peak level of performance thanks in large measure to the women upon whom the navy relied as care providers and care workers. In the war's early stages, Winchilsea's Admiralty linked nurses with what was fundamentally wrong with early modern naval health care: drunken disorderliness. In fact, women were responsible for much of what the system did right during the war against France. Thus, the Royal Navy got its first permanent naval hospital in part because of a willful misapprehension about conditions for care – and the quality of the care workers – on shore.

CHAPTER 8

Conclusion

Toward the end of 1762, Edward Gibbon, a commander in the South Hampshire militia and budding essayist, recorded in his journal a visit to the hospital at Haslar. He noted that, "it is a large convenient and plain structure capable upon emergency of holding 2500 sailors, tho' it has seldom had more than 1100." The same day that Gibbon viewed the Royal Navy's first purpose-built hospital, the "SUSPENSION OF ARMS was solemnly declared at Portsmouth and Gosport." According to Gibbon, news of peace between France and Britain provoked "great regret" in the towns' inhabitants, "who find their account much better in War."[1]

Nearly forty years later, two ships' captains and two ships' surgeons visited the sick quarters for seamen at Yarmouth. They found sick and hurt sailors cared for at "one principal and two lesser Dwelling Houses situated in different parts of the Town, hired by the Agent for the Sick & Hurt Seamen and containing about 150 Men." The householders evidently had contracted with the agent "for Board, Lodging, and Washing" at a rate of six shilling per man per week. The officers deemed two of the houses, one in White Lion Row and the other in Factory Lane, "far too much Crowded." A Mrs Robinson operated the former, Ann Brigs the latter.[2]

These accounts point to seemingly contrasting aspects about naval health care in England in the second half of the eighteenth century. The first one relates to a rupture: Gibbon's journal entry suggests that, by the end of the Seven Years' War, little remained of the early modern system for care that had emerged just over a century earlier. Where once seamen received care at either a privately contracted hospital or in one of many local sick quarters, a single large state-funded, and state-operated, institution provided treatment for thousands of injured and sick sailors. Haslar naval hospital, a massive brick structure standing

188   Early Modern Naval Health Care in England

sentinel-like "near the entrance of Portsmouth harbour," concretized the hopes of medical officials such as Dr Daniel Whistler in the 1650s, John Evelyn in the 1660s, and Dr Richard Lower in the 1690s.[3] The hospital, along with a similar facility erected at Plymouth, remained central to the provision of medical care for Royal Navy seamen for over two and a half centuries. Thus, an early modern system for care, reliant mostly on contractual or informal partnerships between state officials and ordinary people, yielded to one centred on massive and bureaucratically organized institutions. By 1760, naval health care had become modern.[4]

The second aspect of these two accounts concerns continuity in naval health care: the situation that confronted the officers at Yarmouth during Britain's war with Revolutionary France resembled closely what their predecessors faced at coastal communities nearly a century and a half earlier. Seamen received care at private sick quarters. Most of the care providers were women, who contracted for their services with an agent from the sick and hurt board. The early modern system of naval health care on shore thus continued long after the construction of permanent naval hospitals.[5] As late as 1800, modern naval health care existed at Plymouth and Portsmouth only.[6]

Gibbon's journal entry and the officers' report highlight a complex reality about the significance of naval health care in England between 1650 and 1750. The construction of naval hospitals unquestionably shifted the locus of onshore spaces for care from four privately managed hospitals and numerous smaller dwellings belonging to ordinary people to a large, permanent structure directly controlled by the navy. However, the emergence of naval hospitals did not transform the structure of naval health care at a stroke. For one thing, Haslar's construction took years. Secondly, although it and its counterpart at Plymouth were huge, the 1797 officers' report from Yarmouth proves that the permanent hospitals did not care for all sick or injured seamen. Five decades after Haslar's construction, the navy still needed informally managed places to meet its demand for care space. Clearly, even at the turn of nineteenth century, people of coastal communities remained willing to provide space for care and care work in ways that reached back to the Dutch wars. In other words, the system of naval health care in England after 1750 relied on both a modern bureaucratic organization and a series of formal, and informal, contractual agreements between officials and ordinary people. Early-modern naval health care did not end with the emergence of permanent hospitals for seamen.

Conclusion

189

Moreover, naval health care in England took its modern turn for reasons that were not instrumental only.[7] As we saw in the previous chapter, what transpired at Gosport in the summer and autumn of 1744 was an opportunistic and emotional response by the Winchilsea Admiralty to a breakdown of discipline among some seamen and some nurses at the contractor's hospital, stemming from his failure to limit seamen's access to hard liquor. Ultimately, Haslar hospital began because senior Royal Navy officers no longer wanted to collaborate with the people of Gosport over the provision of care of sailors.

During the decades following the emergence of the early modern system, officials' willingness to trust sick and injured seamen to spaces run by local people or hospital contractors ratcheted downward. From the First Dutch War (1652) to the Glorious Revolution (1688), care for seamen happened at town quarters in coastal communities. The core of naval health care fell outside the navy's direct scope of authority. During the Nine Years' War (1689–1697), one hospital emerged at Plymouth, largely to address a problem of a lack of space for care at that town. Otherwise, the heart of the system continued to be sick quarters operated by ordinary women and men. Then, in the early phases of Queen Anne's War (1702–1713), a new commission for sick and hurt expressed great distrust in the quality of care at town quarters. Upon the commissioners' suggestion, private-contract hospitals began operating from 1704 at the great ports, including Portsmouth, Plymouth, Deal, and Rochester. For roughly the following half-century, naval health care operated with spaces for care that were both formally and informally run: contract hospitals for seamen, supplemented by sick quarters at the outports, with sick quarters only at all other places.[8] Then, in 1744, the Admiralty managed to convince the king to give the navy full authority over care conditions – both the space for care and care workers – at Portsmouth. A large, walled building, staffed with naval employees, would better uphold discipline by limiting access to hard liquor by patients and nurses. This was needed, according to the Admiralty, to preserve lives, save money, and keep men in the service in a much better manner than did either Gosport hospital's contractor or its town quarterers. By the 1760s, the system of naval health care consisted of a large permanent institution, several private-contract hospitals, and many town quarters. The latter, once the system's core, now lay at its periphery. Over the final third of the eighteenth century, the centre of naval health care was modern hospitals that fell within the navy's sphere of authority.

At crucial moments, concerns about the quality of care provided to seamen in spaces outside the navy's direct control formed part of the motivation to centralize naval health care. Over the long term, however, naval health care tilted toward institutionalization because of changes in the quality of the relationships between different naval officials and the people of the ports. Certainly, one decisive factor for those relationships was the degree to which key naval officials trusted in the capacity of ordinary people or hospital contractors to provide proper care in ordered contexts. In fact, Commissioner Hills's reports about the conditions at sick quarters and contract hospitals during the final stages of the war with France contradicted officials' pessimism about the capacity of ordinary people to deliver effective care. Contractors and landladies could be trusted to save seamen's lives, but they could not satisfactorily stop them from deserting, nor stop them drinking to excess. If the navy wanted to be sure to preserve sick and injured sailors for itself, it needed, so it seemed, to care for them behind walls.

The shift of naval health care's core from informally operated private quarters to contract hospitals to a permanent naval hospital was not medically or logically necessary, nor was it inevitable. The willingness of naval officers and administrators to entrust seamen's lives to women and men working outside their direct scope of authority drove changes to the naval health care system. Thus, the quality of the relationships between the chief participants within the system, the navy as consumer, and the people as providers of space for care and performing care work, propelled naval health care toward greater formalization and institutionalization. In other words, an institutionalization of English naval health care was an unintended outcome of the state's contractual and informal relationships with local people. This phenomenon mirrored the pattern that emerged in France as the Bourbon monarchy sought to rationalize the provision of care to the sick poor in the provinces over the "classical period."[9] There, the actions of local people modulated a process, undertaken for the sake of efficiency and anti-corruption, of centralizing hospital services. In England, the reactions of naval officials to local people powered the punctual transformations by which a centralized and rationalized health care system for seamen on shore emerged.

It is not surprising that permanent hospitals were one outcome of changes within early modern naval health care. Nonetheless, significant historical changes often occur for reasons distinct from the people who sought them.[10] Naval health care existed within particular social

Conclusion

and natural constraints; and both human minds and material factors imposed themselves on the evolution of naval health care.[11] From at least the 1690s, the administrators of naval health care manifested in word and action a preservative ethos: an official ambition to institute directives or procedures that aimed to save seamen's lives, to save money, and keep seamen from deserting the navy.[12] To realize this goal, naval administrators and officers needed the capacity to control the conduct of seamen and nurses, or at least to believe that their conduct could be known and overseen more thoroughly.[13] Thus, encoded into the official mind of naval health care lay an ambition to know and to master an aspect of the social world. From almost the beginning, the navy's health care system aspired to be modern.[14]

In 1744, the official goal of establishing mastery over care space, care workers, and seamen in need of care at Gosport meshed with the material conditions necessary to make it real. Great Britain's fiscal-naval state found the resources, during an expensive transcontinental war, to construct a massive edifice capable of caring for thousands of men.[15] The capacity of the government to extract sufficient resources to wage war and to provide care depended, in turn, on the strength of the country's capitalist market economy. The emergence of Haslar Hospital is unthinkable absent the advent of Britain's commercial civilization.[16]

Naval health care took a different path toward modernity in comparison to other branches of Britain's fiscal-naval state. Over the course of the seventeenth and eighteenth centuries, naval agencies such as the Victualling Board transformed from networks of patrons and clients to organizations with networks of suppliers who competed for contracts.[17] In the case of the sick and hurt service, officials at first relied on chaotic and informal networks of care providers to meet its demand. Then, from 1704, the number of care providers diminished drastically in those ports allocated a contract hospital: Rochester, Deal, Plymouth, and Gosport/Portsmouth. Yet at the great ports, and at other coastal communities, ordinary people continued to do the necessary work for many thousands of sick and wounded seamen during times of peace and war. These tasks included attending to the needs of patients; administering proper food, drink, and medicine; maintaining the patient's temperature; keeping his surroundings clean; dealing with evacuations of the body; washing his clothes and bedding; and observing his reaction to treatment.[18] With the construction of Haslar Royal Naval Hospital, the navy acquired a permanent treatment institution that eliminated competition over the provision of care at Gosport. This development reflected what happened in Spain, where, over the eighteenth century, the state chose to dampen competition between suppliers to the armed forces to reduce risk.[19] Over the long term, the assumption of direct control over care provision at Gosport, and then at Plymouth, probably served the aggregate interests of both seamen and the navy – and, by extension, the national interest – although not in straightforward and complementary ways.[20] Early-modern and modern states had instrumental reasons for wanting healthy populations, and what constituted health from the government's perspective did not always mesh with their citizens' conceptions of wellness and flourishing.[21]

Naval health care played an important role in the broader history of the Royal Navy during the age of sail.[22] However, the degree to which the Stuart and Georgian navy's performance depended on care workers is difficult to determine because, then as now, care work is mostly invisible. Part of this reality relates to the fact that women did most of the work.

Naval health care relied on a mostly female workforce to an extent not hitherto appreciated by naval historians. Similarly, the navy's demand for care generated economic opportunities for women in coastal communities. At places such as Gosport and Deal, maritime war enhanced the earning potential of women willing to work as care providers or nurses. Indeed, the fiscal-naval state's demands advantaged some women of coastal communities:[23] Mrs Butcher of Deal, who provided lodging and nursing to sailors during the Second Dutch War; Margaret Hicks of Rochester, a quarterer of seamen during Queen Anne's War; Jane Norris of Deal, who cared for two sailors in 1747; along with Mrs Everest, Mary Bailey, Mrs Wisenburn, Ann Tobin, and over thirty other women listed as sick quarterers at Gosport in the summer of the same year. These were dynamic, enterprising people who would have had sound reasons, as Gibbon noted, to regret the coming of peace.

Moreover, it was naval officers' and administrators' occasionally fraught relationships with landladies and nurses, not historical or medical necessity, that sparked significant shifts in the organization of health care for seamen on shore. Contract hospitals arose in Gosport, Deal, and Rochester because the fifth commission for sick and wounded distrusted the capacity of female care providers to attend to seamen without causing mischief. The Winchilsea Admiralty seized on allegations of undisciplined nurses at Forton Hospital to convince the king to centralize care at Gosport under one, navy-controlled, institution. However modern the spaces for care became, Haslar Hospital,

Conclusion

and similar institutions across the globe, depended on women to perform the essential tasks of tending to the recovery of sick and wounded seamen. Many hands extended in care underpinned the projection of British naval power across the globe and the Royal Navy's eventual command of the ocean.

Although only traces of the realities of care work survive in the Admiralty papers and similar archives, sufficient material concerning naval health care exists to suggest that high quality and conscientious nursing did not first emerge in the nineteenth century.[24] Reports about the conditions of care at both hospitals and sick quarters from the war with France indicate that most care providers and care workers offered "due attention" to sick and wounded sailors. No doubt, a few landladies, perhaps for pecuniary reasons, encouraged weakened seamen to consume alcohol in excess, and thereby delayed their recovery. That some nurses employed at contract hospitals occasionally smuggled in spirituous liquor at the behest of their charges, and shared seamen's enjoyment of it, cannot be doubted. However, such disorderly conduct was probably exceptional, and may also be viewed as extreme examples of the typically very good relations between nurses and the seamen in their care. Indeed, in an early modern context, good social relations between carer and patient was a marker of good care.[25] Nurses working within England's early modern naval-health-care system performed much better than the drunken nurse stereotype allows. If all this was not the case, it is difficult to fathom why the late-Georgian navy continued to rely so heavily on women to care for its men, in sick quarters, at its hospitals, and on hospital ships.[26]

Much of this book's account of the system's emergence and transformation focused on the key players whose words and deeds survive as traces in the archive: the admirals and agents, the commissioners for sick and hurt, treasurers, captains, physicians, and surgeons. Along the way, a few of the many thousands of men made sick or injured while serving the Crown at sea appeared as names; more often only numbers in account ledgers or reports represented their experiences. Even fewer of the people who cared for seamen can ever be known, although without them, the system would not have existed. Thus, the most important relationship in the performance of naval health care, that between the carer and patient, remains lost to history.

The importance and near total invisibility of care work to the story of naval health care in early modern England, regretful as it is, forms one of this history's most salient connections to a vital concern of the present: what kind of demand, what sort of need, is care work expected to meet.

The centrality of care work to human flourishing emerged starkly during the last stages of this book's composition. In late March 2020, hundreds of millions of people across the globe willingly surrendered fundamental rights and freedoms out of concern that their national health care systems lacked the capacity to deal effectively with the Covid-19 pandemic. Subsequently, many public discussions focused on the indispensability of care workers to the common good, and the challenges they faced in both extreme and everyday circumstances.[27] Social critics joined scholars in calling for a significant rethinking of the importance of care work in modern societies.[28] Contemporary publics want better-quality health care, and better access to it. Unfortunately, most people also want to keep costs as low as possible.[29] In other words, modern publics want national health-care systems that save lives and save money.

National health-care systems reflect how much citizens care for the vulnerable, a judgment that has both moral and material aspects. The latter is more easier measured through things like infection mortality rates. Similarly, early modern armed forces provided medical care to soldiers and seamen and viewed it as both means and end. Sick and injured seamen were persons in need and resources – manpower – necessary to achieve tactical and strategic, and ultimately political, goals. Likewise prisoners, another population group subject to the oversight of the commissioners for sick and wounded, were often treated well or poorly less out of principled concern and more for pragmatic reasons. Erica Charters shows that reports of prisoners "ill treated" while in enemy hands, which punctuated reports of all eighteenth-century wars between Britain and France, could lead, depending on the strategic situation, either to efforts to improve their conditions or to speed up negotiations for an exchange of men in custody.[30] Toward the end of the eighteenth century, British army medical officers both denigrated their West Indian and West African patients on account of the servicemen's ancestry, yet also argued that the same people deserved "efficacious, compassionate, and humane treatment" as persons serving the Empire.[31] Improving the health of Black troops helped them and aided the army's efforts at economic effectiveness, saving lives and saving money. During wartime, seamen were treated as persons, but most importantly as servicemen in need, and it was in view of the latter that naval officials found, secured, and ordered health care for them. Not

Conclusion

for the last time did a medical establishment help individuals who were trying to preserve a stock of fighting subjects.[32]

Care work is and was necessary, nearly invisible, and often thought to be undervalued.[33] Patriarchy and capitalism usually take the blame for the economic marginalization of care.[34] How a revolutionary transcending of the present economic and gender order would necessarily produce a favourable "transvaluation" of care work is not clear.[35] Care work, as Madeleine Bunting found, demands a "willingness to be present," the embodied and attentive engagement of one person with and for another person.[36] In short, care work calls forth virtue.[37] Thus, care work requires the forging of at least temporary loving interpersonal relationships whose full meaning and import the materialistic terms and conditions of a contract can never fully encompass.[38] Care work underpins and yet escapes the strictures of the state-market relations in which much of what postmodern people count as health care occurs.

During the long and complicated process known to historians as state formation, formal and informal relationships forged connections between social groups and the interest of rulers and governments.[39] The Royal Navy's demand for care fostered many relationships between the state and the people of England's coastal communities.[40] Initially, relations between the navy and the people could be fractious, not least because the state demanded care on credit. As the English state's fiscal situation stabilized, so did most of its interactions with care providers. Underneath these visible relationships of buying and selling care, invisible to history but nonetheless real, percolated many thousands of interpersonal interactions of the most intimate kind. A hand laid on a fevered forehead. A spoon extended toward an open mouth. An attentive gaze fixed on a pain-ridden face.[41] These and other works of care for sick and injured seamen are part of what enabled Britain to make war at sea and helped to make Britain's fiscal-naval state. That state could make war because its people were willing to give good care.

Notes

For acronyms of archival sources, please see the bibliography.

CHAPTER ONE

1 DHC, QS 128/25, 13 January 1674.

2 Bunting, *Labours of Love.*

3 Duffin, *A History of Medicine*, 11.

4 Bunting, *Labours of Love*, 101–02; Murken, "Zur Geschichte der europäischen Marinelazarett," 93–117.

5 Trabut and Weber, "How to Make Care Work Visible," 342–68.

6 Boris and Klein, *Caring for America*, 4; England and Dyck, "Managing the Body Work," 36–49 at 37.

7 Fissell, "Introduction," 1–17; Brown, *Foul Bodies*; Twigg et al., "Introduction," 1–18.

8 Newton, *The Sick Child.*

9 Pelling, 115–37; Nagy, *Popular Medicine*, 54–78 ; Wear, "Caring for the Sick Poor," 41–60; Earle, "Female Labour Market," 328–78; Davies, *Gender and the Professional Predicament*; McPherson, *Bedside Matters.*

10 Himmelweit, "Caring Labor," 27–38; Held, "Care and the Extension of Markets," 1–33; Kathleen Brown, *Foul Bodies: Cleanliness in Early America.*

11 Grell, "War, Medicine, and the Military Revolution," 257–83; Appleby and Hopper, *Battle-scarred*; Obinger et al., *Warfare and Welfare.*

12 North, *Sweet and Clean?* 94–5.

13 Ibid., 110.

14 On the gendered aspects of modern clinical nursing practice see, for example, Davies, *Gender and the Professional Predicament*, and McPherson, *Bedside Matters.*

15 Bennett, "History That Stands Still," 269–83; Des Jardins, "Women's and Gender History," 136–58.

16 Crawford, "Patients' Rights," 381–410 at 400; Smith, "Reassessing the Role of the Family," 327–42.

198 Notes to pages 6–8

17 Himmelweit, "Caring Labor," 27–38; Held, "Care and the Extension of Markets," 19–33; Dooley, "We Gave Loving Care," 229–51.

18 Boris and Klein, *Caring for America*; Buhler-Wilkinson, *No Place Like Home*.

19 McIntosh, "Networks of Care," 72.

20 Hindle, *On the Parish*, 63.

21 Slack, *The English Poor Law*.

22 Wear, "Caring for the Sick Poor," 44–5.

23 Pelling, "Nurses and Nursekeepers," 179–202; Fissell, "Introduction," 13–17.

24 Petty, *The Advice of WP*, 16–17; Gruber von Arni, *Justice to the Maimed Soldier*, 11–13; Harkness, "View from the Streets," 64, 76.

25 Brown, *Foul Bodies*, 7, 215. Water did not become indispensable (again) to cleanliness until the nineteenth century.

26 Pelling, "Nurses and Nursekeepers," 186.

27 Wear, "Caring for the Sick Poor," 47.

28 Boulton, "Welfare Systems and the Parish Nurse," 127–51; Baker, "Parish Nurses and Their Clients."

29 Neufeld and Wickham, "The Care of Sick and Injured," 45–63.

30 Earle, "Female Labour Market," 340–6.

31 Wrightson, *Earthly Necessities*.

32 TNA, SP 18/60/141. The commissioners also had responsibility to find relief for sailors' widows and orphans, and the oversight of prisoners of war.

33 For example, TNA, PC 2/57, fo. 147v-149r, "Order of Councill authorizing … Commissioners for Sick and Wounded Mariners, 11 November 1664; NMM, CLI/31/1, "Instructions to Sir Thomas Clifford," 23 March 1665.

34 RNM, Corbett Manuscripts, 121/13, 9; Magdalene College, Cambridge, Pepys Library (PL), 2867, 628–9, 3 March 1688.

35 LMA, HO1/ST/A/O1/005, fo. 137v, December 1664; SBHA, HA 20/1, 2 May 1674; BL, Harley Manuscripts 6190, Abstract of seamen in care at St Thomas's Hospital, 25 March 1689 to 25 June 1693. Manning the navy was one of the most intractable problems confronting the British state from the mid-seventeenth to the early-nineteenth century: Baugh, "Navy as a National Institution," 133.

36 By state (and Crown) I mean both a framework of institutions with political functions (decision-making powers, resolutions to implement, and social controls to enforce), what one could call the "view from above," and a coordinated and territorially limited network of agents exercising political power, the "view from below"; Reinhard, *Geschichte des Modernen Staates*, 11.

37 Bodl. Lib., Rawlinson Manuscripts A187, fo. 357, Balthasar St Michael at Deal to Samuel Pepys, 11 Sept 1672; BL, Add. MS 11684, fos. 75–82,

Richard Gibson, "A review of the Sick and Wounded Seamen in the several ports of England," 1676; PL, 2867, 629; TNA, ADM 1/3595, Navy Board to Admiralty, 3 March 1703.

38 NMM, ADM/E/1, Admiralty to Sick and Wounded, 16 November 1703.

39 Wimmer, "War," 173–97.

40 Graham, "Credit, Confidence, and Circulation," 63–80.

41 Tilly and Ardant, *Formation of National States*, 6–50; Finer, "State and Nation Building in Europe," 84–163; Downing, "Constitutionalism, Warfare, and Political Change," 44, 50; Foucault, *The Government of Self and Others*.

42 Weber, "Bureaucracy," 126–244; Parker, *The Military Revolution*; Storrs, "War and the Military Revolution," 244–68.

43 North et al., *Violence and Social Orders*, 18–20; Lockwood, *Conquest of Death*, 8–23, 239–45.

44 Grant, *Technology and Justice*, 13–16; Cooter, "Introduction," 1–2; Wegner, *Theorizing Modernity*, 4; Bayly, *Birth of the Modern World*, 10–12.

45 Glete, *Navies and Nations*, 158–61, 178–96; Harding, *Modern Naval History*, 66–77; James, "First Age of Modern Naval Warfare," 38–50.

46 Wheeler, *Making of a World Power*, 43–53; Braddick, *State Formation in Early Modern England*, 202–25; cf. McLean, "Westminster Model Navy."

47 Reinhard, *Geschichte des Modernen Staates*, 76–9; Gorski, *Disciplinary Revolution*; Graham, "War and Society," 91–102.

48 Glete, *War and the State*, 54–5, 217; Asch, "War and State Building," 322–35; Rowlands, *Financial Decline*.

49 Brewer, *Sinews of Power*; Stone, *Imperial State at War*; Storrs, "Introduction," 3–20; O'Brien, "Fiscal Exceptionalism," 245–65.

50 Glete, "Warfare, Entrepreneurship, and the Fiscal-Military State," 300–21; Graham, "Auditing Leviathan," 806–38; Braddick, "State Formation and Social Change," 1–17.

51 Dickson, *Financial Revolution*; Ziegler, "Jacobitism, Coastal Policing, and Fiscal-Military Reform," 1–25.

52 Morriss, *British Military Ascendancy*.

53 Wilkinson, *The British Navy and the State*, 101; Conway, *War, State, and Society*; Torres Sanchez, "The Triumph of the Fiscal-Military State," 13–19, 28.

54 Rodger, "From 'Military Revolution,'" 119–28.

55 An affordance is a concept drawn from perceptual and cognitive psychology; Gibson, "Theory of Affordances," 67–82. Affordances are the properties of things in relation to human action or their environment. Things have objective properties in contingent combinations that exist as affordances in relation to the properties of other perceiving and acting things. Expressed less abstractly, a chair invites a person to sit, but does not determine that the person will sit. Chairs can also serve as doorstops or stepladders. What is crucial is the fact of potentiality: Keane, *Ethical Life*, 27–9.

56 To use another metaphor, English naval health care's early modernity stands in relation to its modernity like English football to successor sports such as rugby and ice hockey and Canadian football. There was nothing inherent in football, as it existed before 1800, to suggest that over the next century it would spawn three very different (albeit similarly high-contact) team sports. Yet football afforded people the potential to develop new modes of collective recreational competition whose common origin and family resemblances are undeniable.

57 Joas, "The Modernity of War," 457–72.

58 Porpora, *Reconstructing Sociology*, 60.

59 Miller, *Fact and Method*, 133–5.

60 Girard, *Battling to the End*, 20–1.

61 Grell, "War, Medicine, and the Military Revolution," 257–83; Obinger et al., *Warfare and Welfare*.

62 Ehrman, *The Navy in the War of William III*; Harding, *Seapower and Naval Warfare*; Harding, *Britain's Global Naval Supremacy*. An exception is Rodger, *Command of the Ocean*.

63 Lloyd and Coulter, *Medicine and the Navy*, 194–7.

64 Gardiner and Atkinson, *Letters and Papers*, 240–1; Bodleian Library, Rawlinson Manuscripts A195, fos. 251–2, Evelyn to Pepys, 23 March 1666; Baugh, *Naval Administration*, 48–52; Crimmin, "British Naval Health," 183–200; Crimmin, "Fit for Purpose," 90–107.

65 Fury, "Health and Health Care at Sea," 193–227; Charters, "'The Intention is Certain Noble,'" 19–37; Convertito, "Mending the Sick and Wounded," 500–33.

66 Crimmin, "Health of Seamen," 48–65; Harland, "First Hospitals."

67 Keevil, *Medicine and the Navy*.

68 Davey, "Navigating State and Society," 1546–62; Blakemore and Davey, *The Maritime World*, 13–35.

69 Wright, *New Testament and the People of God*, 64: "We must renounce the fiction of a god's-eye view of events on the one hand, and a collapsing of events into significance or perception on the other."

70 Collier, *Critical Realism*, 13–14.

71 This distinction is drawn from Hartog, *All This Will Be Yours*, 22.

72 Sources related to Restoration-era naval health care are also found at the Pepys Library, Magdalene College, Cambridge.

73 I engage with these sources in Neufeld and Wickham, "The Care of Sick and Injured."

74 Pool, *Navy Board Contracts*; Rodger, *The Admiralty*, 39–42.

75 TNA, ADM 99/2-11; 99/11, 30 March 1714 shows the final entry in the minute book for twenty-six years; NMM/ADM/E/1-5, 1702 to 1708; 1713–1715.

Notes to pages 14–22

76 TNA, T 1/176/2, List of books and registers kept, 17 May 1714. Had these registers survived, I could have undertaken a finely grained analysis of care work in England during Queen Anne's War.
77 NMM, ADM/E/5, 8 February 1718.
78 That is, a history so long that only a few people would read it.
79 Scheipers, *Prisoners in War*.
80 Brown, *Poxed and Scurvied*, 71–3, 174, 177, 188, 201.
81 Phenomenologically, time has an intrinsically narrative character: Carr, *Time, Narrative, and History*.
82 This label is inspired from Harland's formulation "manning, money, and mercy," "First Hospitals," 181.

CHAPTER TWO

1 Brewer, *Sinews of Power*; Stone, *Imperial State at War*; Storrs, "Introduction," 3–20; Rodger, "From 'Military Revolution,'" 119–28.
2 Brown, *Poxed and Scurvied*, 67.
3 Rommelse, "Role of Mercantilism," 591–611, cf.; Pincus, *Protestantism and Patriotism*. On the operations at sea, see Rodger, *Command of the Ocean*, 11–19, 69–77, 81–8.
4 Braddick, *State Formation in Early Modern England*, 225
5 Thompson, *Making of the English Working Class*, 67–72.
6 See figures 5.1 to 5.4, 121–4.
7 WSHC, 865/422, Bullen Reymes's letter book (December 1664–May 1666), 15–16, January 1665; BL, Add. MS 78320, no. 26, William Doyley to John Evelyn, August 1665; Pelling, "Compromised by Gender," 119.
8 BL, Add. MS 78322, fo. 71, petition to the Commission for Sick and Wounded Seamen from the nurses of Deal (1674); TNA, T1/44, fo. 147 (17 April 1697), a petition to the commission from the "poor widows and other Inhabitants of Dartmouth," 68 per cent of whom were women.
9 BL, Add. MS. 78322, fos. 107v–108, 1676.
10 BL, Add. MS. 78322, fos. 72r–73, no date.
11 Wheeler, *Making of a World Power*, 43–53; Lambert, *Seapower States*.
12 Wettenhall, "Public-Private Interface," 22–43; Wettenhall, "Mixes and Partnerships," 17–42.
13 This distinction between care providers and care workers is evident, for example, from a letter written by a clerk working for the navy at Deal, in which he described a Mr and Mrs Butcher as providing lodging for seamen, with Mrs Butcher taking it upon herself to deal with "her customers our nursese;" BL, Add. MS. 78321, fos. 44–5, Gardner to Evelyn, 30 November 1665.
14 Gabriel, *Between Flesh and Steel*, 53–6.

Notes to pages 22–8

15 Lindemann, *Medicine and Society*, 132.
16 Grell, "War, Medicine, and the Military Revolution," 257–83.
17 Rutherford, "New Kind of Surgery," 57–77; Gruber von Arni, *Justice to the Maimed Soldier*, 42–59.
18 Sandassie, "'Half-Gods,'" 47–8, 51, 58.
19 Lockhart, *Firepower*, 49–55.
20 Lamb, *Scurvy*.
21 Fury, "Health and Health Care at Sea," 193–228.
22 McLean, "Health Provision in the Royal Navy," 107–28.
23 Hudson, "Relief of English Disabled Ex-Sailors," 229–52.
24 Bodl. Lib. Rawlinson MS A209, fos. 18–19, Pensions and Reliefs ordered by the Governors of Chatham's Chest on 22 and 23 April 1662.
25 Hindle, "Civility, Honesty, and Identification," 38–59.
26 Nielson, "Chelsea Out-Pensioners," 18.
27 *FDW*, 3, 288; SA, HD/36/A/189, 1652; SA, HD/36/198, 9 July 1653.
28 SA, HD/36/A/189, n.d., c. 1652.
29 TNA, SP 18/32/8, 4 January 1653. The navy commission was called the navy board before the civil wars.
30 TNA, SP 18/33/110, 25 February 1653; *FDW*, 4, 162; *FDW*, 4, 211, 2 March 1653.
31 SA, HD/36/A/212, 19 September 1653. Gruber von Arni, "Soldiers-at-Sea," 406–19; Capp, *Cromwell's Navy*, 215.
32 BL, Add.. MS 9000, n.d. (c. 1653), fos. 255–6.
33 Volume 40: September 1653, *Calendar of State Papers Domestic: Interregnum, 1653–4*.
34 *FDW*, 4, 89–93; TNA, SP 18/60/14, 29 September 1653.
35 *FDW*, 4, 224.
36 Nicholls, *Almshouses*.
37 Rodger, *Command of the Ocean*, 47; Gruber von Arni, "Who Cared?" 149–82.
38 BL, Add. MS 9300, n.d. (c. 1653), fo. 255; Lambeth Palace Library Archives, MS 951/1, 17 August 1665, fos. 368–86; MS 952, 25 August 1665, items 96–9; MS 639, fo. 355, instructions to conduct a survey of hospitals in the ecclesiastical provinces of Canterbury and York; TNA, PC 2/57, 23 November 1664, fos. 148–9; PC 2/63, 8 March 1672, fo. 99.
39 LMA, HO1/ST/A/001/5, December 1664, fo. 137; SBHA, HA/20/1, 2 May 1672; HA/1/7, 2 September 1689; Neufeld, "Biopolitics," 268–90.
40 Rodger, *Command of the Ocean*, 47; Volume 34: 21 March 1653, *Calendar of State Papers Domestic: Interregnum, 1652–3*.
41 Bodl. Lib., Rawlinson MS A187, fos. 18–42.
42 Hudson, "Relief of English Disabled Ex-Sailors," 229–52.
43 *FDW*, 4, 89–93; TNA, SP 18/60/141.

Notes to pages 28–33

44 TNA, PC 2/57, fos. 147v–149r (November 1664); PC 2/63, fo. 99 (March 1672); PL, 2867, 551–53.

45 This is different from the Republic's commission, which had exercised its responsibilities as a body; Keevil, *Medicine and the Navy*, vol. 2, 97.

46 Sir Thomas Clifford was granted special permission to exercise his office while serving on board a ship; NMM, CLI/39/1, "Instructions to Sir Thomas Clifford," 23 March 1665.

47 TNA, PC 2/57, fo. 148r; PC 2/63, fo. 99v.

48 TNA, PC 2/57, fo. 148v; PC 2/63, fo. 99v; PL, MSS 2867, "General Order to the Governor of the Isle of Wight and all Justices of the Peace, Mayors, Bailiffs Constables and other civil and military officials of Hampshire to assist Commissioner Bullen Reymes and his deputies," 13 March 1672, 542.

49 £25 per month versus 24s. per month; Rodger, *Command of the Ocean*, 61.

50 PL, 2867, 543, 1672, Bullen Reymes, "Instructions to deputies."

51 TNA, SP 25/39/28–31; SP 18/34/28; BL Add MS. 78397, fos. 10–17, Account of Hearne Thurston, Clerk at Gravesend, November 1664 to June 1665.

52 Sharpe, *Early Modern England*, 222.

53 I will discuss such a book in more detail below at pages 60–1.

54 WSHC, 865/422, letter book, no foliation, "Warrant to Fareham Constables."

55 PL, 2867, 542, 13 March 1672, "General Order" to officials of Hampshire and the Isle of Wight.

56 TNA, PC 6/1, 11 October 1665.

57 BL, Add. MS. 78320, fo. 98. On one occasion the commission's agent at Rochester, John Conny, had to put men "in outhouses on straw"; BL Add MS. 78322 fo. 10, 18 June 1673.

58 Bodl. Lib., Rawlinson MS. A187, fo. 357, B. St. Michael to Pepys, 11 September 1672.

59 Shaw, "Commission of Sick and Wounded and Prisoners," 306–27.

60 Rodger, *Command of the Ocean*, 38–41; Harris, *Restoration*, 71–2: Jones, *The Anglo-Dutch Wars*, 93.

61 TNA, PC 2/58, fo. 368, 25 February 1666.

62 BL, Add. MS. 78396, fo. 28.

63 *FDW*, 4, 268; TNA, PC2/65, fo. 107, 21 January 1676.

64 BL, Add. MS. 78320, fos. 90–1, Reymes to Evelyn; 78321, fos. 15 and 20, Mason to Evelyn, October 1665; 78321, fo. 79, Conny to Evelyn, August 1667.

65 BL, Add. MS. 78322, fos. 128–9, St. Michael to Evelyn, May 1673; 78321, fo. 135, E. Smith to Evelyn, May 1673.

66 BL, Add. MS. 78396, fos. 55–6, "Abstract of payments and arrears for sick and injured and prisoners of war in Kent," 14 November 1674; NMM,

204   Notes to pages 33–7

SER/127, Abstract of the accounts of Henry Osborne, treasurer for the sick and wounded.

67 BL, Add. MS 28078, fo. 90, Clifford to Danby on the state of the debt, 1673: total, £344,000; for sick and wounded, £93,000.

68 BL, Add. MS. 78322, fo. 1, Robert Birstall to Mr Bishop, 3 June 1673. Birstall expressed similar fears on 11 and 15 June 1675; BL, Add. MS. 78322, fos 7, 9.

69 TNA, SP 18/35/30, April 1653.

70 BL, Add. MS. 78320, Elnathan Hannan to Evelyn, 24 January 1665; 78320, fo. 82, S. Whitter to Evelyn, June 1665.

71 de la Béydoyère, *Particular Friends*, 45, Evelyn to Pepys, November 1665.

72 BL, Add. MS. 78321, fo. 133, Glover to Evelyn, May 1673; 78321, fo. 116, R. Birstall to Evelyn, February 1673, 78322, fo. 1, Birstall to Evelyn, June 1673; Evelyn to Pepys, August 1673, *Particular Friends*, 79; BL, Add. MS. 78322, fo. 9, Birstall to Evelyn, June 1673.

73 BL, Add. MS. 78321, fo. 133, John Glover to Evelyn, 23 May 1673.

74 BL, Add. MS. 78322, fo. 11, June 1673; fo. 18, September 1673; TNA, ADM 106/293/171, December 1673.

75 BL, Add. MS. 78321, fos. 129, 136; 78322, fo. 11.

76 PL, 2850, fos. 55–6, Pepys to Evelyn, January 1674; fos. 56–7, Pepys to St. Michael, January 1674.

77 BL, Add. MS. 78321, fo. 43, Hannan to Evelyn, 29 Nov 1665.

78 BL, Add MS. 78321, fo. 10, Conny to Evelyn, October 1665; Add MS. 78322, fo. 7, 11 June 1673.

79 In a letter to St. Michael, written in January 1674, Pepys demanded to know the particular reasons why two people at Deal had refused to quarter sick and hurt men; PL, 2850, fo. 44.

80 Coleby, "Military-Civilian Relations," 959; Donagan, *War in England*, 392–3.

81 TNA, PC 2/64, fo. 15; fo. 179.

82 BL, Add. MS. 78320, fos. 68–9, 23 April 1665.

83 Evelyn to Brouncker, 2 September 1672, *Particular Friends*, 80, note 1; TNA, SP 29/328, fo. 140.

84 BL, Add. MS. 78321, fo. 121, copy of letter to Lord Treasurer Danby, March 1673.

85 Braddick, "Administrative Performance," 166-87.

86 The Treasury Board was aware of complaints against Birstall by the summer of 1672; TNA, T 29/4, Treasury Board Minutes, 29 August 1672. By contrast, Evelyn's clerk at Deal during the previous war, Mr Gardner, seems to have been especially conscientious, particularly in his dealings with nurses; BL, Add. MSS 78321, fo. 43v, 30 November 1665.

87 BL, Add MS. 78322, fo. 36, September 1673; fo. 71, Petition of Nurses of Deal, 1674.

Notes to pages 37–44

88 Evelyn to Pepys, 25 March 1666, *Particular Friends*, 60–5, at 65. The original is at the Bodleian Library, Rawlinson Manuscripts A195, fos. 251ff.

89 *FDW*, 4, 240–2; TNA, SP 18/34/48.

90 BL, Add. MS. 78321, fo. 116, February 1673; 78322, fos. 7, 19–20, June 1673.

91 BL, Add. MS. 78322, fo. 46, October 1673; fo. 103, July 1676.

92 DHC, QS1/11, Easter 1666, Easter 1672; KHC, QSO/W3, Easter 1673.

93 PL, 2865, Admiralty Journal, 14 November 1675, 15 July 1675; TNA, SO 8/3-4, Warrants for King's Bills 1667–1669; SO 8/8-11, 1663–1676.

94 PL, 2849, fo. 439, 22 December 1673.

95 BL, Add. MS. 78322, fo. 76, n.d. but before May 1674.

96 BL, Add. MS. 78322, fo. 78, 1 February 1675,

97 *CTB*, iv, 1672–1675, 775.

98 *CTB*, v, part 1, 1676–1679, p. 326;, Richard Gibson, *Publick services in, or relating to the Royal Navy; wherein Mr. Richard Gibson, has been employed since the year of our Lord 1652* (London, c. 1712), 2.

99 *CTB*, v, part 1, 1676–1679, 725, 733; v, part 2, 1676–1679, 869.

100 *CTB*, v, part 2, 1676–1679, 1245, 27 February 1679.

101 *CTB*, vi, 1679–1680, 73, 123–4.

102 *CTB*, vi, 1679-1680, 240; vii, part 2, 1681–1685, 745.

103 TNA, PC 2/71, 92–3, May 1685; *CTP*, viii, part 2, 1685–1689, 1042.

104 Gibson, *Publick Services*, 9–10.

105 SA, HD 36/A/207, Nicholas Philips to General Monck, 16 August 1653.

106 Arrears of pay for medical care were also a feature of casualty care in countries with naval hospitals, such as Spain; Storrs, "Health, Sickness, and Medical Services," 346.

107 BL, Add. MS. 11684, fos. 75–82, at fo. 81.

108 North et al., *Violence and Social Orders*.

109 NMM, CC1/46, "A list of clerks and surgeons" working under commissioners Clifford, Reymes, Doyle, and Evelyn, 1665.

110 PL, 2867, 629, Pearse to Admiralty, 3 March 1688. Pearse was charged with providing care for sick and injured men in "extraordinary cases" when they were set on shore. From 1674 to 1689 the navy's preferred site for care was on ships; Keevil, *Medicine and the Navy*, 2: 131–2.

111 Bruijn, "States and Their Navies," 88.

112 Rodger, *Command of the Ocean*, 110; De Krey, *Restoration and Revolution*, 106–15.

113 Parrott, *Richelieu's Army*, 537.

114 Storrs, "Health, Sickness, and Medical Services," 336; Huard and Niaussat, "Hôpitaux de la Marine Française," 385.

115 Dean, "Charles II's Garrison Hospital," 280–3; Cook, "Practical Medicine," 1–26, at 6.

116 Braddick, "The English Revolution and Its Legacies," 36.

117 Braddick, *State Formation in Early Modern England*, 77–81.

Notes to pages 45–7

CHAPTER THREE

1 Harris, *Revolution*; Sowerby, *Making Toleration*; Cook, "Practical Medicine," 1–26; Harland, "First Hospitals," 108–28.
2 Brewer, *Sinews of Power*, 29–31; Wheeler, *Making of a World Power*, 65.
3 Black, "British Naval Power," 39–59; Ehrman, *The Navy in the War of William III*; J. Jones, "Limitations of British Sea Power," 33–9; Baugh, "Britain's 'Blue Water' Policy," 44.
4 Deringer, *Calculated Values*.
5 TNA, AO 1/1821/490, Auditors of the Imprest, Mr Povey's accompt as treasurer for the sick and wounded to 31 December 1690. A receiver acted as a kind of 'accounts-payable' officer.
6 BL, Add. MS 30999, fo. 1, "Account of war-time expenses according to the Commissioners for Accounts," November 1669.
7 TNA, T 1/18/46, fos. 164–5, 20 May 1692. Four years later, with the French long committed to avoiding large-scale encounters with the Royal Navy, the commissioners projected an annual charge to their service of £35,000; *CTB*, xi, 48, 18 August 1696.
8 The debt for care was still over £61,000 at the end of 1699: *CJ*, House of Commons xiii, 62, "The state of the charge of sick and wounded seamen, and exchange of prisoners of war, from the 11th June 1689 to the 30th September 1699," 14 December 1699. A statement of the commission for sick and wounded's account from May 1700 put the total cost of health care and prisoners of war at £321,684, with the outstanding balance sitting at £61,102; TNA, T 1/68/57, 15 May 1700.
9 Jones, *War and Economy*.
10 I am grateful to the late Aaron Graham for reminding me of this point.
11 Rodger, *Command of the Ocean*, 197–213.
12 TNA, T 38/615, "Moneys received from the Exchequer by the Treasurer of the Royal Navy for particular services from their books from 5 November 1688 to 1 October 1692, 1702." The amounts for sick and injured seamen also covered costs for housing and transporting prisoners of war.
13 Conditions of care for sick and wounded French seamen treated at Rochfort never deteriorated to the same extent as they did at several English ports during the 1690s; de Martel, *Étude sur le recrutement*, 313–21.
14 Dickson and Sperling, "War Finance," 286.
15 TNA, PC 2/72, 181–3: Instructions for the commissioners for the sick and wounded seamen and exchange of prisoners of war, 11 July 1689. Each commissioner received a salary of £300 per year.
16 Hainsworth, *Correspondence of Sir John Lowther*, 433n5; 671; Addison was also a client of Sir Joseph Williamson; *CSPD William*, viii, 276, 329.
17 BL, Add. MS. 42140, fos. 1–2; KHC, PRC/27/33/160-16, Will of J. Nicholes, 25 November 1693.

Notes to pages 47–52

18 The commissioners presented the idea of hospitals for Deal and Portsmouth, and Plymouth, to the Admiralty within a time-frame consistent with Dickinson's narrative: TNA, ADM 3/3, 16 January 1690.

19 The narrative that follows is derived from SRL, MS 129/1, "Mr Dickinson's Paper"; Poynter, *Journal of James Yonge*.

20 TNA, ADM 3/3, 29 January 1690.

21 SRL, MS 129/1.

22 SRL, MS 129/2. Leakie and Baston also alleged that Dickinson embezzled money by charging the crown 8d. per man per day for fuel costs, which was 3d. above the price offered by local suppliers.

23 *CTP*, i, 330, 9 January 1694; 522, 24 June 1696; ii, 6, 29 January 1697.

24 SRL, MS 129/3, 14 April 1694; TNA, PC 2/75, 424, 31 May 1694. The fact that surgeon Berry was rehired in 1692 probably indicates that the Admiralty was not entirely convinced of the agent's uprightness in interacting with the seamen at the hospital or the people of Plymouth.

25 TNA, ADM 99/1, 19 September and 5 December 1698; 6 February 1700.

26 SRL, MS 129/1.

27 Pelling, "Nurses and Nursekeepers," 179–202. Berry evidently returned to the hospital shortly thereafter with impressment officers, who shunted the male nurses back onto naval vessels.

28 Keevil, *Medicine and the Navy*, 2: 199–202; Ehrman, *The Navy in the War of William III*, 441–5; Arnold, *Spaces of the Hospital*.

29 TNA, ADM 1/3997, 2 January 1699; TNA, ADM 3/5, 9 January 1690; ADM 3/6, 10 February 1692; ADM 3/9, 20 December 1693.

30 Stevenson, "Palace to Hut," 227–51; Hudson, "Internal Influences," 253–7.

31 TNA, ADM 3/3, 25 February 1690.

32 TNA, PC 2/76, fo. 116v, 5 September 1695; ADM 1/5249, 200. Commissioner Christopher Kirkby sailed with Sir George Rooke, TNA, PC 2/75, fo. 159, 16 January 1696.

33 TNA, T 61/16, 36, 24 March 1702: £5,614 issued to sick and wounded receiver Povey £2,094 for the West Indies and £1,216 for the Mediterranean. The Treasury papers do not often list the regions for which payments for care were issued.

34 TNA, T 1/78/10, 9 January 1702.

35 Rodger, *Command of the Ocean*, 194.

36 Most of the requests are found in TNA, T 1, Treasury in-letters.

37 Waddell, "Politics of Economic Distress," 318–51.

38 TNA, ADM 3/5, 10 April 1691; ADM 3/6, 14 December 1691.

39 *CTP*, i, 237, 3 May 1692.

40 *CTP*, i, 239, 10 May 1692.

41 TNA, ADM 2/172, fo. 199, 19 May 1692.

42 *CTP*, i, 239–40, 27 May 1692.

208   Notes to pages 52–7

43 *CTP*, i, 240, 3 June 1692; *CTB*, ix, 1666, 7 June 1692.

44 Rodger, *Command of the Ocean*, 158; Helling, "Convoy of Scottish Trade," 109–10.

45 Anderson and Gifford, "Privateering and Private Production," 99–122.

46 *CTP*, i, 450, 26 June 1695; TNA, T 1/32/7, fo. 18, 9 January 1695; *CTB*, x, 1382, 21 November 1695.

47 *CTP*, ii, 14 January 1698.

48 *CTP*, ii, 239, 8 November 1698; TNA, T 29/9, Treasury meeting minutes, 16, 8 November 1698.

49 *CTP*, i, 330, 9 January 1694; *CTB*, x, 450, 11 January 1694.

50 *CTP*, i, 352, 14 March 1694.

51 *CTP*, i, 356, 28 March 1694.

52 *CTP*, i, 368, 5 June 1694; *CTB*, x, 643, 7 June 1694.

53 *CTP*, i, 371, 13 June 1694; *CTB*, x, 656, 15 June 1694.

54 *CTP*, i, 385, 28 August 1694.

55 Duffy, "Establishment of Western Squadron," 60–81; Hattendorf, "The Struggle with France," 80–90.

56 TNA, ADM 1/3997, 8 March 1701.

57 TNA, ADM 1/3997, 6 June 1701; ADM 99/1, 6 June 1701.

58 TNA, ADM 3/3, 28 January 1690. The action was judged "not only a disservice to their Majesties Service but a great discouragement to the Seamen."

59 TNA, ADM 3/3, 31 January 1690; ADM 2/170, fo. 71, 1 February 1690.

60 TNA, ADM 3/3, 6 February 1690.

61 TNA, ADM 3/3, 23 June 1690.

62 TNA, ADM 3/5, 5 December 1690.

63 TNA, T1/21/49, 14 March 1693.

64 TNA, T1/21/65, 10 April 1693.

65 TNA, T1/22/20, 16 May 1693.

66 TNA, T1/22/33, 24 May 1693.

67 TNA, ADM 2/173, 309, 24 May 1693.

68 *CTP*, i, 297, 31 May 1693.

69 *CTP*, i, 303, 28 June 1693; 318, 8 September 1693; 330, 6 December 1693; see also *CTP*, i, 301, 21 June 1693; 310, 27 September 1693; 332, 13 December 1693.

70 *CTP*, i, 319, 27 September 1693.

71 *CTP*, ii, 6, 29 January 1697.

72 TNA, T1/43/24, 29 January 1697.

73 TNA, T1/44/47, 17 April 1697.

74 The "Dartmouth Widows" Petition, as it is listed in the *CTB*, ix, 39, 8 June 1697, included signatures from nineteen men and only one self-declared widow.

75 TNA, ADM 3/13, 14 June 1697.

76 TNA, ADM 3/13, 21 June 1697.

77 *CTP*, ii, 61, 22 June 1697.

78 *CTB*, xii, 217, 30 June 1697.

79 TNA, T1/46/55, 8 July 1697; *CTP*, ii, 84, 31 August 1697.

80 *CTB*, xiv, 237, 9 May 1699.

81 TNA, T 1/61/32, fo. 197, 18 May 1699; PC 2/77, 337. Since most of the signatories were women (eighteen of thirty-one), the "old and infirm" probably included several widows.

82 *CTP*, ii, 335, 20 October 1699: £61,102.

83 Downing, "Constitutionalism, Warfare, and Political Change," 7–56; O'Brien, "England 1485–1815," 65.

84 *CTP*, i, 522, 24 June 1696.

85 *CTB*, xi, 34, 30 June 1696; Roseveare, *The Financial Revolution*.

86 The tallies carried interest as high as 8 per cent, which was 2 per cent above the legal maximum for private loans. Another way to think about tallies is as endorsed, post-dated, interest-bearing cheques. Since the Second Dutch War, tallies were issued as numbered paper standing orders that were linked to specific future revenues; they were supposed to be paid out "in course"; Dickson, *Financial Revolution*, 76; 350; Kleer, "'Fictitious Cash,'" 74.

87 *CTB*, xi, 75, 4 April 1696; xi, 52, 253, 1 and 2 September 1696.

88 *CTP*, i, 556, 27 October 1696. An agent of the Navy Board based at Shoreham reported that his credit with local people was so bad that he did not "know what to do [or] to appear abroad." TNA, ADM 106/485/427, 2 September 1696.

89 Jones, *War and Economy*, 11.

90 Desan, *Making Money*, 13, 296, 328.

91 *CTB*, xii, 70, 24 November 1695; *CTP*, ii, 19, 19 March 1697.

92 TNA, T29/9, 255, 21 July 1697; *CTP*, ii, 77, 27 July 1697; 81, 9 September 1697.

93 *CJ*, xiii, 62, 14 December 1699.

94 11 William III, 2, n. 1, *S.R.*, vii, 1695–1701, 582–6, clause xviii; *CTB*, xv, 105, 26 June 1700; xvi, 8, 31, 15 and 16 October 1700.

95 13 William III, 3, n. 1, *S.R.*, vii, 1695–1701, 716–23; TNA, T61/16, 12 January 1702.

96 TNA, T 1/81/45, 29 July 1702. The bulk of the outstanding charge for sick and wounded/prisoners of war was paid off by February 1702; TNA, T 1/78/51, 24 February 1702.

97 Wheeler, *Making of a World Power*; O'Brien, "Exceptional Fiscal State," 408–46.

98 Hoppit, "Checking the Leviathan," 273.

99 Hoppit, "Checking the Leviathan," 273; Knights, *Trust and Distrust*, 184–222.

210 Notes to pages 60–4

100 Neufeld, "Biopolitics."

101 TNA, ADM 3/6, no fol., 15 June 1696; ADM 3/7, 24 June 1692; ADM 3/8, 3 May and 18 September 1693.

102 TNA, ADM 3/6, 4 March, 1 and 27 April, 17 and 19 May 1692.

103 TNA, ADM 3/7, 22 and 25 July, 30 September 1692.

104 *CTB*, vi, 1209, 30 June 1691; 1295, 7 September 1691.

105 TNA, T 1/28/51, Balance sheet of sick and wounded service, 1689 to 1694, 24 June 1694.

106 TNA, SP 42/2/105, Account of the number of sick and wounded men, 13 June to 30 August, 24 September 1693.

107 TNA, ADM 3/14, 18 and 26 June 1698; NMM, SER/103, 27 February 1697.

108 TNA, ADM 3/13, 27 September 1697; ADM 3/14, 31 December 1697; *CTB*, xiv, 91, 6 June 1699.

109 NMM, SER/102, 2 August 1693.

110 NMM, SER/102, 27 February 1694; SER/103, 28 March 1694.

111 Baston, *Dialogue*, Wing B1056. TNA, PC 2/75/424, 31 May 194; Luttrell, *A Brief Historical Relation*, 307–8, 8 and 10 May 1694; 322, 2 June 1694; BL, Harl. MSS, 1492, fos. 36–8; 1493, fos. 47, 54, 61–3, 77–8.

112 Baston was not satisfied with this verdict and proceeded to carry on in public his unprecedented campaign against the sick and wounded commission for the next two years; Neufeld, "Roots of Whistle Blowing," 410–16.

113 TNA, T1/72/31, 29 January 1701.

114 TNA, ADM 3/3, 11 July 1690.

115 TNA, ADM 3/4, 21 November 1690.

116 TNA, PC 2/73, fo. 40v, 2 December 1690.

117 TNA, ADM 3/5, 5 December 1690.

118 BL, Add. MS 11602, fos 5–6, "Dr Richard Lower's Proposal," 9 December 1690.

119 20,000 men x 30 days in care x 8d. per day per man = £20,000.

120 The non-nursing staff included physicians, surgeons, mates, an apothecary, clerk, purser, cook, and butler.

121 Working three hundred days per year, a nurse would earn £7 10s., roughly half the average annual wage of an agricultural labourer (£15 12s. p.a.); Sharpe, *Early Modern England*, 222.

122 A landlady was owed 4d. per man per day for care, or 3s. 4d. per day for ten men.

123 The instructions directed to the new commission in early 1691 were the same as those from July 1689; BL, Add. MS. 28748, fos. 4–9.

124 TNA, ADM 2/176, fos. 171–2, Navy Board to Admiralty, 8 October 1695; TNA, T 1/77/13, Admiralty to Privy Council, dated 24 December 1695; catalogued in the Treasury in-letters 2 December 1701.

125 Hess and Mendelsohn, "Case and Series," 287–314.

Notes to pages 64–9

126 TNA, PC 2/76, fo. 152r, 9 January 1696.
127 Neufeld, "Biopolitics."
128 TNA, ADM 3/14, 6 May 1698; ADM 1/5249, 12 May 1698; PC 2/77 fo. 90, 12 May 1698.
129 TNA, ADM 3/14, 17 May and 5 June 1698; PC 2/77 fo. 93, 9 June 1698.
130 TNA, ADM 3/14, 15 June 1698.
131 There are at least two extant copies of "Draught Instructions to the Commissioners of the Register in providing for and seeking care of the Sick and Wounded Seamen," one at the National Maritime Museum, which is dated to October 1699 (NMM, CAD/A/16/32), and another at the British Library (BL, Add. MS 28748, fo. 10–18). The NMM catalogue date is implausible because, first, as noted above, the Navy Board was ordered to prepare "draught Instructions" for the registry commissioners in mid-June 1698. Second, the registry commissioners' meeting minutes for 20 June 1698 record their having "no objection to receiving draught Instructions for managing the businesses" of the sick and wounded (TNA, ADM 99/1, 20 June 1698). In late-July 1699, the registry of seamen itself was dissolved and the sick and wounded service assigned to two members of the Navy Board (TNA, ADM 99/1, 22 July 1699).
132 TNA, ADM 1/3997, 16 July 1698.
133 NMM, CAD/A/16/32, item 8 (9).
134 Ibid., item 16.
135 Ibid., item 13.
136 Ibid., items 15 and 12.
137 Ibid., item 19.
138 Ibid., items 21 and 20.
139 Ibid., items 11 and 10.
140 TNA, ADM 2/180, 58–9, 16 July 1699. In May 1699, five Admiralty lords, including Whig grandee Admiral Edward Russell, Lord Orford, resigned under pressure from hostile opponents in parliament.
141 TNA, ADM 2/ 180, 47, 7 July 1699; NMM, SER/104, fos. 170–1, 12 July 1699; TNA, ADM 99/1, 22 July 1699.
142 TNA, T 1/54/5, fos. 22–4, 22 June 1698.
143 See above pages 62–3.

CHAPTER FOUR

1 Watson, "Victualling the Navy"; Crimmin, "Health of Seamen," 48–65; Harland, "First Hospitals," 318, 25, 16.
2 Claydon, *The Making of England*; Satsuma, *Britain and Colonial Maritime War*; Elliott, "Road to Utrecht," 3–8; Schettger, *Der Spanische Erbfolgekreig*; Shovlin, *Trading with the Enemy*.
3 Zahedieh, "Commerce and Conflict," 68–86.

Notes to pages 69–72

4 Although there was tremendous debate in and outside of parliament over the prioritization and goals of domestic and foreign policy, there was broad agreement, especially after 1701, about the constitutional processes by which the governed and the government could settle political differences peacefully; McInnes, "When Was the English Revolution?" 377–92; Rodger, *Command of the Ocean*, 578–82; Taylor, "Afterword," 273–304.

5 TNA, ADM 99/9, 1 and 8 October 1709; ADM 99/11, 26 March 1713.

6 TNA, PC 2/79, 150: Commissioners for sick and wounded seamen, 11 June 1702.

7 TNA, ADM 3/17, 15 June 1702.

8 NMM, ADM/E/5, 24 February 1713.

9 For appointments to the commission see NMM, ADM/E/2, 22 April 1704; TNA, ADM 99/5, 22 April 1704; 99/7, 6 June 1706; 29 April 1707; 28 June 1707; TNA, T 1/103/58, 8 November 1707; ADM 99/8, 27 November 1707.

10 BL, Add. MS. 28748, Catalogue of men employed in the sick and wounded service, fos. 21–23.

11 NMM, ADM/E/1, 11 July 1702.

12 TNA, T 1/80/67, Account of monies due for sick quarters, 24 June 1702. Gosport (£2,949) and Rochester (£997) had drawn the heaviest charges for care over the twelve months prior to the war's outbreak.

13 TNA, T 1/80/46, "Instructions," 20 June 1702, with a copy at NMM, ADM/E/1 (same date). The Admiralty re-issued commissions in the spring of 1704, probably on account of the appointment of several new commissioners; TNA, ADM 3/19, 11 April 1704.

14 NMM, CAD/A/16/32, July 1698; BL, Add. MS. 28748, "Draught of Instructions to the Commissioners of the Register in providing for and seeking care of the Sick and Wounded Seamen," fos. 10–18.

15 TNA, PC 2/72, Instructions for the commissioners for the sick and wounded seamen and exchange of prisoners of war, 11 July 1689.

16 Articles 1, 4, 7, 8, 14, 18, 22, and 24 of the 1689 "Instructions" are replicated in whole or in part in the 1702 version.

17 1689 "Instructions," articles 14, 15, and 16.

18 1689 "Instructions," article 12. See Hudson, "Relief of English Disabled Ex-Sailors," 229–52.

19 Wilcox, "'Poor Decayed Seamen,'" 65–90; Lepka, "Care Work and Nursing."

20 TNA, ADM 3/17, 16 June and 10 July 1702. The commissioners' Westminster office, located at Prince's Court, a short distance from the Admiralty, had a public room, a boardroom, rooms where the clerks wrote, and a hall: TNA, ADM 99/11, no fol., 3 September 1713. TNA, ADM 99/2, 14 July 1702; NMM, ADM/E/1, 7 September 1702.

21 1689 "Instructions," Articles 6, 10, 11.

22 TNA, T1/80/46, 20 June 1702.

Notes to pages 73–7

23 TNA, T 1/170/4, 17 February 1713.

24 Rodger, *Command of the Ocean*, 164–79.

25 TNA, T 1/134/12, 8 June 1711. Foreign bills amounted to £32,634 by early 1712: TNA, T 1/151/3, 13 August 1712; ADM 99/11, 16 August 1712.

26 TNA, ADM 99/9, 30 April 1709.

27 TNA, T 1/111/5D, Debt of Sick and Wounded at Home Ports, 1708.

28 NMM, ADM/E/4, 20 April 1708.

29 TNA, ADM 3/23, 7 May 1708; ADM 99/8, 29 June 1708. The surgeon engaged at Leith, Mr Pringle, unsuccessfully proposed to establish a hospital there. TNA, ADM 99/9, 14 January and 29 June 1710.

30 TNA, ADM 99/9, 9 June, 9 September 1709; 15 July 1710; 1 January 1712.

31 TNA, ADM 99/10, 20 May 1710.

32 HMC, HoL MSS., ns, v., 1702–04, 23 March 1704, 532.

33 TNA, T 1/102/65, Debt of Office, July 1707.

34 Worchester RO, 705:255/1545/49/28, State of the account of Sir Thomas Littleton, Bart., late Treasurer of the Navy, 1699–1709; Account of the whole imprest charge, July 1702 to September 1709, 27 January 1711.

35 TNA, T 1/138/15, State of the Sick and Wounded Debt, 2 October 1711.

36 TNA, T 1/150/8, State of the Sick and Wounded Debt, 24 July 1712.

37 TNA, T1/170/4, Memorials of the commission to the Lord Treasurer dated 17 February and 28 May 1713.

38 TNA, T 1/84/76, 13 February 1703.

39 TNA, T 1/138/15, 18 October 1711.

40 TNA, T1/150/8, 24 July 1712.

41 Five in 1705, three in 1706, four in 1707, five in 1708, two in 1709, and two in 1710.

42 The debt for the final quarter of 1712 reached £10,637; TNA, ADM 106/678/15, 31 January 1713.

43 TNA, T 1/170/4, 28 February and 29 May 1713.

44 TNA, T 1/184/50, State of sick and wounded office charge, 2 December 1714.

45 New style.

46 TNA, T 1/103/14, 14 October 1707.

47 *CTB*, xxii, 268, 14 June 1708.

48 TNA, ADM 99/10, 22 June 1710; *CTB*, xxv, 537, 30 October 1711.

49 TNA, ADM 99/10, 13 May 1711.

50 TNA, ADM 99/10, 15 May 1711.

51 TNA, T 1/134/12, Memorial to Lord Treasurer, 8 June 1711. This is one of the first times the word "government" appears in the commissions' correspondence with the Treasury.

52 TNA, T 1/134/17, 29 June 1711.

53 TNA, ADM 99/10, 25 Sept 1711.

54 TNA, T 1/170/4, Memorial to the Earl of Oxford, 17 February 1713.

214   Notes to pages 77–80

55   *CTB*, xvii, 87, £7,432, 29 July 1702.

56   *CTB*, xviii, 453, £20,000, 17 November 1703; TNA, ADM 99/10, no fol., £20,000, 9 April 1711.

57   *CTB*, xix, 5, £10,000, 21 January 1704.

58   TNA, T 29/19, 2 October 1711; ADM 99/11, 17 November 1711; *CTB*, xxvii, 175, 7 April 1713; *CTB*, xvii, 237, £12,358, 4 June 1713.

59   TNA, ADM 99/11, 16 March 1711; NMM, ADM/E/5, 15 March 1714.

60   Hubbard, *Englishmen at Sea*, 273.

61   Beckett, "Land Tax or Excise," 301. Even Marxist historians concede the English political nation's "unique fiscal responsiveness" to taxation; Teschke, "Revisiting the 'War-Makes-States' Thesis," 55.

62   TNA, ADM 99/2, 25 March 1703; T 27/18, 24 July 1705; ADM 99/9, 31 May and 9 July 1709.

63   That is, of course, the charge of travel on the navy, not the quarterers seeking payment; TNA, ADM 3/27, 2 March 1713.

64   TNA, ADM 99/6, 16 March 1706.

65   TNA, ADM 99/7, 7 June 1707.

66   Rodger, *Command of the Ocean*, 102.

67   TNA, T 1/189/31, "C. Clark's petition," 2 April 1715. The petition concerns a conflict between an undertaker, Mr Colebrook, and his agent at Gosport, Mr Clark. The former could not be paid because the latter refused to endorse the tickets. The dispute originated from "differences lately happened in the family" of Colebrook's former partner and Clark's brother-in-law, one Mr Jackson.

68   TNA, ADM 99/6, 22 December 1705.

69   TNA, ADM 99/7, 18 June 1706.

70   TNA, ADM 99/11, 9 October 1711.

71   TNA, ADM 99/7, 26 May 1707.

72   TNA, T 1/86/115, 14 July 1703; ADM 99/7, 10 May 1707.

73   TNA, ADM 99/11, 27 March 1712.

74   TNA, ADM 99/8, 17 June 1708.

75   TNA, T 61/20, 1 July 1709.

76   TNA, ADM 99/11, 15 March 1712.

77   TNA, ADM 3/19, 30 March 1704; ADM 99/10, 5 May 1711; 99/10, 30 December 1710; 99/11, 27 February 1714; cf. TNA, T 1/173/35A, 4 March 1714.

78   TNA, ADM 3/29, 18 October 1714.

79   See above, 49.

80   TNA, ADM 99/2, 14 October 1702.

81   TNA, ADM 99/2, 24 March 1704.

82   Ibid.

83   TNA, ADM 99/2, 22 October 1703.

84   TNA, ADM 99/9, 8 December 1708, 27 March 1709; cf. 99/10, Submission of debt to September 1710 for the Navy Board for presentation to parliament, 24 August 1710.

Notes to pages 81–5

85 Binney, *British Public Finance*, 140.
86 TNA, T 27/17, 3 September 1703.
87 TNA, T 1/86/115, 14 July 1703.
88 Ibid.
89 TNA, T 29/14, 14 July 1703.
90 TNA, ADM 99/2, 3 August 1703.
91 TNA, ADM 99/ 5, 4 April 1704; 99/7, 24 October 1706.
92 TNA, ADM 99/2, 26 June 1703; ADM 99/8, 25 September 1707. The agent at Pembroke evidently took this directive too much to heart; he was subsequently instructed not to send his "Voluminous Papers for the Christmas quarter to this office by Post," but by some other route: TNA, ADM 99/2, 19 February 1704.
93 TNA, ADM 99/11, 6 November 1711.
94 TNA, ADM 99/6, 15 May 1705.
95 TNA, ADM 99/5, 30 July 1705; TNA, T 1/91/67, Memorial to Lord Treasurer, 30 July 1704.
96 TNA, ADM 99/7, 25 April 1706.
97 TNA, ADM 99/7, 24 May 1707.
98 TNA, ADM 99/10, 24 October 1710.
99 TNA, ADM 99/8, 17 February 1708.
100 RNM, Corbett MSS. 121/13, 6.
101 NMM, ADM/E/4, 1 April 1708.
102 TNA, ADM 2/33, "Instructions to William Churchill," 29 July 1705.
103 https://www.historyofparliamentonline.org/volume/1690-1715/member/churchill-william-1661-1737.
104 TNA, ADM 99/8, 20 July 1708. Churchill evidently proposed a method for better accounting of the sick and wounded service shortly after retiring from the commission; the proposal does not appear to have survived: TNA, T 1/103/58, 8 November 1707.
105 TNA, ADM 2/18; NMM, ADM/E/1, 6 July 1703.
106 TNA, ADM 99/2, 7 July 1703.
107 TNA, ADM 99/5, 15 June 1704.
108 TNA, ADM 99/2, 24 October 1702.
109 TNA, ADM, 99/2, 6 November 1703.
110 TNA, ADM 99/11, 26 August 1712.
111 Tadmor, "Settlement of the Poor," 51.
112 NMM, ADM/E/1, 10 August 1703.
113 TNA, ADM 99/ 2, 18 November 1703.
114 TNA, ADM 99/2, 19 January 1703.
115 TNA, ADM 3/19, 24 December 1703.
116 TNA, ADM 3/21, 21 January 1706; NMM, ADM/E/2, 22 January 1706.
117 TNA, ADM 99/10, 28 September 1710; ADM 97/114/16, "List of men at Lisbon hospital mustered on 2 October 1707."

118 TNA, ADM 99/2, 2 August 1702; ADM 3/22, 8 October 1706. Port Mahon naval hospital had a muster-master, along with a clerk to assist him, three years later, ADM 99/9, 13 September 1709.

119 TNA, ADM 99/2, 20 September 1703.

120 TNA, ADM 99/7, 15 August 1706.

121 TNA, ADM 99/10, 14 December 1710.

122 TNA, ADM 99/6, 13 December 1705.

123 TNA, ADM 99/6, 2 August 1705.

124 TNA, ADM 99/8, 13 December 1707.

125 TNA, ADM 99/10, 20 February 1711.

126 TNA, ADM 99/7, 16 June 1706.

127 NMM, ADM/E/4, 18 July 1708; TNA, ADM 3/23, 21 July 1708.

128 TNA, ADM 99/8, 22 July 1708.

129 TNA, ADM 99/9, 26 July 1709.

130 TNA, ADM 99/9, 8 December 1709. James Berkeley, third earl of Berkeley, known as Lord Dursley in the fleet, served as vice-admiral of the white from 21 December 1708 to 19 December 1709; Hattendorf, "Berkeley, James."

131 TNA, ADM 3/24, 12 December 1709; ADM 99/9, 12 December 1709.

132 TNA, ADM 99/ 9, 18 January 1710.

133 TNA, ADM 99/2, 22 December 1702. Clark of Yarmouth was permitted to answer charges against him in writing; ADM 99/2, 11 May 1703.

134 TNA, ADM 99/5, 28 November 1704.

135 TNA, ADM 99/6, 7 February 1706; ADM 99/7, 21 December 1706; ADM 99/8, 23 March 1708; ADM 99/7, 4 March 1707.

136 TNA, ADM 99/2, 17 February 1704.

137 TNA, ADM 99/2, 8 July 1703.

138 TNA, ADM 99/5, 12 September 1704.

139 TNA, ADM 99/6, 10 November 1705.

140 TNA, ADM 99/9, 9 April 1709.

141 TNA, ADM 99/ 11, 31 July 1712.

142 TNA, T 1/150/20, 31 July 1712.

143 TNA, ADM 3/17, 6 October 1702; NMM, ADM/E/1, 12 November 1702; TNA, ADM 99/2, 12 November 1702.

144 TNA, ADM 99/2, 15 November 1702. The queen had gone on to recommend that there be "no unnecessary expence therein so nothing should be wanting for the relief of those seamen who had served Her Majesty so well."

145 NMM, ADM/E/1, 9 January 1703.

146 Harland, "First Hospitals," 144.

147 Ibid., 181.

148 Finer, "State and Nation Building in Europe," 99; Taylor, *A Secular Age*, 90–143; Hudson, "Internal Influences," 253–72.

Notes to pages 91–9   217

149 Asch, "War and State Building," 322–35.
150 Pihl, "Gender, Labour, and State Formation," 685–710 at 708.
151 Lynn, *Women, Armies, and Warfare*, 8.
152 Wilson, "German Women and War," 134.
153 An undertaker by definition was someone contracted to provide a necessary service for the government; Clay, *Public Finance and Private Wealth*, 32; Parrott, *Business of War*, 20.
154 TNA, ADM 3/17, 2 February 1703.
155 TNA, ADM 99/2, 4 and 11 February 1703.
156 TNA, ADM 1/3595, Navy Board to Admiralty, 2 March 1703.
157 NMM, ADM/E/1, 6 and 22 June 1703.
158 TNA, ADM 99/2, 18 September 1703.
159 TNA, ADM 99/2, 20 September 1703.
160 TNA, ADM 99/2, 19 October 1703.
161 TNA, ADM 99/2, 26 October 1703.
162 TNA, ADM 3/19, 10 November 1703.
163 NMM, ADM/E/1, 16 November 1703.
164 TNA, ADM 99/2, 4 and 14 December; ADM 3/19, 11 December 1703: Mr Sayer at Rochester; Mr Frost at Portsmouth; Mr Saracole at Deal.
165 What follows is drawn from TNA, ADM 1/3595, 2 March 1703.
166 TNA, ADM 99/2, "Mischiefs of the Town Quarters," 20 September 1703.
167 TNA, ADM 99/2, "Mischiefs of the Town Quarters," Items 1, 2, 4, 5, 7, 8, 10, 11.
168 TNA, ADM 99/2, "Mischiefs of the Town Quarters," Items 3, 6, and 9.
169 TNA, T 1/134/66, 27 June 1711.
170 TNA, T 1/150/16, 29 July 1712.
171 NMM, ADM/E/5, 3 March 1713.
172 TNA, ADM 1/3528, Copy of Agreement between John Sayer and the Commission for Sick and Wounded, dated 23 December 1703, 4 December 1727; ADM 99/2, 20 September 1703.
173 Cooter, "War and Modern Medicine," 1536–74; Harrison, "Medicine and Management," 379–410.
174 TNA, T27/18, 30 June 1705.
175 NMM, ADM/E/3, 3 April 1706.
176 TNA, ADM 99/7, 4 April 1706.
177 TNA, ADM 3/17, 8 January 1703. Tutchin, *Treatise of the Navy*.
178 TNA, ADM 1/3528, 4 December 1727.
179 TNA, SP 42/119/247, August 1704.
180 TNA, SP 42/119/269, August 1704.
181 NMM, ADM/E/2, fo. 100, 1 October 1704. A similar complaint was presented in the summer of 1705 against the hospital at Plymouth; Tunstall, *The Byng Papers*, 81–2.
182 NMM, ADM/E/2, fo. 105, 31 October 1704.

218 Notes to pages 100–5

183 TNA, ADM 99/6, 1 December 1705.

184 TNA, ADM 99/6, 15 December 1705.

185 Hacker, "Women and Military Institutions," 643–71.

186 Kopperman, "Medical Services," 428–55.

187 TNA, T 1/189/31a, Copy of proposal dated 23 June 1714 from C. Clark to the commission for sick and wounded, 2 April 1715.

188 TNA, ADM 99/2, 8 December 1702.

189 See above, 98.

190 NMM, ADM/E/2, 4 September 1705; TNA ADM 99/6, 8 September 1705.

191 NMM, ADM/E/2, 1 October 1705; ADM/E/3/, 10 August 1706.

192 TNA, ADM 99/7, 14 December 1706.

193 TNA, ADM 99/9, 26 May 1709.

194 TNA, ADM 99/9, 14 April 1709.

195 TNA, ADM 99/9, 15 September 1709.

196 See above, 99–100. Subsequently, one Captain Jackson of the *Squirrel* complained about the lack both "of care [and] good manners in one of the Nurses" there; TNA, ADM 99/6, 6 February 1705.

197 BL, Sloane MSS 1198, "Account of seamen at Rochester 1703," fo. 130.

198 All data derived from TNA, T 1/145/5, State of Sick and Wounded Debt, 3 April 1712.

199 TNA, ADM 99/9, 24 December 1709 and 17 January 1710.

200 A Margaret Hicks is listed as taking in one man on 26 August and two on 13 November; BL, Sloane MSS. 1198, "Account of seamen at Rochester 1703," fo. 130.

201 TNA, ADM 99/11, 7 April 1713.

CHAPTER FIVE

1 English fleets were active intermittently in the Mediterranean and the Baltic from 1718 to 1721 and defended Gibraltar from the Spanish in 1727. Another fleet suffered notoriously terrible mortality in the Caribbean in 1726–27 under Admiral Hoskins. Peace otherwise obtained over much of the quarter-century after the Treaty of Utrecht, thanks mostly to the British-French alliance of 1716 to 1731 and first minister Robert Walpole's subsequent efforts to avoid war with one of the other two great naval powers. Harding, "British Maritime Strategy," 252–74; Harding, *Hanover and the British Empire*, 80–5; Black, *British Politics and Foreign Policy*, xi, 51–9.

2 One postwar account indicates that since the accession of George I, the biggest draws on the total sick and hurt debt of just over £7,000 were Rochester with 29 per cent (£2,180), Port Mahon at 18.9 per cent (£1,383), Gosport with 10 per cent (£733), and Woolwich at 7.7 per cent (£568); TNA, ADM 1/3638, 25 January 1716.

Notes to pages 105–9   219

3   *CJ*, xviii to xxiii. There is no data for 1732.

4   For example, NMM, ADM/E/5, 20 January 1716; ADM/E/7, 4 December 1730, 2 November 1737.

5   *CJ*, xviii, 374; TNA, ADM 1/3628, 21 January 1716.

6   Between 1702 to 1707, the height of Queen Anne's War, the charge for care was £257,337, over £100,000 more than costs after the change in policies for peacetime; see above, 73–4.

7   Baugh, "Professionalization of the English Navy," 852–66.

8   Crimmin, "British Naval Health," 185.

9   Harland, "First Hospitals," 348–9.

10   Crimmin, "Fit for Purpose," 99–102.

11   RNM, Corbett MSS 121/13, "Sick and Wounded, Prisoners of War, Hospital Ships, Surgeons"; Baugh, *Naval Administration*, 533.

12   Harland, "First Hospitals," 330–4; Collinge, *Office-Holders in Modern Britain*, 89, 92, 100, 103.

13   RNM, Corbett MSS 121/13, 24; TNA, ADM 3/29, 29 April 1715; NMM, ADM/E/5, 9 May 1715.

14   NMM, ADM/E/5, 27 April 1715; NMM, CAD/A/16/32, "Draught Instructions to the Commissioners of the Register in providing for and seeking care of the Sick and Wounded Seamen."

15   TNA, ADM 3/29, 29 April 1715; NMM, ADM/E/5, 6 May 1715.

16   NMM, ADM/E/5, 9, 11 and 20 May 1715.

17   NMM, ADM/E/5/, 27 May 1715.

18   Ibid.

19   NMM, ADM/E/5, 20 May 1715. At that time, the sick and wounded service encompassed sixty-two officials, thirty-five at home and twenty-seven overseas; these figures did not include the hospital undertakers at the great ports.

20   NMM, ADM/E/5, 27 May 1715.

21   TNA, ADM 3/29, 27 May 1715; Alsop, "Sickness in the British Mediterranean Fleet," 57–76.

22   TNA, ADM 7/639, 14 June 1715.

23   TNA, ADM 7/639, 14 June 1715, item 2.

24   TNA, ADM 1/3528, 4 December 1727, Copy of proposal of Thomas Knackston to the commission for sick and hurt "for the better accommodation and preservation of many of the lives of sick and hurt seamen," dated 22 June 1715.

25   NMM, ADM/E/7, 19 and 22 October 1733.

26   TNA, ADM 1/3528, 19 October 1733.

27   TNA, ADM 1/3528, 26 October 1733.

28   NMM, ADM/E/7, 3 December 1733, 4 February 1734; TNA, ADM 106/864/59, 20 January 1734.

29   Knights, *Trust and Distrust*.

Notes to pages 110–13

30 Graham, *Corruption, Party, and Government*; Neu, "Zahlmeister und Kaufmannbankiers."

31 NMM, ADM/E/5, 2 December 1717, Copies of Informations taken by Paul Margarett, JP, at Middlesex quarter session, Michaelmas 1717.

32 NMM, ADM/E/5, Information of Samuel Cloud, 13 November 1717. Three years earlier the same person alleged a fraud of £10,000 against the commission; TNA, ADM 99/11, 1 and 4 March 1714.

33 Neufeld, "Neither Private Contractors nor Productive Partners."

34 NMM, ADM/E/5, Copy of the warrant against Benjamin Dixie for defrauding the government, 22 October 1717.

35 NMM, ADM/E/6, 30 September 1727. Although the undertaker was not named, it was presumably Frederick Hill; TNA, ADM 1/3528, 4 December 1727.

36 NMM, ADM/E/5, 11 December 1717.

37 NMM, ADM/E/5, 20 December 1717.

38 NMM, ADM/E/5, 11 January 1718.

39 NMM, ADM/E/6, 30 September 1727.

40 NMM, ADM/E/6, 21 November 1727.

41 NMM, ADM/E/6, 24 November and 11 December 1727.

42 NMM, ADM/E/7, 12 December 1729.

43 TNA, ADM 1/3644, 17 January 1730. The commissioners did not, for perfectly understandable reasons, mention that it had been they who had in 1727 suggested the switch from the surgeons to the clerks as muster masters.

44 TNA, ADM 1/3644, 29 January 1730.

45 NMM, ADM/E/7, 30 January 1730.

46 NMM, ADM/E/5, 5 June 1716.

47 NMM, ADM/E/5, 27 April 1715.

48 TNA, ADM 3/29, 3 May 1715.

49 Royal Navy, *Instructions*, ESTC no. T132255 (London: 1715?), 9, 24–6.

50 TNA, ADM 1/3640, 2 December 1726.

51 RNM, Corbett MSS 121/13, 7; Baugh, *Naval Administration*, 533, and personal communication, 4 May 2018.

52 TNA, ADM 3/37, 22 April 1729.

53 NMM, ADM/E/7, 26 and 30 April 1729.

54 Royal Navy, *Regulations and Instructions*, ESTC no. T114322 (London: 1731), 58. In the autumn of 1733, the Navy Board proposed new articles and forms for the printed instructions. The article relating to keeping a book of all men sent sick out of the ships "in proper columns" does not include the option of setting a Q next to a man's name. Nonetheless, as we will see below, the practice appears to have continued, or perhaps revived, in a modified form in the 1740s; TNA, ADM 1/3648, 26 October

Notes to pages 113–19   221

1733; ADM 7/339, December 1733, 482; Royal Navy, *Pursers Instructions*, ESTC no. T207298 (London: 1735), 13

55 Royal Navy, *Regulations and Instructions*, ESTC no. T114322 (London: 1731), 55–9.

56 See above, 83.

57 NMM, ADM/E/5, 2 May 1717.

58 TNA, ADM 1/3528, Extract of a letter from Mr Edisbury to the commissioners from Portsmouth, 16 July 1729.

59 NMM, ADM/E/5, 15 December 1719.

60 TNA, ADM 1/3528, 28 November 1727. In late 1727, the commissioners were compelled to admit that in contracting with Hill they had, possibly inadvertently, breached an agreement made between the fifth commission and one Captain Brand in 1710, under which terms Knackston was to operate the hospital on Brand's behalf. ADM 1/3528, 4 December 1727 and NMM, ADM/E/6, 11 November 1727.

61 NMM, ADM/E/7, 2 May 1734.

62 NMM, ADM/E/7, 7 June 1734.

63 See above, 48–9.

64 TNA, ADM 1/3528, 16 June 1734. Edisbury included a census of "distempers" among the seamen quartered at Deal. It shows the typical preponderance of fevers among the men in care: of the 272 under treatment, forty-eight had the Itch (a skin disease traced to mites), seven had smallpox, four suffered the flux, eight had the pox (STI), and 205 were fevered.

65 The 166 men were, Edisbury reported, "in a state of ill health"; thirty-seven had the flux (10.6 per cent), forty-two had scurvy (12.1 per cent), sixty-four had scabies [the itch] (18.4 per cent), 123 either continuous or intermittent fevers (35.4 per cent), fifty-two were lame or hurt (15 per cent). The remainder, twenty-nine, suffered from one of consumption, rheumatism, edema, smallpox, and syphilis.

66 TNA, ADM 1/3528, 16 July 1729.

67 TNA, ADM 1/3528, 17 July 1729; NMM, ADM/E/7, 18 July 1729.

68 TNA, ADM 1/3528, 30 August 1734.

69 NMM, ADM/E/7, 20 September 1737.

70 Spinney, "Naval and Military Nursing," 30–77.

71 NMM, ADM/E/7, 20 November 1734.

72 NMM, ADM/E/7, 23 November 1734.

73 See above, 99–100.

74 NMM, ADM/E/7, Copy of petition from the "Principal Inhabitants of Plymouth," 8 March 1735.

75 NMM, ADM/E/7, 8 March 1735.

76 TNA, ADM 1/3528, 11 March 1735.

77 TNA, ADM 1/3528, 16 March 1735. Gortley reported that the hospital held 140 men, and that there were forty-seven quartered in its immediate

Notes to pages 120–8

neighbourhood of Stonehouse. In Plymouth town were quartered ninety-seven seamen.

78 TNA, ADM 2/33, 29 July 1705, Admiralty Instructions to Commissioner William Churchill to check the musters of sick men and to visit the hospitals.

CHAPTER SIX

1 Lloyd and Coulter, *Medicine and the Navy*, 190–5; Baugh, *Naval Administration*, 48–52; Harland, "First Hospitals," 393–402.
2 NMM, ADM/F/3, 14 March 1744.
3 The Admiralty ordered operations against Spanish shipping in mid-July 1739; Woodfine, *Britannia's Glories*; Harding, *Britain's Global Naval Supremacy*.
4 Peckham, "'A True British Spirit,'" 135; Rodger, "Sea-Power and Empire," 169–83; Harding, "British Maritime Strategy," 254–7. The performance of Spain's royal navy was similarly disappointing after 1741; Storrs, *Spanish Resurgence*, 63, 77.
5 TNA, ADM 1/3528, 24 April 1740.
6 On cleanliness at similar French institutions, see Brockliss and Jones, *The Medical World*, 697–702.
7 TNA, ADM 99/12, 29 July 1740.
8 TNA, ADM 99/13, 10 April 1741.
9 TNA, ADM 99/17, 23 August 1743.
10 TNA, ADM 1/903, 16 September 1741.
11 NMM, ADM/E/10, 24 March 1743.
12 NMM, ADM/F/3, Hawes, surgeon-agent at Rochester, to Commissioners, 28 March 1743.
13 TNA, ADM 3/47, 16 May 1743.
14 See McNeill, *Mosquito Empires*, 152–69, for an account of Admiral Vernon's failures at Cartagena and Santiago del Cuba. He reckons that 11,750 of about 15,000 sailors serving in the West Indies between 1739 and 1742 died of either yellow fever or malaria.
15 CUL, Ch (H), 12/1, Monthly Account of the Number of Seamen on Shore, August 1739 to August 1740; TNA, ADM 1/3528, 10 October 1740, Account of the greatest number of sick on shore at one and the same time since July 1739.
16 CUL, Ch (H), 12/3, Account of the Number of Men put sick ashore at Home, 1 July 1739 to 31 August 1740. The total is 15,868 men. The Kent ports of Rochester and Deal received 19.7 per cent or 2,491 men.
17 *CJ*, xxiii, 26 November 1740, 541; TNA, ADM 99/13, 28 November 1740.
18 April, May, June, July, September, and October 1740.

19 Harding, *Britain's Global Naval Supremacy*, 92–3. The Spanish navy faced similar problems in the Mediterranean in 1743; Navarro's squadron lost 26 per cent of its sailors to sickness en route to Toulon; Storrs, *Spanish Resurgence*, 73, 77.

20 TNA, ADM 1/903, Cavendish to Admiralty, 17 June 1740.

21 TNA, ADM 110/12, Victualling Board to Admiralty, 30 June 1740.

22 Manley, "The Great Winter," 11–17.

23 Baugh, *Naval Administration*, 179; Post, "Climatic Variability," 1–30 at 24.

24 TNA, ADM 99/15, 11 May 1742.

25 NMM, ADM/F/3, 14 March 1744.

26 TNA, ADM 99/14, 25 February 1742.

27 TNA, ADM 99/14, 1 March 1742.

28 TNA, ADM 99/14, 3 March 1742.

29 TNA, ADM 99/15, 7 September 1742.

30 TNA, ADM 99/17, 10 and 14 June 1743.

31 NMM, ADM/B/125, Number of seamen on shore between 31 December 1741 and 31 December 1742: 22,006; cited in Harland, "First Hospitals," 428, n59.

32 TNA, ADM 99/13, 2 June 1741.

33 TNA, ADM 3/46, 17 March 1743. The figure for 1742 turned out to be an even thousand; NMM, ADM/F/3, 18 March 1743.

34 Harland, "First Hospitals," 404.

35 Newton, "Inside the Sick Chambers," 564.

36 TNA, ADM 1/3528, 3 May 1740.

37 TNA, ADM 99/12, 9 July and 10 September 1740.

38 TNA, ADM 99/12, 6 October 1740.

39 TNA, ADM 99/12, 11 February 1741.

40 TNA, ADM 1/905, "Present Conditions of his Majesties Seamen at Forton Hospital, June 8th 1741," 10 June 1741; Barclay reported 357 at the Hospital on 1 May 1740; ADM 1/3528, 3 May 1740.

41 TNA, ADM 1/905, 23 and 27 August 1741.

42 TNA, ADM 99/14, 2 September 1741; TNA 1/3529, 2 September 1741.

43 TNA, ADM 99/14, 18 September 1741.

44 TNA, ADM 1/905, 16 September 1741.

45 CUL, Ch (H), 12/7; TNA, ADM 1/3528, 10 October 1740.

46 TNA, ADM 1/903, 3 June 1740.

47 TNA, ADM 1/903, 15 June 1740.

48 TNA, ADM 99/12, 13 June 1740.

49 CUL, Ch (H), 12/4, "Number of men from Sir Chaloner Ogle's squad put ashore sick at St Helen's 8 July 1740."

50 TNA, ADM 99/12, 21 May 1740. The office was in Broad Street. Payment for the first (Christmas) quarter of 1740 was made from 3 November 1740; ADM 99/12, 22 October 1740.

224 Notes to pages 133–5

51 TNA, ADM 99/13, 27 and 31 August 1741.

52 TNA, ADM 99/12, 2 May 1740.

53 TNA, ADM 99/12, 30 September 1740.

54 TNA, ADM 99/12, 4 June and 16 September 1740.

55 TNA, ADM 99/12, 23 October 1740.

56 A ticket in this case was a form of bill that a quarterer was to receive from seamen in proof of services rendered.

57 TNA, ADM 99/13, 3 July 1741.

58 TNA, ADM 1/3529, 3 July 1741.

59 TNA, ADM 99/13, 8 July and 27 August 1741.

60 TNA, ADM 99/13, 31 August 1741. The agent, Mr Porter, agreed that payments on location would "greatly encourage the people." By contrast, Commissioner Hills, then at Gosport, was more worried that they would not find enough quarters at Gosport.

61 TNA, ADM 99/14, 7 September 1741.

62 TNA, ADM 3/45, 9 January 1742; NMM, ADM/E/9, 9 January 1742. The request was denied because of the "great Desertions that happen ashore."

63 Conway, "British Military Expenditure," 301; Rodger, "Military Revolution at Sea," 60–9; Bowen, "The Contractor State," 239–42.

64 TNA, ADM 99/17, 19 May 1743.

65 TNA, ADM 1/3528, 31 July 1740. Two months later, the commissioners reminded agent Barclay at Gosport to "make a publication that those who will receive the sick men shall be paid 7 shillings per week for each man quarterly"; TNA, ADM 99/12, 22 September 1740.

66 See above 50–8.

67 TNA, ADM 99/13, 28 August 1741; ADM 99/14, 24 September 1741.

68 TNA, ADM 99/12, 7 August 1740; ADM 99/14, 20 November 1741; 19 December 1741; ADM 99/17, 21 April 1743. Brewer, *Sinews of Power*, 95.

69 That a significant portion of the Royal Navy served as the armed division of British West India merchants, including sugar planters, between 1714 and 1763, does not mean that slavery was the essential institution underlying British political economy during the period, as suggested by Beckert, *Empire of Cotton*, xv–xvi, 37–8, 165–6. British merchants wanted unrestricted access to Spanish colonial markets, while planters wanted to eliminate their Caribbean competitors; Pares, *War and Trade*, 83–5, 126, 227; Niedhart, *Handel und Krieg*, 55, 86–7. See also Eltis and Engerman, "The Importance of Slavery and the Slave Trade," 123–44; Shovlin, "War and Peace," 305–27; Hilt, "'New History of Capitalism,'" 511–36; Burnard and Riello, "Slavery and the New History of Capitalism," 224–44; Shovlin, *Trade and Empire*, 277, 26–7

70 *CTP*, iv, 260. Walpole established the sinking fund, which was supposed to receive whatever surplus remained in the national budget each year, in 1717. Intended to pay down the principal of the national debt, the fund

Notes to pages 135–9

was often raided when the government needed money quickly; https://www.historyofparliamentonline.org/periods/hanoverians/walpole-and-national-debt.

71 TNA, ADM 99/13, 15 December 1740.

72 TNA, ADM 99/13, 23 February 1741.

73 TNA, ADM 99/13, 13 April, 5 June, and 13 July 1741.

74 This achievement can be put in a broader context via Conway, "British Military Expenditure," 45–68.

75 Post, "Climatic Variability," 22–4.

76 TNA, ADM 99/12, 15 July 1740. Gashry departed for good in early 1741 and was replaced by Charles Allix; TNA, ADM 99/12, 12 March 1741.

77 NMM, ADM/E/7, 10 November 1739. Barclay had been appointed the previous August: NMM, ADM/E/7, 20 August 1739; TNA, ADM 1/3528, 24 August 1739. Dr Brady was physician at Portsmouth from the late autumn: TNA, ADM 3/43, 27 October 1739.

78 TNA, ADM 1/903, 3 February 1740.

79 TNA, ADM 3/44, 24 April 1740.

80 TNA, ADM 1/903, 27 April 1740.

81 TNA, ADM 1/903, Crawford to Cavendish, 30 April 1740.

82 NMM, POR/H/4, Hughes to Admiralty, 2 May 1740.

83 TNA, ADM 1/3528, 28 April 1740.

84 TNA, ADM 1/3528, Barclay to Commissioners, 27 April 1740.

85 TNA, ADM 1/3528, 3 May 1740, Barclay to Commissioners on 1 May 1740.

86 TNA, ADM 1/3528, Barclay to Commissioners, 27 April 1740.

87 TNA, ADM 1/3528, 3 May 1740, Barclay to Commissioners, 1 May 1740.

88 The fact that the Navy Board put the idea of royal hospitals to the Admiralty within days of Cavendish's complaint suggests Barclay was not entirely wrong to suspect more was going on than concern over his handling of unprecedented demand for care spaces; TNA, ADM 106/2178, Navy Board to Admiralty, 25 April 1740. See also ADM 1/903, Captain Crawford to Cavendish, 30 April 1740.

89 TNA, ADM 1/903, Cavendish to Admiralty, 7 May 1740.

90 TNA, ADM 1/903, Cavendish to Admiralty, 16 and 17 June 1740.

91 Thomas, "Health and Morality," 15–34.

92 NMM, ADM/E/8a, Rules and Instructions for the better Management of the Sick and Hurt service, 3 June 1740.

93 Jussim, "Précis of Social Perception and Social Reality."

94 TNA, ADM 3/45, 8 February 1742; NMM, ADM/E/9, Admiralty to Commissioners, 16 February 1742; TNA, ADM 99/14, 17 February 1742. The previous Instructions were composed in 1715: NMM, ADM/E/5, 27 April and 27 May 1715.

95 TNA, ADM 98/103, Admiralty Instructions to Commissioners, 8 February 1742.

Notes to pages 139–44

96 Barclay lost his position as surgeon-agent after an onsite investigation by Commissioner Hills in late 1740.

97 TNA, ADM 99/12, 11 August 1740.

98 TNA, ADM 99/14, 17, 23, 29 March 1742.

99 TNA, ADM 3/46, 1 May 1742; ADM 99/15, 14 and 17 May 1742.

100 TNA, ADM 99/16, 1 December 1742. The agent insisted that his sick quarters were clean.

101 TNA, ADM 99/12, 15 August 1740.

102 Rodger, *The Wooden World*, 207–10.

103 TNA, ADM 99/12, 6 October 1740.

104 TNA, ADM 99/12, 8 October 1740.

105 Baugh, *Naval Administration*, 183.

106 TNA, ADM 99/15, 11 May 1742.

107 TNA, ADM 99/17, 25 April 1743.

108 TNA, ADM 99/17, 13 September 1743.

109 TNA, ADM 99/17, 14 March 1743.

110 TNA, ADM 99/17, 13 May 1743.

111 TNA, ADM 98/103, Article Six, Admiralty Instructions to Commissioners, 8 February 1742.

112 See above, 13.

113 TNA, ADM 1/903, May 1740: State of the Sick Quarters at Gosport; State of the Sick Quarters at Fareham View'd by Capt Long and Sir Jas. Barclay; An Enquiry into the State of Sick and hurt Seamen in the Hospital at Fortune near Gosport.

114 The sex of the provider was judged from either the title "Mrs" or the first name.

115 One of the twenty-three men at Margaret Esam's house was "violently Pox'd."

116 See above, 117–18.

117 TNA, ADM 1/3528, 28 April 1740, Barclay to Commissioners, 24 April 1740.

118 TNA, ADM 1/3528, Buttall to Commissioners, 27 May 1740.

119 TNA, ADM 98/103, Article Six, Admiralty Instructions to Commissioners, 8 February 1742.

120 TNA, ADM 99/13, 27 April 1741.

121 TNA, ADM 99/13, 23 June 1741; ADM 106/2179, Navy Board to Admiralty, Estimate of the charge of three-storey hospitals at Chatham, Plymouth, and Portsmouth, 15 July 1741.

122 TNA, ADM 1/903, Vincent to Cavendish, 30 April 1740.

123 TNA, ADM 1/903, Cavendish to Admiralty, 28 May 1740.

124 TNA, ADM 99/17, 16 May 1743.

125 TNA, ADM 1/3528, Buttall to Commissioners, 25 July 1740.

Notes to pages 144–51 227

126 TNA, ADM 99/14, 12 March 1742.

127 TNA, ADM 99/16, 28 December 1742 and 3 January 1743; Lepka, "Care Work and Nursing," 62.

128 TNA, ADM 99/13, 27 January 1741.

129 TNA, ADM 99/13, 12 March 1741.

130 TNA, ADM 99/17, 26 and 30 May 1743; NMM, ADM/E/10, 1 June 1743.

131 NMM, ADM/E/10, 24 June 1743, Copy of J. Fowell to Mr Paterson, 7 June 1743; TNA, ADM 99/17, 25 June 1743.

132 NMM, ADM/F/3/ 1 July 1743; TNA, ADM 98/1, 1 July 1743, Vincent and Wyatt to Commissioners, 28 June 1743.

133 TNA, ADM 3/44, 21 May 1740.

134 TNA, ADM 99/12, 23 May 1740.

135 TNA, ADM 1/3528, 27 May 1740.

136 TNA, ADM 1/3528, Buttall to Commission for Sick and Hurt, 30 May 1740.

137 TNA, ADM 1/3528, Vanborough to Commission for Sick and Hurt, 30 May 1740.

138 TNA, ADM 99/12, 2 June 1740.

139 TNA, ADM 3/44, 14 July 1740.

140 TNA, ADM 1/3528, 15 July 1740.

141 TNA, ADM 99/12, 17 July 1740.

142 TNA, ADM 1/3528, 22 July 1740.

143 Oreston is southeast of Plymouth, across the river.

144 TNA, ADM 1/3528, Wyatt to Admiralty, 25 July 1740.

145 TNA, ADM 1/3528, Commissioners to Admiralty, 31 July 1740.

146 TNA, ADM 99/12, 19 August 1740.

147 TNA, ADM 99/12, 28 August 1740.

148 TNA, ADM 99/12, 1 September 1740.

149 TNA, ADM 1/3528, Nathaniel Hills to Admiralty, 17 November 1740.

150 TNA, ADM 99/13, 30 January 1741. The Admiralty allowed Buttall to answer the charges in Hills's report, TNA, ADM 3/45, 24 November 1740. The ex-contractor's statement did not convince, and his dismissal was confirmed the following spring, TNA, ADM 99/13, 24 April 1741.

151 A precursor to gin, Geneva was the Anglicized name for jenever, the juniper-flavored liquor common to northern France, the Low Countries, and northwestern Germany.

152 TNA, ADM 1/3528, Nathaniel Hills to Admiralty, 17 November 1740.

153 TNA, ADM 1/3528, Humphrey Buttall's answers to the articles, 17 November 1740.

154 TNA, ADM 1/3528, Nathaniel Hills to Admiralty, 17 November 1740.

155 TNA, ADM 1/3528, Humphrey Buttall's answers to the articles, 17 November 1740.

228   Notes to pages 151–7

156 TNA, ADM 1/3528, Humphrey Buttall to Admiralty, November 1740; date not listed.

157 TNA, ADM 99/13, 18 November 1740.

158 TNA, ADM 1/3528, Commissioners to Admiralty, 18 November 1740.

159 TNA, ADM 99/13, 25 November 1740.

160 TNA, ADM 1/3529, 13 June 1741.

161 See below, 153–4.

162 Stemming from the reign of William III, the Lords Justices governed the realm in the king's absence; Raymond, "Lords Justices of England," 453–76.

163 Harland thinks the estimated cost of the project, plus the weakness of Walpole's ministry in the second half of 1741, were decisive against it; Harland, "First Hospitals," 422.

164 TNA, ADM 106/2178, Navy Board to Admiralty, 25 April 1740.

165 NMM, ADM/E/8, 2 May 1740.

166 TNA, ADM 106/2178, Navy Board to Admiralty, 3 November 1740. The commissioners' suggestion was evidently prepared by 23 October. Perhaps as an interim measure, the commissioners ordered one of their agents for prisoners to explore the possibility of turning Portchester castle into a naval hospital: TNA, ADM 99/12, 16 September, 1 and 27 October 1740.

167 TNA, ADM 99/13, 23 March 1741.

168 TNA, ADM 99/13, 30 March 1741.

169 NMM, ADM/E/8, 4 April 1741.

170 TNA, ADM 1/3529, Commissioners to Admiralty, 6 April 1741.

171 TNA, ADM 106/2179, Navy Board to Admiralty, 15 July 1741. The cost difference stemmed from the design of the buildings: the two storey structure was envisioned as a quadrangle, while the three storey one conceived in an 'H' formation, which would have needed fewer bricks.

172 NMM, ADM/E/8, 17 July 1741.

173 TNA, ADM 7/339, Admiralty to Lords Justices, 17 July 1741; ADM 1/3529, Commissioners to Admiralty, 21 July 1741.

174 TNA, ADM 7/339, Admiralty to Lords Justices, 17 July 1741.

175 TNA, ADM 1/3529, Commissioners to Admiralty, 21 July 1741. For French officials making similar calculations about care as an inducement to men to serve, see Brockliss and Jones, *The Medical World*, 252–5.

176 TNA, ADM 1/3529, 13 June 1741.

177 The commissioner of Portsmouth's dockyard, Richard Hughes, suggested that a hospital "surrounded with a Brick Wall of a proper Height" would be the best remedy against desertion; NMM, ADM/POR/H/14, Hughes to Admiralty, 26 October 1741.

178 TNA, ADM 99/14, 1 and 22 January 1742.

179 TNA, ADM 99/17, 7 June 1743.

180 TNA, ADM 99/17, 7 March 1743.

Notes to pages 158–61

CHAPTER SEVEN

1 Lloyd and Coulter, *Medicine and the Navy*, 187–90, 191.
2 Crimmin, "Health of Seamen"; Harland, "First Hospitals,"432.
3 Baugh, *Naval Administration*, 51, 185; Harland, "First Hospitals," 422–30; Thomas, "Jack Tar, Mr Sawbones, and the Local Community," 291–302 at 291.
4 See above, 153–6.
5 Between March 1744, when France declared war on Britain, and late December of the same year, the Admiralty was led by Daniel Finch, Earl of Winchilsea. He was replaced by John Russell, Duke of Bedford, who remained First Lord until February 1748, a few months before the war's end. Rodger, *The Admiralty*, 51; Kinkel, "Disorder, Discipline, and Naval Reform," 1451–82.
6 TNA, ADM 1/3528, 10 July 1729.
7 Paquette, *European Seaborne Empires*, 4, 94–5; Plank, *Atlantic Wars*, 229.
8 Niedhart, *Handel und Krieg*; Mimler, *Der Einfluß kolonialer Interessen*; Harding, *Hanover and the British Empire*.
9 Simms, *Three Victories and a Defeat*, 131–48.
10 Pares, *War and Trade*, 179, 268; Scott, *Birth of a Great Power System*, 60; Conway, *War, State, and Society*; Page, *Seventy Years War*.
11 Duffy, "Establishment of Western Squadron," 60–81; Rodger, "Sea-Power and Empire," 174–8.
12 Kinkel, *Disciplining the Empire*, 20–3, 102, 120, 212. The public controversy that this Admiralty's postwar efforts to impose external discipline on naval officers forms, in this view, a prolepsis of the crisis of transatlantic imperial governance beginning fourteen years later: 112.
13 NMM, ADM/F/4, Commissioners to Admiralty, 5 November 1744; ADM/F/5, 3 December 1744, Copy of a letter of the 2nd December from Mr William Hicks, Surgeon and Agent at Sheerness, to the Commissioners.
14 Total figure calculated from the "Accounts shewing how many Men have Run from the Hospitals in England" for the period, dated 16 January, 11 April, 17 July, and 2 October 1745; NMM, ADM/F/5; ADM/F/6; ADM/F/7.
15 TNA, ADM 3/49, 20 November 1744; NMM, ADM/E/11, Admiralty to Commissioners, 20 November 1744.
16 A regulating captain was an officer who certified whether a seaman qualified for release from the navy as an invalid.
17 NMM, ADM/E/11, Admiralty to Commissioners, Extract of a Letter from the Regulating Captain to Mr Corbett dated 19th October 1744.
18 The soldier who tried to evade his duty under the pretence of sickness was first called a malinger in the late-eighteenth century; Grose, *Vulgar*

230   Notes to pages 161–6

Tongue; "malingerer, n.". OED Online. September 2021. Oxford University Press. https://www.oed.com/view/Entry/112945 (accessed 10 November 2021).

19 NMM, ADM/F/4, Commissioners to Admiralty, 2 November 1744.

20 NMM, ADM/E/11, Admiralty to Commissioners, 9 November 1744.

21 TNA, ADM 98/2, Commissioners to Admiralty, 12 November 1744.

22 See Neufeld, "Corruption in the British Naval Healthcare Administration" (forthcoming).

23 TNA, ADM 99/19, 13 March 1746; NMM, ADM/F/7, Commissioners to Admiralty, 13 March 1746; NMM, ADM/E/12, Admiralty to Commissioners, 19 March 1746; NMM, ADM/F/2, Commissioners to Admiralty, 21 March 1746. Porter's case might have been helped when the Admiralty learned that his misdeed happened only once, "and then it was done by his Wife (as it is affirmed) without his Knowledge;" NMM, ADM/E/12, Admiralty to Commissioners, 28 March 1746.

24 TNA, ADM 99/19, 14 December 1747.

25 TNA, ADM 1/915, James Steuart to Admiralty, 2 February 1747; NMM, ADM/E/12, Admiralty to Commissioners, Extract of a letter from Vice-Admiral Steuart to Mr Clevland dated 2nd February 1747.

26 NMM, ADM/E/12, Admiralty to Commissioners, 9 February 1747. On 17 February, Admiral Anson ordered the commissioners to direct their agents at Sheerness, Rochester, and Plymouth likewise to forgo sending seamen to the London hospitals without seeking first the local commanding officer's approval, even when "the Obstinacy of their Diseases requires their being sent"; NMM, ADM/E/12.

27 Neufeld, "Neither Private Contractors nor Productive Partners," 268–90.

28 TNA, ADM 98/4, Commissioners to Admiralty, 16 February 1747; NMM, ADM/F/9, 16 February 1747.

29 NMM, ADM/F/9, Commissioners to Admiralty, 2 March 1747: Extract from Commissioner Hills's letter while at Chatham, 1 March 1747.

30 NMM, ADM/E/12, Admiralty to Commissioners, 28 March 1747.

31 NMM, ADM/E/11, Admiralty to Commissioners, 15 May 1745.

32 TNA, ADM 99/19, 15 May 1745; NMM, ADM/F/6, Commissioners to Admiralty, 15 May 1745.

33 Probably signifying Discharged Sick Query.

34 Thus, if a man entered sick quarters on 15 June and continued there more than a month, his pay stopped on 15 July. Were he released from sick quarters on 20 July, and then reboarded his or another ship on 21 July, his pay would commence from the 21st, meaning that the period from 16 to 20 July did not count toward his wages.

35 Thus, the use of the mark "Q," whereby a man's pay was stopped after thirty days in care, survived in modified form over five decades after its introduction; TNA, ADM 99/19, 16 May 1745; NMM, ADM/F/6, Commis-

Notes to pages 166–8

sioners to Admiralty, 16 May 1745. This corrects Neufeld, "Biopolitics of Manning."

36 NMM, ADM/F/6, Commissioners to Admiralty, 15 May 1745.

37 NMM, ADM/F/8, Commissioners to Admiralty, 10 May 1746; Hills visited Deal hospital on 19 April 1746.

38 NMM, ADM/F/8, Commissioners to Admiralty, 17 September 1746: Hills visited Gosport on 19 May 1746.

39 TNA, ADM 1/915, Steuart to Admiralty, 6 May 1747. The Portsmouth commander did concede that some captains sent ashore men whom the officers disliked, "upon very trifling complaints of illness, that they may be tempted to Run a way from there."

40 NMM, ADM/E/12, Admiralty to Commissioners, 19 May 1750.

41 Twenty-four communities in 1745: NMM, ADM/F/6, Commissioners to Admiralty, 6 July 1745; twenty-three communities in 1747: NMM, ADM/F/7, "Account of Ordinary Standing Charge of the Office and Officers at the Ports," 17 January 1747.

42 TNA, ADM 98/3, Commissioners to Admiralty, 7 February 1746. The commissioners' office was located at Tower Hill.

43 NMM, ADM/F/6, Commissioners to Admiralty, 6 July 1745.

44 TNA, ADM 98/4, Commissioners to Admiralty, 27 October 1747; TNA, ADM 99/19, 28 February 1748; TNA, ADM 99/20. 4 June 1748; NMM, ADM/F/10, Commissioners to Admiralty, 6 June 1748.

45 CTP, v, 741: Order to issue to the treasurer of the Royal Navy £3,000 for bills of exchange and £8,000 for the sick and hurt, 12 December 1745; NMM, ADM/F/9, "Abstract of the Pay of Rochester, Sheerness, and Deal," 17 March 1747; NMM, ADM/F/9, "Abstract of Payments of Sick Quarters at Plymouth," 28 July 1747; NMM, ADM/F/9, "Abstract of Payments for Sick Quarters for Twelve Months end 30 September 1746," 17 March 1747; NMM, ADM/F/9, "Payment of Gosport Quarters, 16 April 1747," 28 July 1747; TNA, ADM 99/20, 16 April 1748.

46 BL Add MS. 33046, fos. 252v–253r, "An Account of Money granted by Parliament to the service of the Royal Navy, 1735 to 1750."

47 Figures calculated from statements of navy debt, abstracts of the disposition of money given for the naval service, and abstracts of ordinary estimates of naval expenses for the years 1743 to 1750, in CJ, xxiv and xxv.

48 CJ, xxiv, 7 February 1744, 549; 13 February 1744, 563; CJ, xxv, 16 December 1747, 467; 7 March 1749, 771; NMM, ADM/B/127, Navy Board to Admiralty, "An Estimate of the Charge of Building an Hospital at Portsmouth" for the House of Commons, 15 November 1744.

49 NMM, ADM/E/11, Admiralty to Commissioners, 28 April 1744.

50 NMM, ADM/F/4, Commissioners to Admiralty, 1 May 1744.

51 TNA, ADM 3/48, 8 May 1744; NMM, ADM/E/11, Admiralty to Commissioners, 8 May 1744.

232 Notes to pages 168–72

52 TNA, ADM 99/19, 19 February 1746; NMM, ADM/F/7, Commissioners to Admiralty, 19 February 1746; NMM, ADM/E/12, Admiralty to Commissioners, 22 February 1746; TNA, ADM 99/19, 25 February 1746.

53 NMM, ADM/F/4, "Extract of a letter of the 24th Nov'r 1744, from the Physician and Surgeon at Gosport, to the Comm'rs for Sick and Hurt," Commissioners to Admiralty, 28 November 1744.

54 NMM, ADM/E/11, Admiralty to Commissioners, "Extract of a Letter from Captain Shirley ... to Mr Corbett dated in Yarmouth Roads the 21st October 1745," 25 October 1745; NMM, ADM/F/7, Commissioners to Admiralty, 22 November 1745. Brown evidently relied too much on his apprentices to care for seamen.

55 NMM, ADM/F/8, Commissioners to Admiralty, Report on the visitation to Kent ports, 5 April and from 9 April to 2 May 1746, 10 May 1746.

56 NMM, ADM/F/8, Commissioners to Admiralty, 10 May 1746; Hills visited Deptford and Woolwich on 5 April 1746.

57 NMM, ADM/F/8, Commissioners to Admiralty, 10 May 1746; Hills visited Deal 17 to 19 April 1746.

58 NMM, ADM/F/8, Commissioners to Admiralty, 10 May 1746; Hills visited Dover on 21–22 April 1746.

59 NMM, ADM/F/8, Commissioners to Admiralty, 10 May 1746; Hills visited Rochester on 26 April 1746.

60 NMM, ADM/F/8, Commissioners to Admiralty, 10 May 1746; Hills visited Sheerness on 28 April 1746.

61 NMM, ADM/F/9, Commissioners to Admiralty, Report of visitation of Woolwich, Rochester, and Sheerness and payment of sick quarters at those places, Deptford and Deal, 17 March 1747. Hills visited Deptford and Woolwich on 23 February 1747.

62 NMM, ADM/F/9, Commissioners to Admiralty, 17 March 1747. Hills visited Rochester/Chatham on 28 February 1747. The flea problem seems to have been solved.

63 NMM, ADM/F/9, Commissioners to Admiralty, 17 March 1747. Hills visited Sheerness on 12–13 March 1747.

64 NMM, ADM/F/8, Commissioners to Admiralty, Report of Mr Hills late Visitation of the Ports and Places to the Westward, 17 September 1746. Hills visited Fareham on 13–14 May 1746.

65 NMM, ADM/F/8, Commissioners to Admiralty, 17 September 1746. Hills visited Gosport on 15 May 1746.

66 NMM, ADM/F/8, Commissioners to Admiralty, 17 September 1746. Hills visited Forton hospital on 19 May 1746.

67 NMM, ADM/F/8, Commissioners to Admiralty, 17 September 1746. Hills visited the *Blenheim* on 21 May, Southampton on 24–30 May, Weymouth on 2–6 June, Plymouth on 10–17 June 1746.

68 NMM, ADM/F/8, Commissioners to Admiralty, 17 September 1746. Hills visited Bristol on 21 July 1746.

69 NMM, ADM/F/9, Commissioners to Admiralty, Visitation to Gosport, etc., 28 July 1747.

70 NMM, ADM/F/11, Commissioners to Admiralty, Commissioner Hills late Visitation and Payment of the Sick Quarters at Gosport, Southampton and Plymouth, 21 September 1749; TNA, ADM 98/5, 21 September 1749.

71 Kinkel, *Disciplining the Empire*.

72 See above, 98–100.

73 Agamben, *Homo Sacer*, 122.

74 de Vries, "Virtue Ethics," 179.

75 "People," referring to seamen, was a common term in naval documents.

76 TNA, ADM 98/1, Commissioners to Admiralty, 20 June 1744; NMM, ADM/F/4, 20 June 1744.

77 TNA, ADM 99/18, 12 July 1744.

78 Ibid.

79 NMM, ADM/E/8, Rules and Instructions for the better Management of the Sick and Hurt service, 3 June 1740.

80 TNA, ADM 99/18, 16 July 1744.

81 TNA, ADM 99/18, 18 and 20 July 1744.

82 TNA, ADM 99/18, 23 July 1744.

83 NMM, ADM/F/4, Copy of letter of 20th July from Mr Hicks, Surgeon and Agent at Sheerness to the Commissioners for Sick and Hurt Seamen, 21 July 1744; TNA, ADM 99/18, 21 July 1744.

84 NMM, ADM/F/4, Commissioners to Admiralty, 21 July 1744.

85 TNA, ADM 99/18, 25 July 1744.

86 TNA, ADM 7/340, Admiralty Memorials and Reports, 15 September 1744, Copy of William Martin to Admiral Sir John Balchen, 24 July 1744.

87 NMM, ADM/F/7, 10 March 1746, Copy of N. Hills, "Report on the particular Enquires I made on my Visitation of the Hospital and Sick Quarters at Gosport," 26 July 1744.

88 NMM, ADM/F/4, 27 July 1744.

89 TNA, ADM 99/18, 14 September 1744.

90 Ibid.

91 Pace Harland, "First Hospitals," 429.

92 Innes, "Governing Diverse Societies," 103–40; Nicholls, *The Politics of Alcohol*, 59, 40–5; Rogers, *Mayhem*, 151–7, 146; Withington, "Introduction," 9–33.

93 Cobbett, *Parliamentary History of England*, 1294.

94 TNA, ADM 7/340, Admiralty Memorials and Reports, Admiralty to the King: Proposal to erect hospitals at Chatham, Portsmouth, and Plymouth, 15 September 1744.

234   Notes to pages 179–83

95 TNA, PC 2/98, 18 September 1744.

96 TNA, PC 2/98, 20 September 1744.

97 TNA, PC 2/98, 7 November 1744.

98 TNA, ADM 1/3529, Commissioners to Admiralty, 21 July 1741.

99 TNA, ADM 99/19, 28 May 1745.

100 Smith, *What Is a Person?* 138.

101 See Innes's argument about the *"real* focus of concern" underlying Hanoverian attempts to regulate gin consumption, "Governing Diverse Societies," 130–1 (italics mine). On expressive individualism, see Taylor, *A Secular Age*, 275.

102 Much as this failure to promote the seaman's right to define his own concept of existence might be taken as a moral failing by many modern scholars, Smith, *The Sacred Project*, 13–16.

103 Foucault, *History of Sexuality*, 78–9.

104 Sienna, *Venereal Disease*, 86–9, 123–5; Charters, *Disease, War, and the Imperial State*, 92.

105 Schoenfeldt, *Bodies and Selves*, 158; Dwyer, *Ordered Society*, 170.

106 Foucault, *Birth of Biopolitics*, 317–25; Foucault, *Society Must Be Defended*, 35, 242–8.

107 Wilson, "German Women at War;" Pelling, "Far Too Many Women?" 695–719.

108 TNA, ADM 98/103, Admiralty Instructions to Commissioners, 8 February 1742.

109 TNA, ADM 7/340, Admiralty Memorials and Reports, 15 September 1744, Copy of William Martin to Admiral Sir John Balchen, 24 July 1744.

110 Swingen, *Competing Visions of Empire*, 159–60, 171.

111 Pace Kinkel, *Disciplining the Empire*; Rodger, *The Wooden World*, 210.

112 O'Brien, "Taxation for British Mercantilism," 295–355.

113 Brewer, *Sinews of Power*; Pincus and Robinson, "Wars and State-Making Reconsidered," 9–34.

114 Kocka, *Capitalism*, 64.

115 NMM, ADM/F/8, 10 May 1746: Commissioner Hills's report: 5 April visit to Woolwich, 19 April visit to Deal, 28 April to Sheerness.

116 NMM, ADM/F/9, 28 July 1747: Commissioner Hills's report: 3–4 April visit to Gosport.

117 NMM, ADM/F/8, 17 September 1746: Commissioner Hills's report: 13–14 May visit to Gosport.

118 NMM, ADM/E/11, Admiralty to Commissioners, 18 June 1745: List of Officers and Servants proposed to have Lodgings in the Hospital at Portsmouth.

119 TNA, ADM 99/18, 25 September and 1 October 1744.

120 TNA, ADM 99/19, 5 and 10 June 1746.

121 TNA, ADM 3/58, 20 October 1747; NMM, ADM/E/12, Admiralty to Commissioners, 20 October 1747.

Notes to pages 183–91

122 NMM, ADM/F/11, Commissioners to Admiralty, 27 May 1754.
123 TNA, ADM 99/19, 29 May 1746; NMM, ADM/F/8, Commissioners to Admiralty, 29 May 1746; TNA, ADM 99/19, 4 June 1746.
124 TNA, ADM 99/19, 18 June 1746.
125 NMM, ADM/F/8, Commissioners to Admiralty, 29 May 1746.
126 NMM, ADM/F/8, 17 September 1746: Commissioner Hills's report: 19 May visit to Gosport.
127 NMM, ADM/F/9, 28 July 1747: Commissioners Hills's report: 27 June visit to *Enterprise* hospital ship.
128 Withington, "Introduction," 14.
129 Spinney, "Servants to the Hospital and State," 3–19.
130 NMM, ADM/F/8, 17 September 1746: Commissioner Hills's report: 13–14 May visit to Fareham.
131 NMM, ADM/F/8, 17 September 1746: Commissioner Hills's report: 19 May visit to Forton; 21 May visit to the *Blenheim*.
132 NMM, ADM/F/9, 28 July 1747: Commissioner Hills's report: 2 April visit to the *Blenheim* and the *Chester*.
133 NMM, ADM/F/8, 17 September 1746; Commissioner Hills's report: 16 June visit to Plymouth.
134 NMM, ADM/F/11, 21 September 1749: Commissioner Hills's report: 21–22 July visit to Gosport.

CONCLUSION

1 Low, *Gibbon's Journal*, 187; Thomas, "Jack Tar, Mr Sawbones, and the Local Community," 291.
2 NMM, ADM/E/46, Admiralty to Commissioners, "Report of the state of Yarmouth hospital," 15 May 1797.
3 *The Gentleman's Magazine*, 408.
4 Harland, "First Hospitals," 436.
5 Lloyd and Coulter, *Medicine and the Navy*, 192.
6 Indeed, at places where no naval medical infrastructure existed, the contract system for care in England endured into the 1970s: Brown, *Poxed and Scurvied*, 68.
7 Instrumental rationality: Eisenstadt, "Multiple Modernities," 8.
8 The great ports were also served by hospital ships from Queen Anne's War.
9 Hickey, *Local Hospitals in Ancien Regime France*, 4.
10 Hacking, *Social Construction of What?* 67–80.
11 Porpora, *Reconstructing Sociology*, 46–57, 118–20.
12 Robinson and Gallagher, *Africa and the Victorians*, 19–21; Cook, "Practical Medicine."
13 Scott, *Seeing Like a State*, 53–83.
14 Wegner, *Theorizing Modernity*, 4.

236   Notes to pages 191–5

15 Rodger, "From 'Military Revolution.'"

16 Wrightson, *Earthly Necessities*, 26.

17 Buchet, *British Navy, Economy, and Society*, 25–46, 90–104; North et al., *Violence and Social Orders*, 183–5.

18 Stobart, *Household Medicine*, 20; Spinney, "Servants to the Hospital and State," 3–19.

19 Torres Sanchez, *Military Entrepreneurs*, 39–40, 230–1.

20 Convertito, "Mending the Sick and Wounded," 500–33.

21 Foucault, *Security, Territory, Population*, 68–72, 104–9; Collins, "The State," 215–41.

22 Haycock, *Health and Medicine at Sea*; McLean, "Health Provision in the Royal Navy," 107–28.

23 Hunt, "Women and the Fiscal-Imperial State," 29–47; Murphy, "'A Water Bawdy House,'" 173–92.

24 Gruber von Arni, "Who Cared?" 121–48; Godden and Helmstadter, *Nursing before Nightingale*.

25 I owe this point to one of this book's anonymous readers.

26 See Spinney, "Naval and Military Nursing," and "Servants to the Hospital and State."

27 An internet search of the term "care work" for the period 1 March to 30 May 2020 brings up over forty million hits.

28 Chatzidakis et al., *The Care Manifesto*; Goodhart, *Head Hand Heart*.

29 Simpson, *Chronic Condition*, 368.

30 Charters, *Disease, War, and the Imperial State*, 176–80.

31 Churchill, "Responses to Non-European Bodies in British Military Medicine, 1780–1815," 149.

32 Mark Harrison, *British Military Medicine in the Second World War*, 24–5.

33 Bunting, *Labours of Love*, viii.

34 Richards, "Women in the British Economy," 337–57; Gamarnikow, "The Sexual Division of Labour," 97–123; Thomas, "Women and Capitalism," 534–49; Hudson and Lee, "Introduction," 2–47; Honeyman and Goodman, "Women's Work, Gender Conflict, and Labour Markets," 608–28; Simonton, *History of European Women's Work*, 17, 63, 73, 82; Whittle and Haliwood, "Gender Division of Labour," 3–32.

35 Del Noce, "Violence and Modern Gnosticism," 20–3; 36, 44–5.

36 Bunting, *Labours of Love*, 26; 250–1.

37 Bachiochi, *Rights of Women*, 269–75.

38 Smith, *Atheist Overreach*, 9–43.

39 Glete, *War and the State*, 51.

40 Graham and Walsh, "Introduction," 34.

41 Newton, "Inside the Sick Chambers," 530, 542.

Bibliography

MANUSCRIPTS AND PRINTED PRIMARY SOURCES

Bodleian Library, University of Oxford (Bodl. Lib.)
MS Rawlinson A

British Library, London (BL)
Additional MS
Harley MS
Sloane MS

Cambridge University Library (CUL)
Cholmondeley (Houghton) MS 12.

Devon Heritage Centre, Exeter (DHC)
QS. Devon Quarter Sessions

Kent History and Library Centre, Maidstone (KHC)
PRC. Canterbury Probate Records, 1396–1895.
QSO. Kent Quarter Sessions, 1595–1973.

London Metropolitan Archives (LMA)
HO1/ST. Saint Thomas' Hospital

The National Archives, London (TNA)
ADM 1. Admiralty. Correspondence and Papers.
ADM 2. Admiralty. Out-Letters.
ADM 3. Admiralty. Minutes.
ADM 7. Admiralty. Miscellanea.
ADM 97. Office of the Commissioners of Sick and Wounded Seamen. In-Letters.
ADM 98. Office of the Commissioners of Sick and Wounded Seamen. Out-Letters.
ADM 99. Office of the Commissioners of Sick and Wounded Seamen. Minutes.

ADM 106. Navy Board. Records.
AO. Auditors of the Imprest and Commissioners of Audit.
PC 2. Privy Council Registers.
PC 6. Privy Council Office. Miscellaneous Books and Correspondence Registers.
SO 8. Signet Office: Warrants for King's Bills, Series I.
SP 18. Council of State, Navy Commission and Related Bodies: Orders and Papers.
SP 42. Secretaries of State. State Papers Naval.
T 1. Treasury. Treasury Board Papers and In-Letters.
T 27. Treasury. General Out-Letter Books.
T 29. Treasury Board. Minutes.
T 38. Treasury. Departmental Accounts.
T 61. Treasury. Disposition Books.

National Maritime Museum, London (NMM)
ADM/B. Board of Admiralty. In-Letters from the Navy Board, 1738–1809.
ADM/E. Sick and Hurt Board. In-Letters and Orders.
ADM/F. Board of Admiralty. In-Letters from the Sick and Hurt Board, 1742–1806.
CAD/A. Central Administration of the Royal Navy. Admiralty Instructions, Papers, and General Accounts.
CLI. Clifford Papers.
POR. Portsmouth Dockyard Manuscripts.
SER. Sergison Papers.

Pepys Library, Magdalen College, Cambridge (PL)
Pepys MS.

Kenneth Spencer Research Library, Lawrence, Kansas (SRL)
MS 129

Royal Navy Museum, Portsmouth (RNM)
Corbett Manuscripts 121

St Bartholomew's Hospital Archives and Museum, London (SBHA)
SBHA/HA/1. Minutes of the Board of Governors.

Suffolk Archives (SA)
HD36. Ipswich Borough Correspondence.

Wiltshire and Swindon History Centre, Chippenham, UK (WSHC)
865. Chafn Grove Family of Zeals. Bullen Reymes Papers.

Bibliography

Baston, Samuel. A Dialogue between a Modern Courtier and an Honest English Gentleman. London: 1696, n.p.

– A Dialogue Between a Modern Courtier, And an Honest English Gentleman. To Which is Added the Author's Dedications to Both Houses of Parliament, To Whom He Appeals for Justice. London: n.p., 1697.

Calendar of State Papers. Domestic series of the reign of William and Mary: Preserved in the Public Record Office. [Vols. 1–11] Edited by William John Hardy. England: H.M. Stationery Office, 1895–1937. (*CSPD*)

Calendar of Treasury Papers, 1556–[1728] Preserved in Public Record Office. [Vols. 1–6] Prepared by Joseph Redington. England: Longmans, Green, Reader, and Dyer, 1868–89. (*CTP*)

Calendar of Treasury Books, 1660–1718. Preserved in the Public Record Office [Vols. 1–32]. England: H.M. Stationery Office, 1904–. (*CTB*)

Gibson, Richard. *Publick services in, or relating to the Royal Navy; wherein Mr. Richard Gibson, has been employed since the year of our Lord 1652* (London, c. 1712).

Journals of the House of Commons, 1547–. Edited by Edgar L. Erickson. England: H.M. Stationery Office. (*CJ*)

Letters and Papers Relating to the First Dutch War, 1652–1654; Volume 3. Edited by Samuel Rawson Gardiner. England: Printed for the Navy Records Society, 1906. (*FDW, 3*)

Letters and Papers Relating to the First Dutch War, 1652–1654; Volume 4. Edited by C.T. Atkinson. England: Printed for the Navy Records Society, 1910. (*FDW, 4*)

"Volume 34: 21 March 1653." In *Calendar of State Papers Domestic: Interregnum, 1652-3*, edited by Mary Anne Everett Green. London: Her Majesty's Stationery Office, 1878. Accessed on *British History Online*, http://www.british-history.ac.uk/cal-state-papers/domestic/interregnum/1652-3.

"Volume 40: September 1653." In *Calendar of State Papers Domestic: Interregnum, 1653-4*, edited by Mary Anne Everett Green. London: Her Majesty's Stationery Office, 1879. Accessed on *British History Online*, http://www.british-history.ac.uk/cal-state-papers/domestic/interregnum/1653-4.

SECONDARY SOURCES

Agamben, Giorgio. *Homo Sacer: Sovereign Power and Bare Life*. Translated by Daniel Heller-Roazen. Stanford, CA: Stanford University Press, 1998.

Alsop, J.D. "Sickness in the British Mediterranean Fleet: The *Tiger*'s Journal of 1706." *War and Society* 11, no. 2 (1993): 57–76.

Anderson, Gary M., and Adam Gifford, Jr. "Privateering and the Private Production of Naval Power." *Cato Journal* 11, no. 1 (1991): 99–122.

Appleby, David J., and Andrew Hopper, eds. *Battle-Scarred: Mortality, Medical Care, and Military Welfare in the British Civil Wars*. Manchester, UK: Manchester University Press, 2018.

Arnold, Dana. *The Spaces of the Hospital: Spatiality and Urban Change in London, 1680–1820*. London: Routledge, 2013.

Asch, Ronald G. "War and State Building." In *European Warfare, 1350–1750*, edited by Frank Tallett and David Trim, 322–37. New York: Cambridge University Press, 2010.

Bachiochi, Erika. *The Rights of Women: Reclaiming a Lost Vision*. South Bend, IN: Notre Dame University Press, 2021.

Baker, Philip. "Parish Nurses and Their Clients: The State of Welfare Provision in Early Modern St Botolph Aldgate." Paper presented at the Economic History Society Conference, Cambridge, 2010.

Baugh, Daniel A. *British Naval Administration in the Age of Walpole*. Princeton, NJ: Princeton University Press, 1965.

– "The Eighteenth-Century Navy as a National Institution, 1690–1815." In *The Oxford Illustrated History of the Royal Navy*, edited by J.R. Hill, 120–60. New York: Oxford University Press, 1995.

– "Great Britain's 'Blue Water' Policy, 1689–1815." *International History Review* 10, no. 1 (1988): 33–58.

– "The Professionalization of the English Navy and Its Administration, 1660–1750." In *The Sea in History: The Early Modern World*, edited by Christian Buchet and Gerard Le Bouedec, 852–66. Woodbridge, UK: Boydell, 2017.

Bayly, C.A. *The Birth of the Modern World: 1780–1914*. Oxford: Blackwell, 2004.

Beckert, Sven. *Empire of Cotton: A Global History*. New York: Knopf, 2014.

Beckett, John V. "Land Tax or Excise: The Levying of Taxation in Seventeenth- and Eighteenth-Century England." *English Historical Review* 100, no. 395 (1985): 285–308.

Bennett, Judith M. "History That Stands Still: Women's Work in the European Past." *Feminist Studies* 14, no. 2 (1988): 269–83.

Binney, John. *British Public Finance and Administration: 1774–92*. Oxford: Clarendon, 1958.

Black, Jeremy. "British Naval Power and International Commitments, 1688–1770." In *Parameters of British Naval Power, 1650–1850*, edited by Michael Duffy, 39–59. Exeter: University of Exeter, 1992.

– *British Politics and Foreign Policy in the Age of George II, 1727–1744*. Farnham, UK: Ashgate, 2014.

Blakemore, Richard J., and James Davey, eds. *The Maritime World of Early Modern Britain*. Amsterdam: Amsterdam University Press, 2020.

Boris, Eileen, and Jennifer Klein. *Caring for America: Home Health Workers in the Shadow of the Welfare State*. New York: Oxford University Press, 2012.

Boulton, Jeremy. "Welfare Systems and the Parish Nurse in Early Modern London, 1650–1725." *Family and Community History* 10, no. 2 (2007): 127–51.

Bowen, H.V. "Forum: The Contractor State, c. 1650–1815." *International Journal of Maritime History* 25, no. 1 (June 2013): 239–42.

Bibliography

Braddick, Michael J. "Administrative Performance: The Representation of Political Authority in Early Modern England." In *Negotiating Power in Early Modern Society: Order, Hierarchy, and Subordination in Britain and Ireland*, edited by Michael J. Braddick and John Walter, 166–87. Cambridge: Cambridge University Press, 2001.

– "The English Revolution and Its Legacies." In *The English Revolution, c. 1590–1720: Politics, Religion, and Communities*, edited by Nicholas Tyacke, 27–44. Manchester, UK: Manchester University Press, 2007.

– "State Formation and Social Change in Early Modern England: A Problem Stated and Approaches Suggested." *Social History* 16, no. 1 (1991): 1–17.

– *State Formation in Early Modern England c. 1550–1700*. Cambridge: Cambridge University Press, 2000.

Brewer, John. *The Sinews of Power: War, Money, and the English State, 1688–1783*. Cambridge, MA: Harvard University Press, 1989.

Brockliss, Laurence W.B., and Colin Jones. *The Medical World of Early Modern France*. Oxford: Oxford University Press, 1997.

Brown, Kathleen. *Foul Bodies: Cleanliness in Early America*. New Haven, CT: Yale University Press, 2009.

Brown, Kevin. *Poxed and Scurvied: The Story of Sickness and Health at Sea*. Annapolis, MD: Naval Institute Press, 2009.

Bruijn, J.R. "States and Their Navies: From the Late Sixteenth to the End of the Eighteenth Centuries." In *War and Competition between States*, edited by P. Contamine, 69–98. Oxford: Oxford University Press, 2000.

Buchet, Christian. *The British Navy, Economy, and Society in the Seven Years War*. Woodbridge, UK: Boydell Press, 2013.

Buhler-Wilkinson, Karen. *No Place Like Home: A History of Nursing and Home Care in the United States*. Baltimore, MD: Johns Hopkins University Press, 2001.

Bunting, Madeline. *Labours of Love: The Crisis of Care*. London: Granta, 2020.

Burnard, Trever, and Giorgio Riello. "Slavery and the New History of Capitalism." *Journal of Global History* 15, no. 2 (2020): 224–44.

Capp, Bernard. *Cromwell's Navy: The Fleet and the English Revolution, 1648–1660*. Oxford: Clarendon Press, 1989.

Carr, David. *Time, Narrative, and History*. Bloomington: Indiana University Press, 1986.

Charters, Erica. *Disease, War, and the Imperial State: The Welfare of the British Armed Forces During the Seven Years' War*. Chicago: University of Chicago Press, 2014.

– "'The Intention Is Certain Noble': The Western Squadron, Medical Trials, and the Sick and Hurt Board during the Seven Years' War (1756–63)." In *Health and Medicine at Sea, 1700–1900*, edited by David Boyd Haycock and Sally Archer, 19–37. Woodbridge, UK: Boydell, 2009.

Chatzidakis, Andreas, Jo Litter, Catherine Rottenberg, and Jamie Hakim. *The Care Manifesto: The Politics of Interdependence*. London: Verso Books, 2020.

Churchill, Wendy. "Efficient, Efficacious, and Humane: Responses to Non-European Bodies in British Military Medicine, 1780–1815." *The Journal of Imperial and Commonwealth History* 40, no. 2 (2012): 137–58.

Clay, C.G.A. *Public Finance and Private Wealth: The Career of Sir Stephen Fox, 1627–1716*. Oxford: Oxford University Press, 1978.

Claydon, Tony. *Europe and the Making of England, 1660–1760*. Cambridge: Cambridge University Press, 2007.

Cobbett, William. *Parliamentary History of England*. Vol. 12. London: R. Bagshaw, 1806–1820.

Coleby, Andrew. "Military-Civilian Relations on the Solent, 1651–1689." *Historical Journal* 29, no. 4 (1986): 949–61.

Collier, Andrew. *Critical Realism: An Introduction to Roy Bhaskar's Philosophy*. London: Verso, 1994.

Collinge, J.M. *Office-Holders in Modern Britain*. Vol. 7: *Navy Board Officials, 1660–1832*. London: Institute for Historical Research, 1978.

Collins, James B. "The State." In *Interpreting Early Modern Europe*, edited by Beat Kümin and C. Scott Dixon, 215–41. London: Taylor and Francis, 2019.

Convertito, Cori. "Mending the Sick and Wounded: The Development of Naval Hospitals in the West Indies, 1740–1800." *Canadian Journal of History* 51, no. 3 (2016): 500–33.

Conway, Stephen. "Checking and Controlling British Military Expenditure, 1739–1783." In *War, State, and Development: Fiscal-Military States in the Eighteenth Century*, edited by Rafael Torres Sanchez, 45–68. Pamplona, Spain: Eusna, 2007.

– *War, State, and Society in Mid-Eighteenth Century Britain and Ireland*. Oxford: Oxford University Press, 2006.

Cook, Harold J. "Practical Medicine and the British Armed Forces after the 'Glorious Revolution.'" *Medical History* 34, no. 1 (1990): 1–26.

Cooter, Roger. "Introduction." In *War, Medicine, and Modernity*, edited by Roger Cooter, Mark Harrison, and Steve Sturdy, 3–18. Stroud, UK: Sutton, 1998.

– "War and Modern Medicine." In *Companion Encyclopedia of the History of Medicine*, edited by Roy Porter and W.F. Bynum, 1536–74. New York: Routledge, 1994.

Coulter, J.L.S., and C. Lloyd. *Medicine and the Navy*. Vol. 3. Edinburgh: E. and S. Livingstone, 1963.

Crawford, Catherine. "Patients' Rights and the Laws of Contract in Eighteenth-Century England." *Social History of Medicine* 13, no. 3 (2000): 381–410.

Crimmin, Patricia K. "British Naval Health, 1700–1800: Improvement over Time?" In *British Military and Naval Medicine, 1600–1830*, edited by Geoffrey L. Hudson, 183–200. Amsterdam: Rodopi, 2007.

– "The Sick and Hurt Board: Fit For Purpose?" In *Health and Medicine at Sea, 1700–1900*, edited by David Boyd Haycock and Sally Archer, 90–107. Woodbridge, UK: Boydell, 2009.

- "The Sick and Hurt Board and the Health of Seamen c. 1700–1806." *Journal of Maritime Research* 1, no. 1 (1999): 48–65.

Davey, James. "Navigating State and Society: New Naval Histories of the Long Eighteenth Century." *English Historical Review* 128, no. 565 (December 2018): 1546–62.

Davies, Celica. *Gender and the Professional Predicament of Nursing*. Briston, PA: Open University Press, 1995.

De Krey, Gary. *Restoration and Revolution in Britain*. Basingstoke, UK: Palgrave, 2007.

de la Béydoyère, Guy, ed. *Particular Friends: The Correspondence of Samuel Pepys and John Evelyn*. Woodbridge, UK: Boydell, 1997.

de Vries, Peer. "Virtue Ethics in the Military: An Attempt at Completeness." *Journal of Military Ethics* 19, no. 3 (July 2020): 170–85.

Del Noce, Augusto. "Violence and Modern Gnosticism." In *The Crisis of Modernity*, by Augusto Del Noce, edited and translated by Carlo Lancellotti, 19–48. Montreal and Kingston: McGill-Queen's University Press, 2014.

Dean, C.G.T. "Charles II's Garrison Hospital, Portsmouth." *Papers and Proceedings of the Hampshire Field Club* 16, no. 3 (1947): 280–3.

Deringer, William. *Calculated Values: Finance, Politics, and the Quantitative Age*. Cambridge, MA: Harvard University Press, 2018.

Des Jardins, Julie. "Women's and Gender History." In *The Oxford History of Historical Writing*. Vol, 5: *Historical Writing since 1945*, edited by Axel Schneider and Daniel Woolf, 136–58. Oxford: Oxford University Press, 2011.

Desan, Christine. *Making Money: Coin, Currency, and the Coming of Capitalism*. Oxford: Oxford University Press, 2014.

Dickson, P.G.M. *The Financial Revolution in England: A Study of the Development of Public Credit, 1688–1756*. London: Macmillan, 1967.

Dickson, P.G.M., and John Sperling. "War Finance, 1689–1714." In *The New Cambridge Modern History*. Vol. 6: *The Rise of Great Britain and Russia, 1688–1715/25*, edited by J.S. Bromley, 284–315. Cambridge: Cambridge University Press, 1971.

Donagan, Barbara. *War in England, 1642–1649*. Oxford: Oxford University Press, 2004.

Dooley, Chris. "'They Gave Their Care, but We Gave Loving Care': Defining and Defending Boundaries of Skill and Craft in the Nursing Service of a Manitoba Mental Hospital during the Great Depression." *Canadian Bulletin of Medical History* 21, no. 2 (2004): 229–51.

Downing, Brian M. "Constitutionalism, Warfare, and Political Change in Early Modern Europe." *Theory and Society* 17, no. 1 (January 1988): 7–56.

Duffin, Jacalyn. *A History of Medicine: A Scandalously Short Introduction*. Basingstoke, UK: Macmillan, 2004.

Bibliography

Duffy, Michael. "The Establishment of Western Squadron as the Linchpin of British Naval Strategy." In *Parameters of British Naval Power, 1650–1850*, edited by M. Duffy, 60–81. Exeter: Exeter University Press, 1992.

Dwyer, Susan. *An Ordered Society: Gender and Class in Early Modern England*. New York: Columbia University, 1993.

Earle, Peter. "The Female Labour Market in London in the Late Seventeenth and Early Eighteenth Centuries." *Economic History Review* 42, no. 3 (1989): 328–78.

Ehrman, J. *The Navy in the War of William III*. Cambridge: Cambridge University Press, 1953.

Eisenstadt, S.N. "Multiple Modernities." *Daedalus* 129, no. 1 (2000): 1–29.

Elliott, John H. "The Road to Utrecht: War and Peace." In *Britain, Spain, and the Treaty of Utrecht, 1713–2013*, edited by Trevor J. Dadson and J.H. Elliott, 3–8. London: Routledge, 2014.

Eltis, David, and Stanley L. Engerman. "The Importance of Slavery and the Slave Trade to Industrializing Britain." *Journal of Economic History* 60, no. 1 (2000): 123–44.

England, Kim, and Isabel Dyck. "Managing the Body Work of Home Care." In *Body Work in Health and Social Care*, edited by Julia Twigg, Carol Wolkowitz, Rachel Lara Cohen, and Sara Nettleton, 36–49. Malden, MA: Wiley-Blackwell, 2011.

Finer, Samuel. "State and Nation Building in Europe: The Role of the Military." In *The Formation of National States in Western Europe*, edited by Charles Tilly and Gabriel Ardant, 84–163. Princeton, NJ: Princeton University Press, 1975.

Fissell, Mary E. "Introduction: Women, Health, and Healing in Early Modern Europe." *Bulletin of the History of Medicine* 82, no. 1 (2008): 1–17.

Foucault, Michel. *The Birth of Biopolitics: Lectures at the Collège de France, 1978–79*. Translated by Graham Burchell. Basingstoke, UK: Palgrave, 1999.

– *The Government of Self and Others: Lectures at the Collège de France, 1982–1983*. Translated by Graham Burchell. Basingstoke, UK: Palgrave Macmillan, 2011.

– *The History of Sexuality*. Vol. 2: *The Uses of Pleasure*. Translated by Robert Hurley. New York: Pantheon, 1985.

– *Security, Territory, Population: Lectures at the Collège de France, 1977–78*. Edited by Michel Senellart. Translated by Graham Burchell. New York: St Martin's Press, 2007.

– *"Society Must Be Defended": Lectures at the Collège de France, 1975–76*. Edited by Mauro Bertani and Allesandro Fontana. Translated by David Macey. New York: St Martin's Press, 2003.

Fury, Cheryl. "Health and Health Care at Sea." In *The Social History of English Seamen, 1485–1649*, edited by Cheryl Fury, 193–227. Woodbridge, UK: Boydell, 2012.

Gabriel, Richard A. *Between Flesh and Steel: A History of Military Medicine from the Middle Ages to the War in Afghanistan*. Lincoln, NB: Potomac Books, 2013.

Bibliography

Gamarnikow, Eva. "The Sexual Division of Labour: The Case of Nursing." In *Feminism and Materialism: Women and Modes of Production*, edited by Annette Kuhn and Ann Marie Wolpe, 97–123. London: Routledge and Kegan Paul, 1978.

The Gentleman's Magazine 21 (1751): 408.

Gibson, James J. "The Theory of Affordances." In *Perceiving, Acting, and Knowing: Toward an Ecological Psychology*, edited by R. Shaw and J. Bransford, 67–82. Hillsdale, NJ: Lawrence Erlbaum, 1977.

Girard, René. *Battling to the End: Conversations with Benoît Chantre*. Translated by Mary Baker. East Lansing: Michigan State University Press, 2010.

Glete, Jan. *Navies and Nations: Warships, Navies, and State Building in Europe and America, 1500–1860*. Vol. 2. Stockholm: Almqvist and Wiksell, 1993.

– *War and the State in Early Modern Europe: Spain, the Dutch Republic, and Sweden as Fiscal-Military States*. New York: Routledge, 2002.

– "Warfare, Entrepreneurship, and the Fiscal-Military State." In *European Warfare, 1350–1750*, edited by Frank Tallett and David Trim, 300–21. New York: Cambridge University Press, 2010.

Godden, Judith, and Carol Helmstadter. *Nursing before Nightingale, 1815–1899*. London: Taylor and Francis, 2016.

Goodhart, David. *Head Hand Heart: The Struggle for Dignity and Status in the 21st Century*. London: Penguin Books, 2021.

Gorski, Philip. *The Disciplinary Revolution: Calvinism and the Rise of the State in Early Modern Europe*. Chicago: University of Chicago Press, 2003.

Graham, Aaron. "Auditing Leviathan: Corruption and State Formation in Early Eighteenth-Century Britain." *English Historical Review* 128, no. 533 (August 2013): 806–38.

– *Corruption, Party, and Government in Britain, 1702–1713*. New York: Oxford University Press, 2015.

– "Credit, Confidence, and the Circulation of Exchequer Bills in the Early Financial Revolution." *Financial History Review* 26, no. 1 (2019): 63–80.

– "War and Society in Early Modern Europe." In *The Routledge History of Global War and Society*, edited by Matthew S. Muehlbauer and David J. Ulbrich, 91–102. London: Routledge, 2018.

Graham, Aaron, and Patrick Walsh. "Introduction." In *The British Fiscal-Military States, 1660–c. 1783*, edited by Aaron Graham and Patrick Walsh, 1–26. London: Routledge, 2016.

Grant, George. *Technology and Justice*. Toronto: House of Anansi Press, 1991.

Grell, Ole Peter. "War, Medicine, and the Military Revolution." In *The Healing Arts: Health, Disease, and Society in Europe*, edited by Peter Elmer, 257–83. Manchester: Manchester University Press, 2004.

Grose, F. *A Classical Dictionary of the Vulgar Tongue*. 1st ed. London: S. Hooper, 1785.

Bibliography

Gruber von Arni, Eric. *Justice to the Maimed Soldier: Nursing, Medical Care, and Welfare for Sick and Wounded Soldiers and Their Families during the English Civil War and Interregnum, 1642–1660*. Burlington, VT: Ashgate, 2001.

– "Soldiers-at-Sea and Inter-Service Relations during the First Dutch War." *Mariner's Mirror* 87, no. 4 (2001): 406–19.

– "Who Cared? Military Nursing during the English Civil Wars and Interregnum, 1642–60." In *British Military and Naval Medicine, 1600–1830*, edited by Geoffrey Hudson, 149–82. Amsterdam: Rodopi, 2007.

Hacker, Barton C. "Women and Military Institutions in Early Modern Europe." *Signs* 6, no. 4 (1981): 643–71.

Hacking, Ian. *The Social Construction of What?* Cambridge, MA: Harvard University Press, 2000.

Hainsworth, D.R., ed. *The Correspondence of Sir John Lowther of Whitehaven, 1693–1698: A Provincial Community in Wartime*. Records of Social and Economic History, n.s., 7. London: Published for the British Academy by the Oxford University Press, 1983.

Harding, Nick. *Hanover and the British Empire, 1700–1837*. Woodbridge, UK: Boydell and Brewer, 2007.

Harding, Richard. "British Maritime Strategy and Hanover." In *The Hanoverian Dimension in British History, 1714–1837*, edited by Brendan Simms and Torsten Riotte, 252–74. Cambridge: Cambridge University Press, 2007.

– *The Emergence of Britain's Global Naval Supremacy: The War of 1739–1748*. Woodbridge, UK: Boydell, 2010.

– *Modern Naval History: Debates and Prospects*. London: Bloomsbury Academic, 2016.

– *Seapower and Naval Warfare, 1650–1830*. Annapolis, MD: Naval Institute Press, 1999.

Harkness, Deborah E. "A View from the Streets: Women and Medical Work in Elizabethan London." *Bulletin of the History of Medicine* 82 no. 1 (2005): 52–85.

Harland, Kathleen. "The Establishment and Administration of the First Hospitals in the Royal Navy, 1650–1745." PhD diss., University of Exeter, 2003.

Harris, Tim. *Restoration: Charles II and His Kingdoms, 1660–1685*. London: Allen Lane, 2005.

– *Revolution: The Great Crisis of the British Monarchy, 1685–1720*. London: Penguin, 2007.

Harrison, Mark. "Medicine and the Management of Modern Warfare." *History of Science* 34, no. 4 (1996): 379–410.

– *Medicine and Victory : British Military Medicine in the Second World War*. New York: Oxford University Press, 2004.

Hartog, Hendrik. *Someday All This Will Be Yours: A History of Inheritance and Old Age*. Cambridge, MA: Harvard University Press, 2012.

Bibliography

Hattendorf, John B. "Berkeley, James, third earl of Berkeley (1680–1736), naval officer." In *Oxford Dictionary of National Biography*. Oxford: University of Oxford Press, 2004. https://www-oxforddnb-com.cyber.usask.ca.

– "The Struggle with France, 1690–1815." In *Oxford Illustrated History of the Royal Navy*, edited by J.R. Hill, 80–119. Oxford: Oxford University Press, 1995.

Held, Virginia. "Care and the Extension of Markets." *Hypatia* 17, no. 2 (2002): 19–33.

Helling, Colin George. "Convoy of Scottish Trade by the English Royal Navy on the Eve of the Union of 1707." *Journal of British Studies* 59, no. 1 (2020): 101–20.

Hess, Volker, and Andrew Mendelsohn. "Case and Series: Medical Knowledge and Paper Technology, 1600–1900." *History of Science* 48, nos 3–4 (2010): 287–314.

Hickey, Daniel. *Local Hospitals in Ancien Regime France: Rationalization, Resistance, and Renewal, 1530–1789*. Montreal and Kingston: McGill-Queen's University Press, 1997.

Hilt, Eric. "Economic History, Historical Analysis, and the 'New History of Capitalism.'" *Journal of Economic History* 77, no. 2 (2017): 511–36.

Himmelweit, Susan. "Caring Labor." *Annals of the American Academy of Political and Social Science* 561, no. 1 (1999): 27–38.

Hindle, Steve. "Civility, Honesty, and the Identification of the Deserving Poor in Seventeenth Century England." In *Identity and Agency in England, 1500–1800*, edited by Henry French and Jonathan Barry, 38–59. Basingstoke, UK: Macmillan, 2004.

– *On the Parish? The Micro-Politics of Poor Relief in Rural England, c. 1550–1750*. Oxford: Oxford University Press, 2004.

Honeyman, K., and J. Goodman. "Women's Work, Gender Conflict, and Labour Markets in Europe, 1500–1900." *Economic History Review*, new series 44, no. 4 (November 1991): 608–28.

Hoppit, Julian. "Checking the Leviathan, 1688–1832." In *The Political Economy of British Historical Experience, 1688–1914*, edited by Donald Winch and Patrick O'Brien, 267–94. Oxford: Published for the British Academy by Oxford University Press, 2002.

Huard, P., and P. Niaussat. "Les hôpitaux de la marine française au XVIIIe siècle." In *La médécine hospitalière français au XVIIIe siècle: Colloque de l'Institut d'histoire de la médecine et de la pharmacie de l'Université René Descartes, Paris, 6 Octobre 1977*. Strasbourg: Université Louis Pasteur, 1980.

Hubbard, Eleanor. *Englishmen at Sea: Labor and the Nation at the Dawn of Empire, 1570–1630*. New Haven, CT: Yale University Press, 2021.

Hudson, Geoffrey L. "Internal Influences in the Making of the English Military Hospital." In *British Military and Naval Medicine, 1600–1830*, edited by Geoffrey L. Hudson, 253–72. New York: Rodopi, 2007.

– "The Relief of English Disabled Ex-Sailors, c. 1590–1680." In *The Social History of English Seamen, 1485–1649*, edited by Cheryl Fury, 229–52. Woodbridge, UK: Boydell and Brewer, 2012.

Hudson, Pat, and W.R. Lee. "Introduction." In *Women's Work and the Family Economy in Historical Perspective*, edited by Pat Hudson and W.R. Lee, 2–47. Manchester, UK: Manchester University Press, 1990.

Hunt, Margaret. "Women and the Fiscal-Imperial State in the Late Seventeenth and Early Eighteenth Centuries." In *A New Imperial History: Culture Identity, and Modernity in Britain and the Empire, 1660–1840*, edited by Kathleen Wilson, 29–47. Cambridge: Cambridge University Press, 2006.

Innes, Joanna. "Governing Diverse Societies." In *The Eighteenth Century: 1688–1815*, edited by Paul Langford, 103–40. New York: Oxford University Press, 2002.

James, Alan. "The Seventeenth Century: A First Age of Modern Naval Warfare." In *European Navies and the Conduct of War*, edited by A. James, C.A. Zaforteza, C.A. Murfett, and M. Murfett, 38–50. London: Routledge, 2018.

Joas, Hans. "The Modernity of War: Modernization Theory and the Problem of Violence." *International Sociology* 14, no. 4 (December 1999): 457–72.

Jones, D.W. *War and Economy in the Age of William III and Marlborough*. Oxford: Basil Blackwell, 1988.

Jones, J.R. *The Anglo-Dutch Wars of the Seventeenth Century*. London: Longman, 1996.

– "The Limitations of British Sea Power in the French Wars, 1689–1815." In *The British Navy and the Use of Naval Power in the Eighteenth Century*, edited by J. Black and P. Woodfine, 33–49. Leicester, UK: Leicester University Press, 1988.

Jussim, Lee. "Précis of Social Perception and Social Reality: Why Accuracy Dominates Bias and Self-Fulfilling Prophecy." *Behavioral and Brain Sciences* 40 (2017): e1.

Keane, Webb. *Ethical Life: Its Natural and Social Histories*. Princeton, NJ: Princeton University Press, 2016.

Keevil, John Joyce. *Medicine and the Navy, 1200–1900*. Vol. 1: *1200–1649*; Vol. 2: *1649–1714*. Edinburgh: E. & S. Livingstone, 1957.

Kinkel, Sarah. *Disciplining the Empire: Politics, Governance, and the Rise of the British Navy*. Cambridge, MA: Harvard University Press, 2018.

– "Disorder, Discipline, and Naval Reform in Mid-Eighteenth-Century Britain." *English Historical Review* 128, no. 535 (2013): 1451–82.

Kleer, Richard. "'Fictitious Cash': English Public Finance and Paper Money, 1689–97." In *Money, Power, and Print: Interdisciplinary Studies on the Financial Revolution in the British Isles*, edited by Charles Ivar McGrath and Chris Fauske, 70–114. Newark, NJ: University of Delaware Press, 2008.

Knights, Mark. *Trust and Distrust: Corruption in Office in Britain and Its Empire, 1600–1850*. Oxford: Oxford University Press, 2022.

Bibliography

Kocka, Jürgen. *Capitalism: A Short History*. Princeton, NJ: Princeton University Press, 2018.

Kopperman, Paul E. "Medical Services in the British Army, 1742–1783." *Journal of the History of Medicine and Allied Science* 34, no. 4 (1979): 428–55.

Lamb, Jonathan. *Scurvy: The Disease of Discovery*. Princeton, NJ: Princeton University Press, 2018.

Lambert, Andrew. *Seapower States: Maritime Culture, Continental Empires, and the Conflict That Made the Modern World*. New Haven, CT: Yale University Press, 2018.

Lepka, Lesya. "Care Work and Nursing in Greenwich Hospital, 1705–1714." MA thesis, University of Saskatchewan, 2019.

Lindemann, Mary. *Medicine and Society in Early Modern Europe*. Cambridge: Cambridge University Press, 2004.

Lockhart, Paul. *Firepower: How Weapons Shaped Warfare*. New York: Basic, 2021.

Lockwood, Matthew. *The Conquest of Death: Violence and the Birth of the Modern English State*. New Haven, CT: Yale University Press, 2017.

Low, D.M., ed. *Gibbon's Journal to January 28th, 1763*. London: Chatto and Windus, 1929.

Luttrell, Narcissus, ed. *A Brief Historical Relation of State Affairs from September 1678 to April 1714*. Vol. 2. Cambridge: Cambridge University Press, 2011.

Lynn, John A. *Women, Armies, and Warfare in Early Modern Europe*. Cambridge: Cambridge University Press, 2007.

Manley, Gordon. "The Great Winter of 1740." *Weather* 13, no. 1 (1958): 11–17.

Martel, Marie-Thérèse de. *Étude sur le recrutement des matelots et soldats des vaisseaux du Roi dans le ressort de l'intendance du port de Rochfort (1691–1697): Aspects de la vie des gen de mer*. Vincennes: Service Historique de la Marine, 1982.

McInnes, Angus. "When Was the English Revolution?" *History* 67, no. 221 (1982): 377–92.

McIntosh, Marjorie K. "Networks of Care in Elizabethan English Towns: The Example of Hadleigh, Suffolk." In *The Locus of Care: Families, Communities, Institutions, and the Provision of Welfare since Antiquity*, edited by Peregrine Horden and Richard Smith, 71–89. London: Routledge, 1998.

McLean, David. "Health Provision in the Royal Navy, 1650–1815." In *The Social History of English Seamen: 1650–1815*, edited by Cheryl Fury, 107–28. Martlesham, UK: Boydell and Brewer, 2017.

McLean, Samuel A. "The Westminster Model Navy: Defining the Royal Navy, 1660–1749." PhD diss., University of London, 2017.

McNeill, J.R. *Mosquito Empires: Ecology and War in the Greater Caribbean, 1620–1914*. New York: Cambridge University Press, 2010.

McPherson, Kathryn. *Bedside Matters: The Transformation of Canadian Nursing, 1900–1990*. Toronto: Oxford University Press, 1996.

Miller, Richard W. *Fact and Method: Explanation, Confirmation, and Reality in the Natural and Social Sciences*. Princeton, NJ: Princeton University Press, 1987.

Mimler, Manfred. *Der Einfluß kolonialer Interessen in Nordamerika auf die Strate-gie und Diplomatie Großbritanniens während des 18. Jahrhunderts*. Hildesheim: Georg Olms, 1983.

Morriss, Roger. *The Foundations of British Military Ascendancy: Resources, Logistics, and the State, 1755–1815*. Cambridge: Cambridge University Press, 2011.

Murken, Axel Hinrich. "Zur Geschichte der europäischen Marinelazarett: Ihr Einfluß auf das Krankenhauswese des 19. Jahrhunderts." In *Geschichte der Schiffahrtsmedizin*, edited by Heinz Goerke, 93–117. Koblenz: Bernard und Graefe, 1985.

Murphy, Elaine. "'A Water Bawdy House': Women and the Navy in the British Civil Wars." In *The Maritime World of Early Modern Britain*, edited by Richard J. Blackmore and James Davey, 173–92. Amsterdam: Amsterdam University Press, 2020.

Nagy, Doreen Evenden. *Popular Medicine in Seventeenth-Century England*. Bowling Green, OH: Bowling Green University Press, 1988.

Neu, Tim. "Zahlmeister und Kaufmannbankiers: Zur politischen Ökonomie der britischen Finanzlogistik in der Frühen Neuzeit." In *Administration, Logistik, und Infrastrukturen des Krieges in der Frühen Neuzeit*, edited by Jutta Nowosadtko, Kai Lohsträter, and Sebastian Pranghofer. In preparation.

Neufeld, Matthew. "The Biopolitics of Manning the Royal Navy in Late Stuart England." *The Journal of British Studies* 56, no. 3 (2017): 506–31.

– "Corruption in the British Naval Healthcare Administration during the War of the Austrian Succession." Forthcoming.

– "Neither Private Contractors nor Productive Partners: The English Fiscal-Naval State and London Hospitals, 1660–1715." *International Journal of Maritime History* 28, no. 2 (2016): 268–90.

– "Parliament and Some Roots of Whistle Blowing during the Nine Years War." *The Historical Journal* 57, no. 2 (2014): 397–420.

Neufeld, Matthew, and Blaine Wickham. "The State, the People, and the Care of Sick and Injured Sailors in Late Stuart England." *Social History of Medicine* 18, no. 1 (2015): 45–63.

Newton, Hannah. "Inside the Sick Chambers in Early Modern England: The Experience of Illness through Six Objects." *English Historical Review* 136, no. 580 (June 2021): 530–67.

– *The Sick Child in Early Modern England, 1580–1720*. Oxford: Oxford University Press, 2012.

Nicholls, Angela. *Almshouses in Early Modern England: Charitable Housing in the Mixed Economy of Welfare, 1550–1725*. Woodbridge, UK: Boydell and Brewer, 2017.

Nicholls, James. *The Politics of Alcohol: A History of the Drink Question in England*. Manchester, UK: Manchester University Press, 2009.

Niedhart, Gottfried. *Handel und Krieg in der britischen Weltpolitik, 1738–1763*. Munich: Wilhelm Fink Verlag, 1979.

Nielson, Caroline L. "The Chelsea Out-Pensioners: Image and Reality in Eighteenth-Century and Early Nineteenth-Century Social Care." PhD diss., University of Newcastle upon Tyne, 2014.

North, Douglass C., John Joseph Wallis, and Barry R. Weingast. *Violence and Social Orders: A Conceptual Framework for Interpreting Recorded Human History.* Cambridge: Cambridge University Press, 2009.

North, Susan. *Sweet and Clean? Bodies and Clothes in Early Modern England.* Oxford: Oxford University Press, 2020.

Obinger, Herbert, Klaus Petersen, and Peter Starke. *Warfare and Welfare: Military Conflict and the Welfare State Development in Western Countries.* New York: Oxford University Press, 2018.

O'Brien, Patrick. "England 1485–1815." In *The Rise of the Fiscal State in Europe c. 1200–1815,* edited by Richard Bonney, 53–100. Oxford: Oxford University Press, 1999.

– "Fiscal Exceptionalism: Britain and Its European Rivals from Civil War to the Triumphs at Trafalgar and Waterloo." In *The Political Economy of British Historical Experience, 1688–1914,* edited by D. Winch and P.K. O'Brien, 245–65. Oxford: Oxford University Press for the British Academy, 2002

– "The Nature and Historical Evolution of an Exceptional Fiscal State and Its Possible Significance for the Precocious Commercialism and Industrialization of the British Economy from Cromwell to Nelson." *Economic History Review* 64, no. 1 (2011): 408–46.

– "Taxation for British Mercantilism from the Treaty of Utrecht (1713) to the Peace of Paris (1783)." In *War, State, and Development: Fiscal Military States in the Eighteenth Century,* edited by Rafael Torres Sanchez, 295–355. Pamplona, Spain: Eusna, 2007.

Page, Anthony. *The Seventy Years War: Enlightenment, Revolution, and Empire.* Basingstoke, UK: Palgrave, 2015.

Paquette, Gabriel. *The European Seaborne Empires: From the Thirty Years' War to the Age of Revolutions.* New Haven, CT: Yale University Press, 2019.

Pares, Richard. *War and Trade in the West Indies, 1739–1763.* London: F. Cass, 1963.

Parker, Geoffrey. *The Military Revolution: Military Innovation and the Rise of the West, 1500–1800.* Cambridge: Cambridge University Press, 1988.

Parrott, David. *The Business of War: Military Enterprise and Military Revolution in Early Modern Europe.* Cambridge: Cambridge University Press, 2012.

– *Richelieu's Army: War, Government, and Society in France, 1624–1642.* Cambridge: Cambridge University Press, 2001.

Peckham, Madeleine. "'A True British Spirit': Admiral Vernon, Porto Bello, and British National Identity, 1730–1745." MA thesis, University of Saskatchewan, 2015.

Pelling, Margaret. "Compromised by Gender: The Role of the Male Medical Practitioner in Early Modern England." In *The Task of Healing: Medicine,*

Religion, and Gender in England and the Netherlands, 1450–1800, edited by H. Marland and M. Pelling, 101–33. Rotterdam: Erasmus Press, 1996.

– "Far Too Many Women? John Graunt, the Sex Ratio, and the Cultural Determination of Number in Seventeenth-Century England." *The Historical Journal* 59, no. 3 (2016): 695–719.

– "Healing the Sick Poor: Social Policy and Disability in Norwich, 1550–1640." *Medical History* 29, no. 2 (1985): 115–37.

– "'Nurses and Nursekeepers': Problems of Identification in the Early Modern Period." In *The Common Lot: Sickness, Medical Occupations, and the Urban Poor in Early Modern England*, by Margaret Pelling, 179–202. New York: Longman, 1998.

Petty, William. *The Advice of WP to Mr. Samuel Hartlib for the Advancement of Some Particular Parts of Learning*. London: n.p., 1648.

Pihl, Christopher. "Gender, Labour, and State Formation in Sixteenth-Century Sweden." *Historical Journal* 58, no. 3 (2015): 685–710.

Pincus, Steven. *1688: The First Modern Revolution*. New Haven, CT: Yale University Press, 2008.

– *Protestantism and Patriotism: Ideologies and the Making of English Foreign Policy, 1650–1668*. Cambridge: Cambridge University Press, 1996.

Pincus, Steven, and James Robinson. "Wars and State-Making Reconsidered: The Rise of the Developmental State." *Annales. Histoire, Sciences Sociales: English Edition* 71, no. 1 (2016): 9–34.

Plank, Geoffrey. *Atlantic Wars: From the Fifteenth Century to the Age of Revolution*. New York: Oxford University Press, 2020.

Pool, Bernard. *Navy Board Contracts, 1660–1832: Contract Administration under the Navy Board*. London: Longmans, 1966.

Porpora, Douglas V. *Reconstructing Sociology: The Critical Realist Approach*. Cambridge: Cambridge University Press, 2015.

Post, John D. "Climatic Variability and the European Mortality Wave of the Early 1740s." *The Journal of Interdisciplinary History* 15, no. 1 (Summer 1984): 1–30.

Poynter, F.N.L., ed. *The Journal of James Yonge, 1647–1721, Plymouth Surgeon*. London: Longmans, 1963.

Raymond, Edward. "The Lords Justices of England." *English Historical Review* 29, no. 115 (July 1914): 453–76.

Reinhard, Wolfgang. *Geschichte des Modernen Staates: Von den Anfängen bis zur Gegenwart*. München: C.H. Beck, 2007.

Richards, Eric. "Women in the British Economy since about 1700: An Interpretation." *History* 54, no. 197 (1974): 337–57.

Robinson, Ronald, and John Gallagher, with Alice Denny. *Africa and the Victorians: The Official Mind of Imperialism*. New York: Macmillan, 1961.

Rodger, N.A.M. *The Admiralty*. Lavenham, UK: T. Dalton, 1979.

Bibliography

- *The Command of the Ocean: A Naval History of Britain, 1649–1815.* London: Penguin, 2006.
- "From the 'Military Revolution' to the 'Fiscal-Naval State.'" *Journal for Maritime Research* 13, no. 2 (2011): 119–28.
- "The Military Revolution at Sea." In *Essays in Naval History, from Medieval to Modern*, edited by N.A.M. Rodger, 59–76. Aldershot, UK: Ashgate Press, 2009.
- "Sea-Power and Empire, 1688–1793." In *The Oxford History of the British Empire*. Vol. 2: *The Eighteenth Century*, edited by P.J. Marshall, 169–83. Oxford: Oxford University Press, 1998.
- *The Wooden World: An Anatomy of the Georgian Navy.* New York: Norton, 2009.

Rogers, Nicholas. *Mayhem: Post-War Crime and Violence in Britain, 1748–1753.* New Haven, CT: Yale University Press, 2012.

Rommelse, Giljs. "The Role of Mercantilism in Anglo-Dutch Political Relations, 1650–74." *The Economic History Review* 63, no. 3 (2010): 591–611.

Roseveare, Henry. *The Financial Revolution, 1660–1760.* London: Longmans, 1991.

Rowlands, G. *The Financial Decline of a Great Power: War, Influence, and Money in Louis XIV's France.* Oxford: Oxford University Press, 2012.

Rutherford, Stephen M. "A New Kind of Surgery for a New Kind of War: Gunshot Wounds and Their Treatment in the British Civil Wars." In *Battle-scarred: Mortality, Medical Care, and Military Welfare in the British Civil Wars*, edited by David J. Appleby and Andrew Hopper, 57–77. Manchester, UK: Manchester University Press, 2018.

Sandassie, Samantha. "'Half-Gods Good Surgeons May Be Called': Surgery's Quest for Occupational Credit in England, 1590–1715." PhD diss., Queen's University, 2014.

Satsuma, Shinsuke. *Britain and Colonial Maritime War in the Early Eighteenth Century: Silver, Seapower, and the Atlantic.* Woodbridge, UK: Boydell and Brewer, 2013.

Scheipers, Sibylle, ed. *Prisoners in War.* Oxford: Oxford University Press, 2010.

Schettger, M. *Der Spanische Erbfolgekreig, 1701–1713/14.* Munich: C.H. Beck, 2014.

Schoenfeldt, Michael. *Bodies and Selves in Early Modern England: Physiology and Inwardness in Spenser, Shakespeare, Herbert, and Milton.* New York: Cambridge University Press, 1999.

Scott, Hamish. *The Birth of a Great Power System, 1740–1815.* New York: Pearson Longman, 2006.

Scott, James C. *Seeing Like a State: How Certain Schemes to Improve the Human Condition Have Failed.* New Haven, CT: Yale University Press, 2020.

Sharpe, J.A. *Early Modern England: A Social History.* London: Arnold, 1997.

Shaw, J.J. "The Commission of Sick and Wounded and Prisoners, 1664–1667." *Mariners Mirror* 25 no. 3 (1939): 306–27.

Bibliography

Shovlin, John. "War and Peace: Trade, International Competition, and Political Economy." In *Mercantilism Reimagined: Political Economy in Early Modern Britain and Its Empire*, edited by Philip J. Stern and Carl Wennerlind, 305–27. Oxford: Oxford University Press, 2014.

– *Trading with the Enemy: Britain, France and the 18th-Century Quest for a Peaceful World Order*. New Haven, CT: Yale University Press, 2021.

Sienna, Kevin. *Venereal Disease, Hospitals, and the Urban Poor: London's 'Foul Wards,' 1600–1800*. Manchester, UK: Manchester University Press, 2004.

Simms, Brendan. *Three Victories and a Defeat: The Rise and Fall of the First British Empire, 1714–1783*. London: Allen Lane, 2007.

Simonton, Deborah. *A History of European Women's Work: 1700 to the Present*. London: Routledge, 1998.

Simpson, Geoffrey. *Chronic Condition: Why Canada's Health Care System Needs to Be Dragged into the 21st Century*. Toronto: Penguin, 2012.

Slack, Paul. *The English Poor Law, 1531–1782*. New York: Cambridge University Press, 1995.

Smith, Christian. *Atheist Overreach: What Atheism Can't Deliver*. Oxford: Oxford University Press, 2018.

– *The Sacred Project of American Sociology*. New York: Oxford University Press, 2014.

– *What Is a Person? Rethinking Humanity, Social Life, and the Moral Good from the Person Up*. Chicago: University of Chicago Press, 2010.

Smith, Lisa W. "Reassessing the Role of the Family: Women's Medical Care in Eighteenth-Century England." *Social History of Medicine* 16, no. 3 (2003): 327–42.

Sowerby, Scott. *Making Toleration: The Repealers and the Glorious Revolution*. Cambridge, MA: Harvard University Press, 2013.

Spinney, Erin. "Naval and Military Nursing in the British Empire, c. 1763–1830." PhD diss., University of Saskatchewan, 2018.

– "Servants to the Hospital and the State: Nurses in Plymouth and Haslar Naval Hospitals, 1775–1815." *Journal for Maritime Research* 20, no. 1–2 (2018): 3–19.

Stevenson, Christine. "From Palace to Hut: The Architecture of Military and Naval Medicine." In *British Military and Naval Medicine, 1600–1830*, edited by Geoffrey L. Hudson, 227–251. New York: Rodopi, 2007.

Stobart, Anne. *Household Medicine in Seventeenth-Century England*. London: Bloomsbury Publishing, 2016.

Stone, Lawrence, ed. *An Imperial State at War: Britain from 1689–1815*. London: Routledge, 1994.

Storrs, Christopher. "Health, Sickness, and Medical Services in Spain's Armed Forces, c. 1665–1700." *Medical History* 50, no.3 (2006): 325–50.

– "Introduction: The Fiscal-Military State in the 'Long' Eighteenth Century." In *The Fiscal-Military State in Eighteenth-Century Europe: Essays in Honour of*

P.G.M. Dickson, edited by Christopher Storrs, 3–20. Aldershot, UK: Ashgate, 2009.

– *The Spanish Resurgence, 1713–1748*. New Haven, CT: Yale University Press, 2010.

– "War and the Military Revolution." In *Interpreting Early Modern Europe*, edited by C. Scott Dixon and Beat Kümin, 244–68. London: Routledge, 2020.

Swingen, Abgail L. *Competing Visions of Empire: Labor, Slavery, and the Origins of the British Atlantic Empire*. New Haven, CT: Yale University Press, 2015.

Tadmor, Naomi. "The Settlement of the Poor and the Rise of the Form in England, c. 1662–1780." *Past & Present* 236, no. 1 (2017): 43–97.

Taillemite, E. "Une bataille de l'Atlantique au XVIIIe siècle: La Guerre de Succession d'Autriche." In *Guerres et Paix: 1660–1815: 1 Colloque franco-anglaises d'histoire de la Marine*. (1987): 131–48.

Taylor, Charles. *A Secular Age*. Cambridge, MA: Harvard University Press, 2007.

Taylor, Stephen. "Afterword: State Formation, Political Stability, and the Revolution of 1688." In *The Final Crisis of the Stuart Monarchy: The Revolutions of 1688–91 in Their British, Atlantic, and European Contexts*, edited by Tim Harris and Stephen Taylor, 273–304. Woodbridge, UK: Boydell and Brewer, 2013.

Teschke, Benno. "Revisiting the 'War-Makes-States' Thesis: War, Taxation, and Social Property Relations in Early Modern Europe." In *War, the State, and International Law in Seventeenth-Century Europe*, edited by O. Asbach and P. Schroeder, 36–59. Farnham, UK: Ashgate, 2010.

Thomas, James. "Jack Tar, Mr Sawbones, and the Local Community: The Impact of Haslar Hospital, Gosport, 1750–1800." *Hatcher Review* 26, no. 3 (1988): 291–301.

Thomas, Janet. "Women and Capitalism: Oppression or Emancipation? A Review Article." *Comparative Studies in Society and History* 30, no. 3 (July 1998): 534–49.

Thomas, Keith. "Health and Morality in Early Modern England." In *Morality and Health*, edited by Allan M. Brandt and Paul Rozin, 15–34. New York: Routledge, 1997.

Thompson, E.P. *The Making of the English Working Class*. Harmondsworth, UK: Penguin, 1968.

Torres Sanchez, Rafael. *Military Entrepreneurs and the Spanish Contractor State in the Eighteenth Century*. Oxford: Oxford University Press, 2016.

– "The Triumph of the Fiscal-Military State in the Eighteenth Century. In *War, State, and Development: Fiscal-Military States in the Eighteenth Century*, edited by Rafael Torres Sanchez, 6–28. Pamplona, Spain: EUNSA, 2007.

Tilly, Charles, and Gabriel Ardant, eds. *The Formation of National States in Western Europe*. Princeton: Princeton University Press, 1975.

Trabut, Loïc, and Florence Weber. "How to Make Care Work Visible? The Case of Dependence Policies in France." *Economic Sociology of Work: Research in the Sociology of Work* 18 (2009): 343–68.

Bibliography

Tunstall, Brian. *The Byng Papers*. Vols 67 and 68. London: Navy Records Society, 1930.

Tutchin, John. *An Historical and Political Treatise of the Navy*. London: n.p., 1704.

Twigg, Julia, Carol Wolkowitz, Rachel Lara Cohen, and Sara Nettleton. "Introduction: Conceptualising Body Work in Health and Social Care." In *Body Work in Health and Social Care*, edited by Julia Twigg, Carol Wolkowitz, Rachel Lara Cohen and Sara Nettleton, 1–18. Malden, MA: Wiley-Blackwell, 2011.

Waddell, Brodie. "The Politics of Economic Distress in the Aftermath of the Glorious Revolution, 1689–1702." *The English Historical Review* 130, no. 543 (2015): 318–51.

Watson, P.K. "The Commission for Victualling the Navy: The Commission for Sick and Wounded Seamen and Prisoners of War and the Commission for Transport, 1702–1714." PhD diss., University of London, 1965.

Wear, Andrew. "Caring for the Sick Poor in St Bartholomew's Exchange, 1580–1676." Supplement, *Medical History* 35, no. S11 (1991): 41–60.

Weber, Max. "Bureaucracy." In *From Max Weber: Essays in Sociology*, edited by H.H. Gerth and C. Wright Mills, 126–244. London: Routledge, 1991.

Wegner, Peter. *Theorizing Modernity: Inescapability and Attainability in Social Theory*. London: Sage, 2001.

Wettenhall, Roger. "Mixes and Partnerships through Time." In *International Handbook on Public-Private Partnerships*, edited by G.A. Hodge, C. Greve, and A.E. Boardman, 17–42. Northampton, MA: Edward Elgar Publications, 2010.

– "The Public-Private Interface: Surveying the History. In *The Challenge of Public-Private Partnership: Learning from International Experience*, edited by Graeme Hodge and Carsten Greve, 22–43. Northampton, MA: Edward Elgar Publications, 2005.

Wheeler, J.S. *The Making of a World Power: War and the Military Revolution in Seventeenth-Century England*. Stroud, UK: Sutton, 1999.

Whittle, Jane, and Mark Haliwood. "The Gender Division of Labour in Early Modern England." *Economic History Review* 73, no. 1 (2020): 3–32.

Wilcox, Martin. "The 'Poor Decayed Seamen' of Greenwich Hospital, 1705–1763." *International Journal of Maritime History* 25, no. 1 (2013): 64–90.

Wilkinson, C. *The British Navy and the State in the Eighteenth Century*. Woodbridge, UK: Boydell and Brewer, 2004.

Wilson, Peter H. "German Women and War, 1500–1800." *War in History* 3, no. 2 (1996): 127–60.

Wimmer, Andreas. "War." *Annual Review of Sociology* 40, no.1 (2014): 173–97.

Withington, Phil. "Introduction: Cultures of Intoxication." *Past & Present* 222, Supplement 9 (2014): 9–33.

Woodfine, Philip. *Britannia's Glories: The Walpole Ministry and the 1739 War with Spain*. Woodbridge, UK: Boydell and Brewer, 1998.

Bibliography

Wright, N.T. *The New Testament and the People of God. Christian Origins and the Question of God*. Vol. 1. London: SPCK, 1992.

Wrightson, Keith. *Earthly Necessities: Economic Lives in Early Modern Britain*. New Haven, CT: Yale University Press, 2000.

Zahedieh, Nuala. "Commerce and Conflict: Jamaica and the War of the Spanish Succession." In *The Caribbean and the Atlantic World Economy: Circuits of Trade, Money, and Knowledge, 1650–1914*, edited by Adrian Leonard and D. Pretel, 68–86. London: Palgrave Macmillan, 2015.

Ziegler, Hannes. "Jacobitism, Coastal Policing, and Fiscal-Military Reform in England after the Glorious Revolution, 1689–1702." *Journal of British Studies* 61, no. 2 (2022): 290–314.

Index

Page numbers with (f) refer to maps.

accounting systems: overview, 60–5, 72, 79–86, 108, 120, 164–6; agents' duties, 29–31, 65; certificate of injury or illness, 29–30; desertions overview, 112–13, 161–4; discharges, 129; effectiveness of systems, 88, 164–6; Instructions (1698, 1702, 1731), 64–6, 71–2, 113–14, 117, 220n54; ordered care's dependence on, 105, 108; paper technologies, 30–1, 63–5, 80, 83–4, 108; payment procedures, 30, 65–7, 78–9, 133–5; prevention of corruption and waste, 109–13; "Q" for query, 112–13, 220n54, 230n35; registry of seamen, 63–5, 72, 108; sick frauds, 29, 72, 93, 160–1, 164–6, 231n39; tallies, 58–9, 209n86; tickets, 224n56. *See also* desertions; mustering

Adams, Richard, 70–1, 73, 94, 98–9, 103

Addison, Thomas, 47, 61, 66, 206n16

affordance, as term, 199n55

agents for commissioners: overview, 8, 28–31, 106–7; accounting systems, 29–31, 60–5, 82–6; co-operation with local people, 31–2, 35–6, 43–4; dishonesty and irregularities, 37, 48–9, 61, 82–3, 86; duties, 28–31, 66, 106–7; muster masters, 83–5, 87–8, 111,

220n43; payments to quarterers, 30, 65–6; payments to surgeons, 30; statistics, 71; trust relationships with local people, 29–31, 88. *See also* surgeon-agents for commissioners

alcohol use: overview, 166–7, 177–82, 184–6, 193; alcohol in seamen's provisions, 184; as analgesic, 184; care worker's authority, 11; disorderly conduct, 184–5, 193; exaggeration of disorderly conduct, 160; gin's popularity, 160, 227n151; impact on ordered care, 166–7; public anxiety over abuse, 177–8; rationale for permanent hospitals, 176–83, 185–7; regulations (1740), 138–9; by women care workers, 144–5, 184–6

Aldborough, 33, 121(f)

Allix, Charles, 136, 225n76

Anne, Queen, 89

apothecaries, 8, 12, 26, 210n120

arrears in care payments. *See* care payments in arrears

Bailey, Ralph, 34

Balchen, John, 131, 137, 176, 177

Barclay, James, 130–1, 133, 135–8, 143, 223n40, 224n65, 225n77, 225n88, 226n96

Baston, Samuel, 61, 207n22, 210n112

Beachy Head, Battle of (1690), 51, 62, 73

Bedford, Duke of (John Russell), 162, 164, 168, 229n5
Beers, Mr, 141
Bell, William, 136
Berkeley, James, 216n130
Berry, Mr (Plymouth attorney), 47–50, 207n24, 207n27
Birkby, Oliver, 108–9, 115
Birstall, Robert, 34, 37–8, 204n86
Blenheim hospital ship, 130–1, 134, 137, 140–1, 143–5, 172, 175, 185
Brady, Dr (Portsmouth), 116–17, 125, 225n77
Bristol, 122(f), 123(f), 172, 233n68
Brownjohn, Rawlins, 91–4
Bunting, Madeleine, 4, 195
Burchett, Josiah, 14, 115
Burton, Edward, 140
Burton, Richard, 107
Butcher, Mrs, 192
Butler, John, 129, 156–7, 162, 177
Buttall, Humphrey, 131–2, 134–5, 144, 146–7, 149–53, 227n150

care payments in arrears: overview, 19–20, 32–41, 45, 54–8, 76–9; advocacy for unpaid care providers, 37–40, 46, 52–8, 66–7, 102; broken trust relations, 21, 32–3, 38–42, 55–8, 102; emergency actions (1711), 76–7; hardships from debt, 38–41, 46, 51, 54–8, 76–7; payment procedures, 30, 65–7, 78–9, 81, 133–5; prioritizing of groups, 38, 78–9; resistance by care workers, 20, 101–2; Treasury's rationale for delays, 45. *See also* resistance and protests
care providers. *See* quartering system
care systems. *See* health-care systems; health-care systems, naval
care work: overview, 4–5, 11–12, 41–2, 101, 191–5; carer/patient relationship, 4–5, 11, 193–5; continuity of system, 188–90, 235n6; hierarchy of sites, 90, 101, 106–7, 134;

historiography, 12–13; invisibility of care work, 192–5; male care workers, 5, 20–1, 44, 49–50, 201n8; mutual benefits, 43–4; ordinary people, 12; as paid labour, 6–7; power relations, 11–12, 145, 183–4; quality of care, 72–3, 113–20, 191; ratio of nurses to patients, 117, 141, 143; requirement for relief recipients to work, 6–7; shift from involuntary to voluntary, 6–7; workers vs providers, 201n13
care workers, women: overview, 5, 20–1, 44, 141–6, 182–6, 192–5; continuity of system, 188–90, 235n6; distrust by naval officials, 143–5; importance of, 17–18, 50, 182–6, 192–5; invisibility of care work, 192–5; as moral dangers, 17, 86, 90, 93–6, 98–9, 139, 181; paid vs domestic duties, 5–6; power relations, 11–12, 144–5, 183–4; private vs public spheres, 5; quality of care, 141–4; rates per day, 145, 210n121; terms for, as widows or landladies, 21; typhus (Great Sickness), 142–4
Cavendish, Philip, 112, 117, 126, 128, 131, 137, 142–4, 146, 225n88
Champainge, Francis, 49
Charles II, King, 19–20, 28–9, 32–6
Charters, Erica, 194
Chatham: accounting systems, 85; care payments in arrears, 40, 53; contagious diseases, 35, 89; hardships from debt, 56; map, 121(f); transfers to London, 164
Chatham, permanent hospital: proposal (1741), 153–8, 226n121, 228n171; proposal (1744), 177–9
Chatham's Chest, 24, 28, 46, 72
Churchill, William, 83, 215n104, 222n78
Clark, Christopher, 100
cleanliness: overview, 5; clothes and bedding, 5, 23, 125–6, 141–4; contagious diseases, 138–40; instructions

Index

and regulations (1702, 1740, 1742), 73, 138–9; lice in bedding (typhus), 129, 130; on ships, 23; water usage, 198n25

Cleaveland, William, 107

Clifford, Thomas, 28, 203n46

clothing for patients. *See* ordered care

Cole, Mrs Beate, 103

colonial ports. *See* overseas colonial and foreign ports

commissioners, agents for. *See* agents for commissioners; surgeon-agents for commissioners

commissioners (1650–1688), Dutch Wars: overview, 8, 25–30, 41–4; accounting systems, 29–30; advocacy for unpaid care providers, 37–40, 46; agents' reports to, 29–30; compensation, 28, 206n15; co-operation with local people, 31–2, 35–6, 43–4; duties, 8, 26, 27–8, 198n32; first commission, 8, 25–30; hospitals-first plan, 26–7; Instructions, 28–30, 31; London as care site, 25, 27, 121(f); members, 26; mutual benefits, 43–4; ports as care sites, 27–9. *See also* Dutch Wars (1652–1654, 1665–1667, 1672–1674); history of naval care (1650–1688), Dutch Wars

commissioners (1689–1701), Nine Years' War: overview, 15–16, 46; accounting systems, 60–5, 211n131; advocacy for unpaid care providers, 46, 52–8, 66–7; archives and sources, 14; central office, 71; commission's reconstitution (1691), 63; compensation, 63, 206n15; duties, 66–8; Instructions, 64–6, 71–2, 210n123, 211n131; members, 47, 63, 75; Navy Board postwar (1697–1702), 54, 63, 107, 202n29, 211n131; preservative ethos, 62–8; recommendations by (1698), 66–8; resistance and protests, 51–8; for West Indies and Mediterranean,

50. *See also* history of naval care (1689–1701), Nine Years' War; Nine Years' War (1689–1697)

commissioners (1702–1713), Queen Anne's War: overview, 16, 69–73; accounting systems, 72, 79–80, 82–6; advocacy for unpaid care providers, 89, 102; archives and sources, 14, 73; care payments in arrears, 76–9, 81, 101–2; central office, 71–2, 107, 212n20; commissioners' staff, 219n19; contract hospitals, 69–70, 76–7, 90–100, 104; contract hospitals, proposals (1703), 91–4; gendered trust, 103–4; Instructions, 70, 71–2, 92; members, 70–1, 75; mustering, 83–5, 87–8, 114; Navy Board prewar (1697–1702), 54, 63, 107; payment procedures, 78–9; preservative ethos, 16, 86, 89, 92–100; reports, 95–6; standards of care, 83. *See also* history of naval care (1702–1713), Queen Anne's War; Queen Anne's War (1702–1713)

commissioners (1715–1739), Georgian Era: overview, 105–6, 120; accounting systems, 109–13; agents, 106–7; central office, 107; corruption and waste in system, 109–13, 120; epidemics, 118–19, 221nn64–5; inspections of care, 114–20; Instructions and regulations, 107, 113–14, 120, 220n54, 225n94; members, 107; Navy Board, 107; preservative ethos, 105–7, 120. *See also* Georgian Era (1715–1739); history of naval care (1715–1739), Georgian era

commissioners (1739–1744), War with Spain: overview, 17, 125–7, 155–7; archives and sources, 15, 127; care payments in arrears, 133–4; evaluation of care, 125, 130, 132, 136, 155–7; financial status of navy, 135–6, 157; Instructions and regulations, 125–6, 138–9,

262 Index

143, 175, 220n54; members, 136; Navy Board, 153; ordered care, 125–7, 136–41; payment procedures, 133–5; permanent hospital proposal (1741), 153–8, 177, 178, 228n171; Plymouth scandal, 146–53; preservative ethos, 125–7; prompt care payments, 133–5; women care workers, 141–6. *See also* history of naval care (1739–1744), War with Spain

commissioners (1744–1748), War against France: overview, 17, 124(f), 158–60; accounting systems, 164–6; evaluation of care, 166–7, 173, 186; map, 124(f); oversight of contract hospitals, 158–60; prisoners of war, 167; reports on conditions, 158–60, 164, 169–73, 175–9, 182, 184–6, 231nn37–8, 232nn56–67, 233nn68–70; sick-frauds, 160–1; women care workers, 182–6. *See also* France, War against (1744–1748); Gosport, Haslar naval hospital

contagious distempers, 100, 111, 119, 125, 139–40, 175m 221nn64–5

contract hospitals. *See* hospitals, contract

Cooper, Samuel, 26

Corbett, Thomas, 83, 113

Cornwall, 28, 74

Coulter, Jack L.S., 158

Crawford, Captain, 137

Crimmin, Patricia, 12, 158

Crown. *See* state and Crown

Danby, Lord Treasurer, 39–41

Dartmouth, 50, 53, 56–7, 122(f), 123(f), 208n74

Deal: overview, 169–70; alcohol use, 166; care payments in arrears, 34, 35, 39, 57, 76–7, 79, 115–16, 133; continuity of system, 188–90; dishonesty in agents, 37; Dutch Wars care, 20–1, 32, 34, 35, 37, 121(f), 192; maps, 121(f), 122(f), 123(f);

Nine Years' War care, 47, 53–4, 57; ordered care, 116, 169–71; Queen Anne's War care, 71, 74, 76–7, 79, 116; resistance and protests, 37, 57; typhus (Great Sickness), 130, 222n16; War against France care, 169–71, 192; women care workers, 182–3, 192

Deal, contract hospital: overview, 90–1, 104, 169–70, 192; care payments in arrears, 76–7, 79, 115–16; contract proposals, 91–4; corruption and waste, 106, 116; disorderly conduct, 166, 170

debt. *See* care payments in arrears; Treasury

Deptford, 36, 50, 78, 88, 122(f), 123(f), 169–71, 232n56, 232n61

deputies. *See* agents for commissioners

desertions: overview, 112–13, 160, 163–6; accounting systems, 87–8, 112–13, 120, 128, 129, 161–6, 223n33; from care on shore, 112–13, 155–6, 160, 163–4, 177–8, 224n62, 228n177; from hospital ships, 126, 164; to merchant marine, 164, 177; from permanent hospitals, 155; preservative ethos, 120, 126, 163, 191; statistics, 128, 160, 163, 177, 223n33; typhus (Great Sickness), 128

Devon, 3, 28, 145

Dickinson, George, 47–50, 58, 80, 207n18, 207n22

Dilkie, Lieutenant, 117

diseases and illnesses: overview, 22–3, 221nn64–5; care in epidemics, 118–19, 221nn64–5; injuries and wounds, 22; living conditions, 23, 129, 149–50; sick-frauds, 160–1; typhus epidemic overview, 127–32. *See also* typhus epidemic (Great Sickness) (1739–1742)

diseases and illnesses, specific: overview, 221nn64–5; contagious distempers, 100, 111, 119, 125, 139–40,

175m 221nn64–5; dysentery (flux), 23, 140, 175, 221nn64–5; malaria, 23, 222n14; plague, 31, 35, 37; scurvy, 23, 175, 221n65; smallpox, 109, 118–20, 221nn64–5; yellow fever, 23, 222n14
Dixie, Benjamin, 110, 220n34
Dorset, 28, 36, 57
Dover, 21, 33, 53, 57, 79, 89, 121(f), 122(f), 123(f), 170, 171
Doyley, William, 28
drunkenness. *See* alcohol use
Dunwich, 33
Dursley, Lord, 87, 216n130
Dutch Wars (1652–1654, 1665–1667, 1672–1674): overview, 15, 19; archives and sources, 14, 31; care sites, 19–20, 27–9, 32, 121(f); co-operation with local people, 31–2, 35–6, 43–4; costs and debt for care, 32–6, 45; financial status of navy, 4, 19, 32–6, 42–3, 45; first naval health commission, 8, 25–30; legitimacy in civilian-military relations, 35–6; professionalization of navy, 10. *See also* commissioners (1650–1688), Dutch Wars; history of naval care (1650–1688), Dutch Wars
dysentery (flux), 23, 140, 175, 221nn64–5

Earle, Peter, 7
early Georgian era. *See* Georgian Era (1715–1739)
East Anglia, 74
economy: financial crises (1693–94), 51; financial revolution (1690s), 76–9; loss of merchant ships in Nine Years' War, 52; recoinage (1696), 51; slavery issues, 224n69; South Sea Company, 69, 77. *See also* Treasury
Edisbury, Kendrick, 107, 109, 115–17, 221nn64–5
Elder, David, 48, 61, 66

Elizabeth I, Queen, 43
Ely House, 27
England, as focus of this study, 15
Erith, 34, 35
Essex, 20
Europe: health-care system, 180, 190. *See also* France; France, War against (1744–1748); Spain; Spain, War with (1739–1744)
Evelyn, John: archives, 13–14, 30; authority for Kent and Sussex, 28; care payments in arrears, 33–40; hospital proposal, 37, 43, 90, 188; quarterers' protests, 36–40

Fareham, 31, 88, 142, 171–2, 182, 185
Faversham, 34–5, 39–40
Fawler, John, 107, 109, 125, 136–7, 140
financial records. *See* accounting systems
Finch, Daniel. *See* Winchilsea, Earl of (Daniel Finch)
Firth, Captain, 146
food for patients. *See* ordered care
foreign ports. *See* overseas colonial and foreign ports
Forton contract hospital. *See* Gosport, Forton Hospital (contract)
Fowell, John, 145
France: coercion of care workers, 43; Nine Years' War, 52; Treaty of Utrecht (1713), 16, 105, 218n1
France, War against (1744–1748): overview, 17, 124(f), 158–60; accounting systems, 164–6; alcohol use, 166–7, 177–82, 184–6; archives and sources, 15; centralizing vision of empire, 159; desertions, 160, 177; evaluation of care, 166–7, 173, 186; financial stability of navy, 160, 167–74, 181–2, 191; map, 124(f); prisoners of war, 167, 170, 171, 172; War of the Austrian Succession, 159; Western Squadron approach, 159. *See also* commissioners

(1744–1748), War against France; history of naval care (1744–1748), War against France

Gashry, Francis, 107, 125, 135–7, 140, 225n76

gender: contract hospital entrepreneurs, 93–4, 98–104; male care workers, 5, 20–1, 44, 49–50, 201n8; medical care as gendered sphere, 94; power relations in care, 11–12, 145, 183–4; trust relations, 103–4. *See also* care workers, women; women

George II, King, 158

Georgian Era (1715–1739): overview, 16, 105–6, 120; archives, 14–15; Baltic Sea (1718–1721), 106, 218n1; corruption and waste, 109–13; Mediterranean (1726–1727), 106, 218n1; in peacetime, 16, 106–9; Treaty of Utrecht (1713), 16, 105, 218n1; West Indies (1726–1727), 106. *See also* commissioners (1715–1739), Georgian Era; history of naval care (1715–1739), Georgian era

Gibbon, Edward, 187

Gibraltar, 145, 218n1

Gibson, Richard, 39–41

Gillett, Edward, 49

gin's popularity, 160, 227n151. *See also* alcohol use

Glorious Revolution, 14, 15, 45, 67–8

Glover (agent), 34

Godolphin, Treasurer, 81–2, 97

Gortley, Dr (Plymouth), 119, 146–9, 151, 153, 221n77

Gosport: accounting systems, 86, 129, 133, 161–2; agents, 106, 177; alcohol use, 160, 166, 172, 174, 176–82; care payments in arrears, 40, 53–7, 76–7, 79, 131, 133, 135; continuity of system, 188–90; costs and

debt for care, 218n2; desertions, 161–3, 177; Dutch Wars care, 20, 121(f); maps, 121(f), 122(f), 123(f); mustering, 161–2; Nine Years' War care, 53–7; Queen Anne's War care, 71, 74, 76–7, 86, 98–9, 101, 212n12; survey (1740), 142–3; transfers from outports to London, 162–4; typhus (Great Sickness), 127–32, 142–4, 222n16; War against France care, 161–4, 166, 172–5; women care providers, 142–3, 173, 182, 192

Gosport, Forton Hospital (contract): overview, 90–1, 104, 120, 142–3, 158–9, 167; accounting systems, 129, 161–2; alcohol use, 166, 173, 176–82, 184, 185–6; Brownjohn's proposal, 91–4; care payments in arrears, 76–7, 79; corruption and waste, 106; disordered care, 17, 158, 160, 161–2; disorderly conduct, 166, 172, 174; gendered consequences, 91, 98–100, 104; ordered care, 115–18, 125–6, 137–40, 143–4, 169, 172–3, 175, 185; resistance to (1704), 98–9, 101; trust in care workers, 9, 17, 100, 192; typhus (Great Sickness), 127–32, 142–4; women as moral dangers, 17, 181; women entrepreneurs, 101

Gosport, Haslar naval hospital: overview, 17, 185–9, 191–2; continuity of system, 188–90; cost of, 179; financial stability of navy, 17, 168, 181–2, 191; navy's rationale, 158, 160, 168, 174, 176, 179–83, 185–7, 191, 193; preservative ethos, 181, 189; proposal (1741), 153–8, 177, 178, 228n163, 228n171; proposal (1744), 177–80, 189; women care workers, 17–18, 182–6, 193

Grafton, 147–8

Gravesend, 32, 34, 35, 37–8, 121(f)

great ports. *See* Deal; Plymouth; Portsmouth; Rochester

Great Sickness. *See* typhus epidemic
(Great Sickness) (1739–1742)
Greenwich, 36
Greenwich Naval Hospital, 50, 72,
144

Hampshire, 25, 28, 31, 36, 187
Hardy, Charles, 175
Harland, Kathleen, 12, 90, 158,
201n82, 228n163
Harley, Robert, 74, 77, 80, 89, 95
Harwich, 56–7, 74, 82–3, 85, 121(f),
123(f)
Haslar naval hospital. *See* Gosport,
Haslar naval hospital
Hastings, 122(f), 123(f)
Hawk, 169
health-care systems: overview, 4–8,
194–5; apothecaries, 8, 12, 26,
210n120; biopolitics, 180, 234n102;
commercialization of care work,
7; disordered conditions as enemy,
174; in Europe, 180, 190; historiography, 11–12; lack of military
discipline, 140–1; non-nursing staff,
210n120; women's participation
as healers, 7. *See also* care work;
surgeons and physicians
health-care systems, naval: overview,
8–11, 90–1, 174, 191–5; centralization in hospitals, 90–6, 100,
118, 155–7, 188–90; continuity of
system, 105, 120, 188–90, 235n6;
hierarchy of care sites (greater/
lesser), 90; honour of the Crown,
24, 38, 67; importance of women
care workers, 17–18, 50, 182–6,
192–5; "manning, money, and
mercy," 90, 201n82; ordered care
overview, 9, 174; preservative ethos
overview, 10–11, 16, 89; public/
private co-operation, 10; on ships,
23; transfers from outports to
London, 55, 162–4; warfare orientation, 9–10. *See also* care work;

care workers, women; hospitals;
hospitals, contract; hospitals,
permanent; ordered care; preservative ethos; quartering system; trust
relations
health-care systems, naval, commissioners. *See entries beginning with*
commissioners
health-care systems, naval, history.
See entries beginning with history of
naval care
Henry VIII, King, 43
Herbert, Philip, 70–1, 73, 103
Hervey, John, 177–8
Hicks, Margaret, 103, 192, 218n200
Hildesley, Captain, 135, 140, 144,
147–9
Hill, Frederick, 115, 220n35, 221n60
Hills, Nathaniel: overview, 159,
185–6; commissioner and surgeon,
136, 153; inspection reports, 131,
157, 164, 169–73, 175–9, 182, 184–6,
190, 224n60, 226n96, 227n150,
231nn37–8, 232nn56–67, 233nn68–
70; Plymouth scandal, 140, 149–51
historiography: archives and sources,
12–14, 193, 200n72; financial
records, 13; invisibility of women
care workers, 192–5; lack of full
analysis of care work, 11–12, 31; loss
of registers after 1688, 14, 201n76;
narrative and time, 201n81; third-
party observers of care work, 13
history of naval care (1650–1688),
Dutch Wars: overview, 3–4, 15,
19–22, 28–32, 41–4; accounting
systems, 29–31, 209n86; advocacy
for unpaid care providers, 37–40,
46; agents for commissioners, 8,
28–31; archives and sources, 14;
care payments in arrears, 19–20,
32–41, 45; care sites, 4, 20–1,
27–9, 42, 121(f), 205n110; care
work by relief recipients, 15; care
workers, men, 20–1; care workers,

women, 4, 20–1, 201n8; continuity of system, 188–90; costs and debt for care, 39–40, 45; county pension scheme, 19; early health system, 19, 22–5, 43; evaluation of care, 41–4, 82; financial status of navy, 4, 15, 19, 32–6, 42–3, 45; first commission, 8, 25–30; hardships from debt, 38–41, 46; legitimacy in civilian-military relations, 35–6; moral economy, 20, 21–2; mutual benefits for all, 43–4; professionalization of navy, 10; resistance and protests, 32–41, 55; ships as preferred site, 205n110; trust relations, 21–2, 31–3, 38–42. *See also* commissioners (1650–1688), Dutch Wars; Dutch Wars (1652–1654, 1665–1667, 1672–1674)

history of naval care (1689–1701), Nine Years' War: overview, 4–5, 15–16, 45–6, 50–8; accounting systems, 60–5; advocacy for unpaid care providers, 46, 52–8, 66–7; archives and sources, 14; care payments in arrears, 45–6, 50–8; care sites, 67–8; continuity of system, 188–90; contract hospitals, 47–50; costs and debt for care, 45–6, 52–3, 67, 74, 106, 206nn7–8; evaluation of care, 16, 46, 58, 67–8, 82; financial irregularities, 48–50; financial status of navy, 16, 45–6, 51, 58–60, 74; fiscal innovations, 58–60; hardships from debt, 51, 54–8; peacetime plan (1698), 64–8; poor quality of care, 54–6; preservative ethos, 62–8; proposals to improve care, 62–8; resistance and protests, 51–8; trust relationships with local people, 55–8, 61–2, 66–8. *See also* commissioners (1689–1701), Nine Years' War; Nine Years' War (1689–1697)

history of naval care (1702–1713), Queen Anne's War: overview, 16, 69–70, 89, 123(f); accounting systems, 72, 82–6; care payments in arrears, 76–9, 81, 101–2; care sites, 71, 74–5, 90, 123(f); central office, 71–2, 107, 212n20; continuity of system, 188–90; contract hospitals, 16, 69–70, 76–7, 104; contract hospitals overview, 90–100, 103–4; costs and debt for care, 73–5, 95, 209n96, 212n12, 213n42, 219n6; decline in quarterers, 102–3; evaluation of care, 100–4; financial status of navy, 4, 59, 69, 75–9; fiscal innovations, 16, 76–9; hierarchy of care sites (greater/lesser), 90, 123(f); map, 123(f); moral dangers, 86, 90, 93–6, 98–9; mustering, 83–5, 87–8, 114; ordered care, 70, 72–3; overseas costs, 73, 75; payment procedures, 78–9; preservative ethos, 16, 69–70, 73, 86, 89, 90, 92–100; standards of care, 83; trust relationships with local people, 69, 77–8, 88–9. *See also* commissioners (1702–1713), Queen Anne's War; hospitals, contract; Queen Anne's War (1702–1713)

history of naval care (1715–1739), Georgian era: overview, 105–6, 120; accounting systems, 109–13; continuity of system, 105, 120, 188–90; corruption and waste, 109–13; costs and debt for care, 105–6; desertions, 112–13; epidemics, 118–19, 221nn64–5; evaluation of care, 105, 118, 120; hierarchy of care, 107; Instructions and regulations, 113–14, 117, 120, 220n54; mustering, 111–14; ordered care, 105–9, 113–20; peacetime care, 106–9; preservative ethos, 105–7, 120; trust relationships with local people, 16.

See also commissioners (1715–1739), Georgian Era; Georgian Era (1715–1739)

history of naval care (1739–1744), War with Spain: overview, 125–7, 141–6, 155–7; archives and sources, 15, 127; care payments in arrears, 133–4; continuity of system, 188–90; evaluation of care, 125, 130, 132, 136, 155–7; financial status of navy, 135–6, 157; Instructions and regulations, 138–9, 143; lack of resistance by care workers, 132; ordered care, 125–7, 136–41; permanent hospital proposal (1741), 153–8, 177, 178, 228n171; Plymouth scandal, 146–53; preservative ethos, 125–7, 153–7; trust relationships with local people, 132–6; women care workers, 141–6. *See also* commissioners (1739–1744), War with Spain; typhus epidemic (Great Sickness) (1739–1742)

history of naval care (1744–1748), War against France: overview, 17, 124(f), 158–60; accounting systems, 164–6; alcohol use, 166–8, 177–82, 184–6; continuity of system, 188–90; costs and debt for care, 167; desertion, 160–6, 231n39; disorderly conduct, 170; evaluation of care, 166–7, 173, 186; financial stability of navy, 160, 167–74, 181–2, 191; inspection reports, 164, 169–73, 175–9, 182, 184–6; map, 124(f); ordered care, 168–73; preservative ethos, 181; prisoners of war, 167, 170, 171, 172; proposals for permanent hospitals (1741, 1744), 153–8, 177–82, 189, 228n171; transfers from outports to London, 162–4, 168; women as moral dangers, 181; women care workers, 182–6. *See also* France, War against

(1744–1748); Gosport, Haslar naval hospital

hospitals: centralization of care, 90–6, 100, 118, 188–90; continuity of system, 188–90; evaluation of care, 155–7; Greenwich hospital, 50, 72, 144; hierarchy of care, 90, 101, 106–7, 134; inspections by commissioners, 67; "manning, money, and mercy," 90, 201n82; moral dangers, 90, 93–6, 98–9; preservative ethos, 62–3, 67–8, 90; quality of care, 90, 100. *See also* hospital ships

hospitals, contract: overview, 4, 47–50, 69, 90–104, 120; care payments in arrears, 76–9, 81; continuity of system, 188–90, 235n6; contract provisions, 76; corruption and waste, 106; cost savings, 47–9; entrepreneurs, 91–4, 98–104; evaluation of care, 100–4, 118, 130, 155–7, 186; financial irregularities, 48–9; gendered consequences, 93–4, 98–104; hardships from debt, 76–7; male entrepreneurs, 94, 103–4; ordered care, 70, 93–4, 113–20; payment procedures, 134–5; Plymouth scandal, 146–53; preservative ethos, 92–100; proposals for, 27, 47–8, 82; resistance to (1704), 98–9, 101; sample agreement (1703), 96–8; staff, 49; women care workers, 182–6. *See also* Deal, contract hospital; Gosport, Forton Hospital (contract); Plymouth, contract hospital; Rochester, contract hospital

hospitals, contract, proposals and planning: arguments for/against, 90–5, 99–100; Brownjohn's proposal (1703), 91–4; commissioners' proposal (1703), 91, 93–4, 96; commissioners' reports (1711–1712),

95–6; early proposals, 37, 43, 90; Lower's proposal (1690), 62–3, 67–8; moral dangers, 90, 93–6; women entrepreneurs' proposals, 103, 218n200

hospitals, permanent: overview, 90–1; continuity of system, 188–90; in France and Spain, 43; ordered care, 12; Port Mahon, 73, 77, 129, 144, 216n118, 218n2. *See also* Gosport, Haslar naval hospital; Greenwich Naval Hospital

hospitals, permanent, proposals and planning: arguments for/against, 154–7; commissioners' views (1741, 1744), 17, 153–8, 174, 179; navy's plan (1744), 4, 174, 177–82; navy's rationale for, 179–83, 185–7; navy's request (1741), 17, 153–8, 174, 177, 178, 228n171; preservative ethos, 153–7, 181

hospital ships: *Blenheim* (Portsmouth), 130–1, 134, 137, 140–1, 143–5, 172, 175, 185; *Britannia,* 183; desertions from, 126, 164; *Enterprise,* 235n127; Queen Anne's War care, 235n8; staff quarters, 183; typhus (Great Sickness), 128; women nurses, 183–4, 185, 193

Hughes, Richard, 117, 137, 228n177

Hull, 79, 103, 122(f), 123(f)

hygiene. *See* cleanliness

illnesses. *See* diseases and illnesses

injuries and wounds, 22

intoxication. *See* alcohol use

Ipswich, 25, 26, 33, 40, 121(f)

Isle of Wight, 31, 126, 131–2, 138

James II, King, 40

Kent: care payments in arrears, 33, 36–9, 53–5, 79, 80; Dutch Wars care, 20–1, 28, 34, 36–7; ordered care, 169–71; resistance and protests, 35, 37–8, 55; typhus

(Great Sickness), 222n16; women care workers, 182. *See also* Deal; Rochester

Kirkby, Christopher, 66, 207n32

Knackston, Thomas, 108–9, 115, 219n24, 221n60

Ladyday, 75

Langley (agent in Harwich), 82–3, 85

Larke, Joseph, 26

Leakie, John, 48–9, 207n22

Lee, Henry, 70

Leigh, Edward, 47

Lidderdale, James, 117

liquor. *See* alcohol use

Littleton, Thomas, 74

Liverpool, 122(f)

Lloyd, Christopher, 158

London hospitals: overview, 27; care during Nine Years' War, 55; Dutch wars care, 25, 27, 121(f); maps, 121(f), 122(f); plague (1665), 31; St Bartholomew's, 27, 55, 110, 168; St Thomas's, 27, 55, 168; transfers from outports, 55, 86, 162–4, 168, 230n26; War against France care, 162–3, 168

Lower, Richard, 55, 62–3, 67, 188

Lowther, John, 47

Mahon, Port, naval hospital, 73, 77, 129, 144, 216n118, 218n2

malaria, 23, 222n14

male care workers, 5, 20–1, 44, 49–50

malingerers and sick frauds, 29, 31, 72, 93, 160–1, 164–6, 229n18, 231n39

Margate, 34, 36, 79, 121(f), 122(f), 123(f)

Martin, William, 173, 176–81, 186

Marwich, 122(f)

medical care. *See* health-care systems; ordered care; surgeons and physicians

Mediterranean: costs for care, 207n33; Gibraltar, 145, 218n1; Nine

Years' War, 50; Port Mahon naval hospital, 73, 77, 129, 144, 216n118, 218n2
Melcombe Regis, 57
merchant ships, 9, 23, 52, 164, 177, 224n69
Milton, 40, 121(f)
modernization theory, 10–11. *See also* ordered care
Monck, George, 34, 40
Monmouth, HMS, 54
Morley, Charles, 70, 94, 98–9
mustering: accounting system, 83–5, 87–8, 108, 111–13, 161–2; muster masters, 83–5, 108, 111–13, 114, 162, 216n118, 220n43; *Regulations* (1731), 113, 114; resistance to, 111–12, 114, 162

naval health care. *See* health-care systems, naval
Newcastle, 88, 101–2, 122(f)
Nicholes, Josias, 47
Nine Years' War (1689–1697): overview, 15–16, 45–6, 58–60; accounting systems, 60–4; archives and sources, 14; battle near Barfleur and La Hougue (1692), 51–2; costs and debt for care, 51–3, 58, 67, 74, 106; financial status of navy, 16, 45–6; statistics on seamen, 45; West Indies and Mediterranean, 50. *See also* commissioners (1689–1701), Nine Years' War; history of naval care (1689–1701), Nine Years' War
Norfolk, 28
Norris, Jane, 183, 192
Norris, John, 115, 117
nurses and nurse keepers. *See* care work; care workers, women

Ogle, Chaloner, 130–1, 223n49
ordered care: overview, 4, 9, 11, 70, 90–1, 105, 113–20, 136–41, 174; accounting systems for, 105, 108, 114;

centralization in hospitals, 90–6, 100, 118, 188–90; epidemic disease, 118–20; evaluation of care, 118, 120, 125, 130, 155–7, 173, 186; food, clothing, and bedding, 113–20, 125–6; as goal of naval health-care system, 4, 9, 90–1, 174; inspections for, 72–3, 114–20; Instructions and regulations (1731, 1740, 1742), 117, 120, 138–9, 143; "manning, money, and mercy," 90, 201n82; medical treatment, 114; Plymouth scandal, 146–53; prevention of corruption and waste, 109–13; quality of care, 72–3, 113–20; ratios of nurses to patients, 117, 141, 143. *See also* preservative ethos
overseas colonial and foreign ports: accounting systems, 165–6; costs and debt for care, 73, 75, 213n25. *See also* Mediterranean; West Indies

payments in arrears. *See* care payments in arrears
peacetime and care, 64–8, 74, 95, 106–9, 192
Pearse, James, 42, 205n110
Pembroke, 122(f), 123(f), 215n92
Penn, William, 34
pensions. *See* relief for seamen
Pepys, Samuel, 33, 35, 39, 204n79
permanent hospitals. *See* Gosport, Haslar naval hospital; hospitals, permanent
physicians. *See* surgeons and physicians
Pinder, Charity, 39–40
plague, 31, 35, 37
Plymouth: accounting systems, 87–8, 162; alcohol use, 166; care payments in arrears, 76–7, 79; continuity of system, 188–90; desertions, 87, 162; Dutch Wars care, 20; Georgian era care, 118–19, 221n77; maps, 122(f), 123(f), 124(f); Nine Years' War care, 47–50, 51,

53–4, 56–7; payment procedures, 78–9, 134–5, 150; prisoners of war, 166, 172; Queen Anne's War care, 71, 74, 76–7, 87; smallpox epidemic, 118–20, 221n77; trust in local people, 151–3; typhus (Great Sickness), 127–32, 148, 157, 222n16; War against France care, 162, 167, 172, 175

Plymouth, contract hospital: overview, 47–50, 90–1, 120, 146–53, 167; accounting systems, 84, 87–8, 162; care payments in arrears, 76–7, 79; George Dickinson as agent, 47–50, 58, 80, 207n18, 207n22; irregularities and corruption, 48–9, 106, 127, 134–5, 140, 146–53, 162; repairs (1733), 109; scandal over care conditions (1740–1741), 146–53; women care workers, 144, 185

Plymouth, permanent hospital: overview, 9, 188, 192; continuity of system, 188–90; naval control, 9; proposal (1741), 153–8, 177, 178, 228n171; proposal (1744), 177–9; restoration of old hospital, 166

poor people and care work, 6–7

Porter, Richard, 134, 162, 175, 224n60, 230n23

Port Mahon naval hospital, 73, 77, 129, 144, 216n118, 218n2

Portsmouth: agents, 29–30, 162; *Blenheim* hospital ship, 130–1, 134, 137, 140–1, 143–5, 172, 175, 185; care payments in arrears, 52, 54–7, 76–7, 133; commissioners for, 29; continuity of system, 188–90; Dutch Wars care, 20, 27, 35, 121(f); maps, 121(f), 122(f); Nine Years' War care, 50, 52, 53–7; Queen Anne's War care, 71, 76–7, 102; War against France care, 162, 167, 175; War with Spain, 125. *See also* Gosport

Portsmouth, hospitals. *See* Gosport, Forton Hospital (contract); Gosport, Haslar naval hospital

preservative ethos: overview, 10–11, 16, 62–8, 89, 105, 120, 191; accounting systems, 63–6, 82–6; care site procurement, 66, 89; continuity of system, 188–90; contract hospitals overview, 90–100; hospital proposals, 62–3, 67–8, 92–8; impact on modernization, 11; Instructions, 64–6, 71–2; "manning, money, and mercy," 90, 201n82; payment procedures, 65–7; peacetime care, 64–8, 106–9; permanent naval hospitals, 153–7; recommendations by former commissioners, 66–8; retention of seamen, 10–11, 89; saving Crown money, 10–11, 89; saving seamen's lives, 10–11, 89; trust relationships with local people, 66–8, 89. *See also* desertions; mustering; ordered care; Treasury

prisoners of war: overview, 194; accounting systems, 60; archives and sources, 14; commissioners' responsibilities, 15, 71, 72, 73, 83, 167, 170, 194, 198n32; costs for custody and care, 73, 74, 81, 167, 206n8, 206n12, 209n96; foreign ports, 73; hospitals for, 172; lack of emphasis in this book, 15; payments in arrears, 59, 81; during Queen Anne's War, 71, 72, 73, 74, 75, 81; during War against France, 167, 170, 171, 172

private-contract hospitals. *See* hospitals, contract

protests. *See* resistance and protests

public relief. *See* relief for poor people; relief for seamen

"Q" for query in accounting systems, 112–13, 220n54, 230n35

quality of care. *See* ordered care

quartering system: overview, 8, 153–60, 191; blended system with contract hospitals, 101, 129, 132, 151–3, 179; care payments in arrears (1711), 76–9; continuity of system, 188–90, 235n6; co-operation with commissioners, 31–2, 35–6, 43–4; corruption and waste, 118; debt for care, 32–6; decline in spaces, 102–3, 191; disease as threat to, 35; evaluation of care, 118, 120, 130, 155–8, 186; hierarchy of care, 90, 101, 106–7, 134; local regulations, 66; mutual benefits, 43–4; payments directly by agents, 30; procurement by commissioners, 66; providers, as term, 201n13; rates per day, 30, 49, 109, 150–1, 167, 210n122; shift to contract hospitals overview, 90–104, 188–90, 191; shift to permanent hospitals overview, 153–60, 187–90; trust relations, 9, 29, 31–3, 38–42, 61–2, 66–8, 77–9, 88–9, 103, 151–3; women care workers, 182–6

Queen Anne's War (1702–1713): overview, 16, 69–70, 123(f); archives and sources, 14; care payments in arrears, 76–9, 81, 101–2; costs and debt for care, 73–5; financial status of navy, 59, 69, 75–8; foreign care costs, 73; peacetime, 74, 95; preservative ethos, 16, 73, 89; prisoners of war, 71, 72, 73, 74, 75; Treaty of Utrecht (1713), 16, 105, 218n1. *See also* commissioners (1702–1713), Queen Anne's War; history of naval care (1702–1713), Queen Anne's War

Queenborough, 102, 115

records. *See* accounting systems
regulating captain, as term, 229n16
relief for poor people: overview, 6; care work as paid labour, 15;

involuntary care work by poor people, 6–7; requirement for care work, 6–7; taxes and levies to raise money, 6; women's care work, 6–7

relief for seamen: overview, 24; Chatham's Chest pensions, 24, 28, 46, 72; county pensions, 24, 28, 38; county pensions, exemptions, 38; double cost of care during war, 38; Dutch Wars care, 38; elderly veterans, 24; hardships from debt, 38; honour of the Crown, 24, 38, 67; injured seamen, 24; war-related disability as meritorious, 24

resistance and protests: overview, 8, 36–41, 100–2; advocacy by commissioners, 37–40, 46, 66–7; against contract hospitals, 98–9; dishonest agents, 37; during Dutch Wars, 32–41, 55–8; epidemic diseases, conditions, 118–19; hardships from debt, 38–41, 46, 51, 54–8; just compensation complaints, 36; vs mustering, 111–12; during Nine Years' War, 51–8; poor care for seamen, 54–6; during Queen Anne's War, 98–102; seamen transferred to London hospitals, 55. *See also* care payments in arrears

resistance to Portsmouth hospital (1704), 98–9, 101

retention of seamen, 4, 10–11, 28. *See also* preservative ethos

Revell, Russell, 144

Reymes, Bullen, 13, 28–31, 33, 36, 38, 40

Rochester: care payments in arrears, 34, 40, 56–7, 76–7, 79, 133; continuity of system, 188–90; costs and debt for care, 218n2; Dutch Wars care, 34, 203n57; Georgian era care, 114–15; hardships from debt, 56; maps, 122(f), 123(f); Nine Years' War care, 50, 53, 56–7; Queen Anne's War care, 71,

74, 76–7, 102, 192, 212n12; surgeon-agents, 108–9; typhus (Great Sickness), 130, 222n16; women care workers, 191

Rochester, contract hospital: overview, 90–1, 104, 114–15, 192; care payments in arrears, 76–7, 79; contract proposals, 91–4; corruption and waste, 109–10; desertions, 126; disorderly conduct, 171; gendered consequences, 91, 104; ordered care, 108–9, 114–15, 170, 171; sample agreement (1703), 96–8; transport of patients to, 102, 115

Rooke, George, 57, 207n32

royal naval hospitals. *See* hospitals, permanent

Royal Navy: global pre-eminence (1650–1750), 8

Russell, Edward (Earl of Orford), 52, 241n140

Russell, John (Duke of Bedford), 162, 164, 168, 229n5

Rycaul, Captain, 149

sailors. *See* seamen

Sandwich, 21, 88, 122(f), 123(f)

sanitary conditions. *See* cleanliness

Savoy Hospital, 27

Sayer, John, 96–8

Scotland, 74

scurvy, 23, 175, 221n65

seamen: accounting systems, 60–5, 72, 211n131, 230n34; alcohol in basic provisions, 184–5; compensation, 28, 230n34; discipline, 174, 180, 181; dishonest conduct, 30, 72, 96; disorderly conduct, 184–5; gendered power relations, 183–4; "people" as term for, 233n75; preservative ethos, 60–8; quality of care, 72–3, 113–20, 194–5; sick frauds and malingerers, 29, 72, 93, 160–1, 164–6, 229n18, 231n39. *See also* accounting systems; preservative ethos

Sergison, Charles, 14

Seymour, Dr (Plymouth), 119, 147

Sheerness, 79, 87, 98, 102, 123(f), 124(f), 169–71, 176, 182, 230n26

shelter providers. *See* quartering system

Shepherd, Anthony, 47, 61

Sherrard, William, 70

ship fever, 23. *See also* typhus epidemic (Great Sickness) (1739–1742)

ships, hospital. *See* hospital ships

Shirley, Captain, 169

sick and hurt service. *See entries beginning with* commissioners *and* history of naval care

sick frauds and malingerers, 29, 31, 72, 93, 160–1, 164–6, 229n18, 231n39

sinking fund (reserves), 135, 224n70

smallpox, 109, 118–20, 221nn64–5

sobriety. *See* alcohol use

Somerset, 74

Southampton, 103, 122(f), 123(f), 172

South Sea Company, 69, 77

Southwold, 33, 121(f)

Spain: naval care system, 192, 205n106, 223n19

Spain, War with (1739–1744): overview, 17, 125–7, 155–7; archives and sources, 15, 127; evaluation of care, 125, 130, 132; financial status of navy, 135–6, 157; typhus (Great Sickness) overview, 127–32; West Indies theatre, 127. *See also* commissioners (1739–1744), War with Spain; history of naval care (1739–1744), War with Spain

spirits. *See* alcohol use

Spry, John, 3

St Albans, 131

standards for care. *See* ordered care

Starkey, John, 47

state and Crown: formation as top-down and bottom-up, 21; legitimacy in civilian-military

Index

relations, 35–6; modernization of institutions, 9; moral economy of health system, 20, 21–2, 37; mutual benefits for upholding authority, 43–4; public-accounts commission, 80; as terms, 198n36; trust relations with ordinary people, 21, 31–3, 38–42, 61–2, 66–8, 77–8. *See also* trust relations

St Boltoph Aldgate, 7, 110

Steuart, James, 163–4, 166, 173

St Leger, Edward, 54

St Martin-in-the-Fields, 7

St Michael, Balthasar, 33, 37, 204n79

Strood, 40

Suffolk, 25, 28, 34

surgeon-agents for commissioners: accounting systems, 108, 111; duties, 108, 111, 160; muster masters, 111, 114; rate per day, 165, 167

surgeons and physicians: overview, 12, 22–3; accounting systems, 60–5, 79–80, 82–6; appointments by commissioners, 28, 47; as commission members, 63, 71, 94, 107; compensation, 23, 30, 47, 71; derelictions of duty, 88; diagnosis of sick-frauds, 160–1; gendered sphere, 94; mustering, 85, 111–12; shipboard surgeons, 19, 23, 64–5; statistics on, 42; status in armed forces, 94; training and apprenticeships, 22. *See also* diseases and illnesses; surgeon-agents for commissioners

Sussex, 28, 37

systems. *See* health-care systems; health-care systems, naval; hospitals; quartering system

tallies, 58–9, 209n86

Tilbury, 87

Torrington, Lord, Admiral of the Fleet, 110–11, 113, 114

town quarterers. *See* quartering system

Treasury: overview, 58–60; accounting systems, 60–5, 79–81; Bank of England, 51, 59; lotteries, 59, 135; revenue streams, 16, 58–60, 76–9, 135; sinking fund (reserves), 135, 224n70; tallies as credit mechanism, 58–9, 209n86; taxes and duties, 59, 77, 135, 214n61. *See also* accounting systems; care payments in arrears

Treaty of Utrecht (1713), 16, 105, 218n1

Trevanion, Nicholas, 109

trust relations: overview, 8–9, 21–2, 31–3, 38–42, 61–2, 66–8, 190; capacity of care providers, 9, 132; Crown authority and local people, 31–2, 35–6, 43–4; gender and distrust, 101, 103–4; hardships from debt, 38–41, 46, 55–8, 76–7; legitimacy in civilian-military relations, 35–6; in peacetime, 106–9; preservative ethos, 66–8; prompt care payments, 133–5; quartering system, 9, 29, 31–3, 38–42, 61–2, 66–8, 77–9, 88–9, 103, 151–3; trends in, 8–9, 77–8, 88–9, 132–3, 151–3; typhus (Great Sickness), 157

Turner, Methuselah, 26

Tutchin, John, 98

typhus epidemic (Great Sickness) (1739–1742): overview, 23, 125, 127–32, 136; desertions, 128, 130; evaluation of care, 136; lice in bedding, 23, 129, 130; Plymouth scandal, 146–53; quality of care, 136, 142–4, 157, 158; statistics, 127–8, 222n16; trust relations, 157; women care providers, 142–4

undertakers, as term, 69, 217n153. *See also* hospitals, contract

Vallack, Mr (Plymouth agent), 47

Vanborough, Philip, 146–7

Vane, Henry, 37

274   Index

Vincent, Captain, 126, 131, 138, 143–6
Vincent, Thomas (Plymouth physician), 145

Wager, Charles, 116, 181
Walpole, Robert, 127, 156, 218n1, 224n70, 228n163
War against France. *See* France, War against (1744–1748)
Ward, Samuel, 26
warfare: health care's orientation to, 9; impact on modern political formations, 9; modernization of, 9; power concentration in government, 10; public/private co-operation, 10; Western Squadron approach, 159; women as moral dangers, 91
War of the Austrian Succession, 159. *See also* France, War against (1744–1748)
War with Spain. *See* Spain, War with (1739–1744)
Wear, Andrew, 7
Welwood, James, 63
West Indies: costs for care, 207n33; diseases, 222n14; navy as armed division of merchants, 224n69; Nine Years' War care, 50; war with Spain (1726–1727), 106, 127

Weymouth, 51, 57, 78, 122(f), 123(f), 172
Whistler, Daniel, 27, 37, 43, 188
Wight, Isle of, 31, 126, 131–2, 138
William III, King, 46, 58, 62–3, 71
Williams, George, 145
Williams, Samuel, 29–30
Willoughby, Francis, 25
Winchilsea, Earl of (Daniel Finch), 129, 160–1, 168, 172, 179–81, 186, 189, 192–3, 229n5
Withington, Phil, 184
women: alcohol use, 184–6, 193; contract hospital entrepreneurs, 101, 103; importance of women care workers, 17–18, 50, 182–6, 192–5; invisibility of care work, 192–5; as moral dangers, 17, 86, 90–1, 93–6, 98–9, 139, 181; power relations, 11–12, 145, 183–4. *See also* care workers, women
Woolwich, 74, 103, 123(f), 140, 169–71, 182, 218n2, 232n55, 232n61, 234n115
Wyatt, William, 140–1, 145, 147–50, 156

Yarmouth, 78, 121(f), 122(f), 123(f), 169, 187–8
yellow fever, 23, 222n14